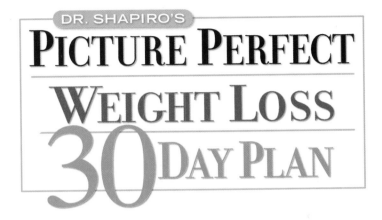

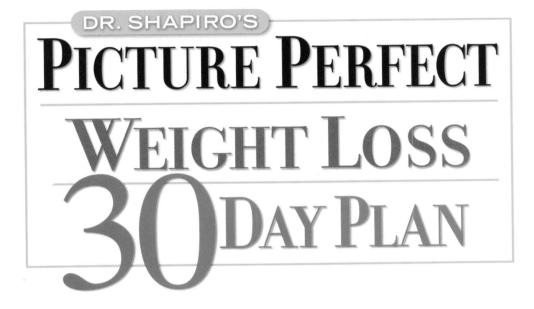

DR. SHAPIRO'S
PICTURE PERFECT
WEIGHT LOSS
30 DAY PLAN

Dr. Howard M. Shapiro

RODALE®

Notice

This book is intended as a reference volume only, not as a medical manual. The information given here is designed to help you make informed decisions about your health. It is not intended as a substitute for any treatment that may have been prescribed by your doctor. If you suspect that you have a medical problem, we urge you to seek competent medical help.

Mention of specific companies, organizations, or authorities in this book does not imply endorsement by the publisher, nor does mention of specific companies, organizations, or authorities in the book imply that they endorse the book.

Cover and interior design by Christina Gaugler

Interior photographs by Kurt Wilson, except pp. 7 (after) and 82 (after) by Hilmar; p. 317 (after) by Mitch Mandel/Rodale Images; p. 1 (children) by Ryan McVay/PhotoDisc; p. 303 (before) by Michael Metzger; pp. 303 (after), 314 (after), and 324 (after) by Scott Olson; pp. 289 (fireman) and 295 (after) by Todd Plitt; p. 82 (before) courtesy of Michael Carter; p. 7 (before) courtesy of Tom Kontizas; p. 314 (before) courtesy of Heidi McInerney; pp. 1 (adults at table) and 289 (chefs) courtesy of Dr. Howard Shapiro; p. 324 (before) courtesy of David Taylor; p. 317 (before) courtesy of WPN International Studio

Cover author photograph by Hilmar

Cover food photographs by Kurt Wilson

Food styling by Diane Vezza

For more information about Picture-Perfect Weight Loss, log on to www.drshapiropictureperfect.com

ISBN 1-57954-417-7

To Kay von Bergen
With deep appreciation and great respect
Simply put, thank you . . .

In memory of Paul Pansini and Raymond Meisenheimer
and in honor of their brethren, New York City's firefighters—
"The Bravest"—who responded to the tragedy of
September 11, 2001 with uncommon valor,
reclaiming for us all a sense of human decency
and exemplifying the true meaning of heroism.

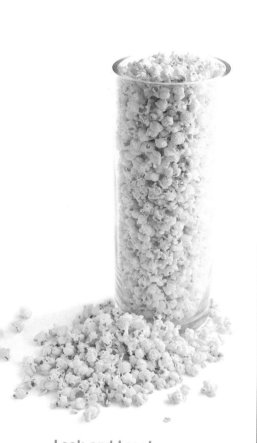

Look and Lose!
Popcorn is a treat that kids and teens love, and it's a smart choice in the Picture-Perfect Plan. See page 179.

For more information about Picture-Perfect Weight Loss, log on to www.drshapiropictureperfect.com.

Contents

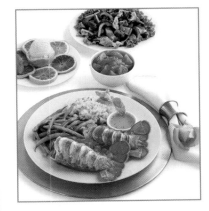

Look and Lose!
Just because you want to lose a few pounds doesn't mean you can't enjoy a special occasion. See page 281.

Look and Lose!
Looking for dessert? You could have one cookie or all of these luscious berries and whipped topping. See page 189.

Acknowledgments

*M*any of the people who helped make the *Picture-Perfect Weight Loss 30-Day Plan* a reality appear in the pages of the book—some of them in its photographs. But many more people were involved in the effort, and I am glad to acknowledge them here.

Thanks, above all, to Phyllis Roxland for guidance on non–meat eating and on the food demonstrations. Roz Siegel, my editor at Rodale Press, provided wisdom, expertise, and humor in shepherding the manuscript through to its completion. She even went so far as to provide her vacation phone number, a gesture above and beyond the call of duty. I am grateful also to Susanna Margolis, my editorial collaborator, who possesses an uncanny ability to translate my thoughts into clear and compelling language. And Mel Berger, my agent at the William Morris Agency, remains the "godfather" of my book-writing. Everyone assures me that with Mel, I am "well looked after." Everyone is absolutely right.

Food stylist Diane Vezza and her assistants Joan Parkin and Rose Holden and photographer Kurt Wilson and his assistant Troy Schnyder brought to life with great style the wonderful demonstrations that tell the Picture-Perfect Weight-Loss story so vividly. Book designer Christina Gaugler dealt cheerfully, on this book as on the last, with my questions and suggestions and created a uniquely user-friendly book for users of all ages. Thanks also to art director Darlene Schneck and to the rest of the Rodale design and production staff, including Tom Aczel, Dan MacBride, Diane Meckel, and Denise Millios.

Those Rodale staffers who labored in the editorial and research vineyards of the *30-Day Plan*—Jennifer Bright, Lois Hazel, and Carrie Havranek—added incalculable value.

I also want to thank Rodale's senior management: Steve Murphy and Marc Jaffe, for believing in the message I bring and granting me the opportunity to articulate it; Amy Rhodes and Tammerly Booth for overseeing the process; and marketing gurus Leslie Schneider, Denyse Corelli, Karen Taus, and Lorraine Rodriguez.

I cannot say enough about Cindy Ratzlaff and Mary Lengle of Rodale and Vanessa Menkes, Kara Cohen, and Judy Drutz of Dan Klores Communications. Together, they are surely the most creative, effective, and supportive publicity team in the history of the world. They instantly understood the book's message and its potential audience—and they have worked diligently and relentlessly to get the message out. I'm grateful.

A word of thanks also to Rodale's direct-sales representatives, the people who are truly the front line of the Picture-Perfect Weight-Loss message; their enthusiastic efforts make everything else possible.

I'm also grateful, on this book as on the original *Picture-Perfect Weight Loss*, to my friend Anne-Laure Lyon, fashion stylist, for the vision, direction, and expertise she provided for the cover of the book. And to Hilmar and Adrienne Bearden: my thanks for the world-class job, as always, in bringing the cover to life.

Thanks also as always to the staff at my New York office, who somehow make it possible for me to pursue two busy careers—one as physician, one as author. Gerri Pietrangolare, Alexandra Lotito, and Catherine Fallon keep the office running smoothly, and nutritionists Sharon Richter, M.S., R.D., and Marcia Cohen, M.S., R.D., along with physical therapist Les Koch, provide essential services to my patients.

Special thanks to a number of psychology experts who offered their expertise for the *30-Day Plan*. Psychologist Adele Fink, Ph.D., shares my office space in New York and generously shared her considerable knowledge of the psychology of weight loss. Esther Altmann, Ph.D., a New York–based practitioner specializing in adult and child psychotherapy, provided thoughtful and important insights in the writing of the chapters on childhood and teenage overweight, as did clinical psychologists Dr. Lynn Vinnick Kaller and Dr. Maria LaPadula Perez, who maintain a joint private practice in New York specializing in child and family therapy. And to my staff psychotherapist Susan Amato, C.S.W., who served as counselor to the Chicago 7 and provided substantial input on how to deal with some of the psychological issues raised in the *30-Day Plan*, I express heartfelt thanks.

My family has rendered me unswerving support throughout the writing process: my brother and sister-in-law, Michael and Andee Shapiro; my sister and brother-in-law, Marilyn and Michael McLaughlin; my mother, Eleanor, and her husband, Chuck DeWalt. A daily presence during the writing of the book was the memory of my father, whose often-repeated philosophy that "If it's worth doing, it's worth doing well" has been a constant guide.

The heroes and heroines of this book are the people you'll meet in its pages. The Chicago 7, the Stamford 250, members of the New York Police Department, and several of the many New York City firefighters I've treated let me tell their stories in the book. I am grateful to them all, but I want in particular to mention four members of the New York Fire Department: Mike Carter, department chaplain Father John Delendick, Tom Kontizas, and John Rohr. They have traveled with me to tell the Picture-Perfect Weight-Loss story, have become familiar faces on television, and serve as representatives of the fire department's advocacy of the program and as models of the program's success. Like so many of my patients and readers, they are living proof that anyone can change his or her way of eating and lose considerable weight—even in 30 days. I applaud their success, and I am grateful to them for serving as inspiration to others.

New York, September 2001

Dr. Shapiro's Picture-Perfect Weight Loss Food Pyramid

No menus, no measuring, no schedule, no portion sizes. You won't achieve Picture-Perfect Weight Loss—and you certainly won't maintain it—by weighing food portions, eating a certain number of servings at a certain time of day, or combining foods in mandated menus. That's not what fundamental weight loss—Picture-Perfect Weight Loss—is all about.

Instead, Picture-Perfect Weight Loss is about change and choice. You change your relationship with food by expanding your eating options, choosing the option that is lowest in calories, most nutritious, and tastiest, and then by eating until satisfied.

The Picture-Perfect Weight-Loss Food Pyramid is a guide to those choices. It maps the proportionate amounts of foods in an overall eating plan. Here's what it tells you:

Make fruits and vegetables the foundation of your eating. Just as the pyramid is necessarily widest at the base, let fruits and vegetables be the foods you eat most—most often, most regularly, and most of.

Next, go for protein. But as often as possible, get your protein in beans and other legumes, seafood, and soy products rather than in meats, poultry, and dairy. (*Note:* The FDA recommends avoiding shark, swordfish, tilefish, and king mackerel during pregnancy because of their high mercury content.)

When you take in grain products, choose whole grain or light versions if possible.

Where fats and oils are concerned, choose nuts, seeds, olives, avocados, and either olive or canola oil wherever possible.

For sweet treats, stick with hard candies and fat-free frozen desserts.

If you don't see your favorite food category on my pyramid, keep in mind that no food is forbidden with Picture-Perfect Weight Loss. The pyramid presents my recommendations for a healthy way of eating that will provide all the nutrients you need as you lose weight and maintain your weight loss.

Make the pyramid your guide, and you will be thin for life.

Hard candies, fat-free frozen desserts
SWEETS

Nuts, seeds, olives, avocados, and olive and canola oil
FATS AND OILS

Preferably whole grains or light versions
GRAIN PRODUCTS

Soy products, beans, legumes, seafood
PROTEIN FOODS

Any and all—fresh, frozen, canned, packaged—as much as possible, as often as possible
FRUITS AND VEGETABLES

PART I

THE PICTURE-PERFECT
WEIGHT-LOSS PLAN
IS FOR EVERYONE

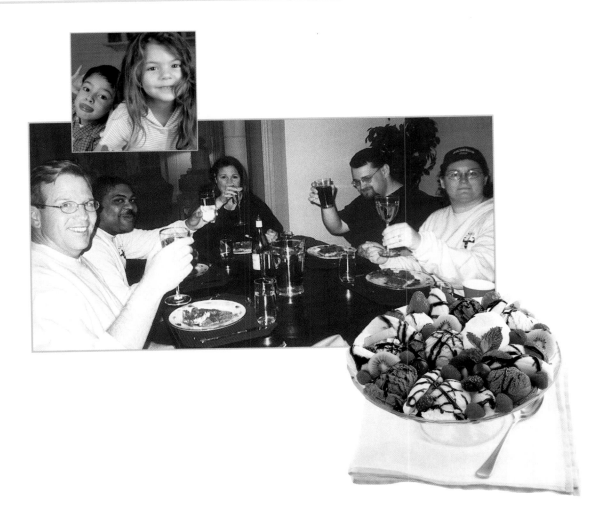

One New York City firefighter lost 80 pounds as a result
of changing his eating habits to adhere to the principles
of Picture-Perfect Weight Loss.
He has maintained that weight loss ever since.

～

A police detective brought a postpregnancy weight
of 170 pounds down to 118 pounds—and keeps it off
despite endless stakeouts and frustrating paperwork.

～

Seven Chicago-based men and women, after a weeklong
cram course in Picture-Perfect Weight Loss, went on to lose
a total of 282 pounds in the course of 9 months.
As this book goes to press, they are still losing weight.

～

*None of these people changed their lives.
What they changed is their relationship with food.*

Chapter 1

WEIGHT LOSS AND REAL LIFE— *Your* REAL LIFE

You're reading this book because you're overweight—or someone in your family is overweight—and you're unhappy about it. You can put an end to that situation. Right now.

For nearly 25 years, I've treated patients who claimed they had "tried everything" and been unable to lose weight. I've treated those who gained back all the weight they had lost on popular diet programs. I've worked with patients who have followed every fad from hypnosis to fasting, patients who have measured portions and counted grams of fat, patients who have deprived themselves of foods they love, forced themselves to eat foods they didn't particularly like, eaten meals when a book or diet guru told them to, and beaten themselves up every time they had a cookie or asked for a second helping.

I've worked with children and the elderly, high-powered executives, celebrities, politicians, and stay-at-home moms, people who eat on the run and people who regularly dine at the world's finest restaurants. I've helped them understand why diets don't work, why deprivation is counterproductive, why fasting can

actually harm you. I've taught them what this book will teach you in 30 days: There is a way of eating—eating what you enjoy eating and eating it until you feel satisfied—that actually helps you lose weight and keep it off.

I call it Picture-Perfect Weight Loss. Yes, that's partly because you can see the difference in yourself as you lose weight. But mostly, Picture-Perfect Weight Loss refers to the method I use in my practice for teaching this way of eating. The nutritionists on my staff continually create food comparison demonstrations that show patients a range of food options and allow them to compare the weight-loss consequences of each. As you'll see, we've reproduced our food demos in the photographs in this book. They provide vivid lessons in how you can eat healthfully and deliciously for the rest of your life and still lose weight and keep it off.

How can I be so sure? Because Picture-Perfect Weight Loss has worked for the thousands of patients I've treated in my New York practice. They've all lost weight, and they've maintained the weight loss. All without diets or deprivation, without starving themselves or scheduling their meals by the clock or carrying around scales to measure what they're eating—and without being angry with themselves or feeling like failures because they went out for pizza or "slipped" at a party.

The first thing you need to know about your will to lose weight is that it will happen. You are about to embark on a weight-loss program that *will* succeed.

A Worldwide Problem

You are not alone in feeling unhappy about your weight. In fact, you can join a growing, worldwide crowd.

From Trenton to Tokyo, from Seattle to Samarqand, in country after country and in just about every region of the planet, more and more people today are either overweight (defined as weighing 10 to 15 percent above an ideal weight), or obese (20 percent over an ideal weight), or even morbidly obese (30 percent or more above an ideal body weight). It may be small consolation for the dismay you feel when you stand on a scale, but you're part of a global trend.

The trend is both recent and fast-moving. Around the world, the number of obese people has doubled in the last 2 decades. Even in China, which maintains one of the world's lowest incidences of overweight people—just 14 percent of men and 17 percent of women—and an even lower measure of obese

The Weight of the World . . .

Obesity has become "a global epidemic," according to a 2000 report from the International Obesity Task Force. Here's how some countries around the globe weigh in.

Country	Percentage of Men Who Are Overweight	Percentage of Women Who Are Overweight	Percentage of Men Who Are Obese	Percentage of Women Who Are Obese
Australia	45.2	28.8	18	18
Canada	56	41	15	15
China	14	17	2	6
England	44	33	19	21
Italy	37.9	24.9	9	9.9
Japan	24	20	1.8	2
Mexico	48	36	15	21
Romania	38	28	17	23
Russia	35	31	10	25
United States	39.3	24.8	20	25

Welcome to the United States, Welcome to Weight Gain

Researchers tracking 24 immigrants to the United States from all over the world found that the new residents each put on 2 pounds in their first 10 weeks here, and another pound 10 weeks after that. Those figures represent the average. A man from Colombia gained 20 pounds, and a woman from Italy gained 12.

The reason? The researchers concur: fast food. It's cheap, it's convenient, and it's *American*. It's also full of calories, especially in the popular new supersized portions.

people—2 percent of men and 6 percent of women—even there, the growth rate in the numbers of overweight and obese people is increasing. Give the Chinese time, and weight gain will do what government policy has long tried to do—decrease the billion-person population, not through population planning, but through increased occurrence of diabetes, stroke, high blood pressure, and even some forms of cancer.

One of the countries leading the way in this unhappy, unhealthy spiral is the United States—a dubious distinction if ever there was one. More than half of us—about 55 percent, in fact—are overweight or obese, up from 44 percent in 1990. What's more, the rise in the number of people in the obese category is proceeding at a fast clip. According to the International Obesity Task Force, in 1973, 12 percent of American men and 16 percent of American women were obese; today, 20 percent of men and a quarter of women are obese—some 3 to 5 percent of them morbidly obese. So our national weight gain must be measured not just in the numbers of people gaining weight, but also in the amount of weight they are gaining.

Further, this weight gain is everywhere. In a pivotal study, the Centers for Disease Control and Prevention (CDC) found that obesity occurred in *all of the 50 states, in every region, across all demographic groups.* It is, therefore, a national public health problem, inevitably linked to the nation's number one killer, heart disease, as well as to diabetes, respiratory problems, some cancers, and a range of chronic and debilitating conditions. In fact, the CDC concluded that obesity was a threat to millions of lives, and that it "should be taken as seriously as any infectious disease or epidemic."

Chances are you know all this already. You don't really need the statistics to measure the problem. You can see it—in the office, at the mall, walking along Main Street, in your own reflection in the mirror. And you probably don't need the dire warnings to be reminded of the ill effects of being overweight. You can feel it—in the clothes that suddenly feel tight, in your shortness of breath when you climb the stairs, in a sense of discomfort with your own body.

That discomfort is something else you share with millions. It is estimated that more than two-thirds of Americans are either on a diet in an attempt to lose weight or are "watching what they eat" so they don't gain weight. As a people, we spend some $30 billion to $50 billion *per year* trying to lose weight—on diets, with pills and supplements, by measuring out portions, counting calories, combining certain foods with certain other foods, listening to tapes, and fasting. As you know, those "solutions" simply don't work. That's why you're reading this book.

The Causes of Overweight and Obesity

How did it happen? How did we get this way? How did *you* get this way?

There is one reason for becoming overweight, and there are many contributing causes. The reason is metabolic, and it is absolutely unique to the individual. Your metabolism is the particular combination of chemical processes occurring inside you. That combination, in turn, depends on the interactions between genetic and environmental factors. Just what those factors are and just how they interact are as distinctive to you as your fingerprint; no one else has just that combination working in just that way. Yet it is the sum total of all those factors and their interactions that pretty much directs how your body handles calories, what foods taste good to you, and even how you think about food. In a sense, you've been dealt your very own metabolic hand of cards. While you have no control over what's in the hand, you do control how you play the hand.

Enter a range of additional contributing causes. These are the cultural, sociological, and psychological factors that drive the lifestyle choices we all make every day—the different ways we each play our own metabolic hand of cards. These include things like the foods we eat, whether or not we exercise, and our levels of everyday stress.

Even anthropology plays a role. One important cause contributing to today's global epidemic of overweight may simply be that, as a species, we are outstripping our own evolution. Biological anthropologists tell us that at an earlier stage of human development, the ability to form fat was an advantage. When our ancestors were subject to uncontrollable cycles of feast and famine, bodies that could store fat for the lean times were "fitter" bodies. They're the ones that survived, and as happens in evolution, the traits that kept the organism alive were the traits imprinted on the genetic code passed to descendants. Result? Humans in general evolved into organisms programmed for high-calorie foods they could store efficiently as fat.

Today, however, at least in the industrialized world, we aren't threatened by famine. (In those parts of the world where famine is a threat, the causes are more often than not manmade—typically, politics and civil strife.) In fact, for most of us in developed countries, life is an almost endless feast. But since our bodies have evolved to deal with famine—to take in lots of calories and expend very few—our era's very abundance is a surefire formula for weight gain.

Other aspects of our current culture exacerbate the problem. We live in a high-stress, high-tech world. With both parents working—often long hours in high-pressure jobs—with kids on schedules that would tire a marathoner, with families in a constant state of arranging and rearranging plans for getting each family member here, there, and everywhere, the notion of sitting down together for a relaxing family dinner has gone the way of the dodo. There simply isn't time for such a dinner, and even if there were, everybody is either too busy or too exhausted to enjoy it. It's easier, more convenient, and even less costly for each family member to just pop a frozen dinner in the microwave and eat it on the run.

Meanwhile, we're increasingly equipped with cell phones, pagers, Internet access, and the all-in-one remote control. Together, they let us gratify any wish instantly—without even getting up out of a chair, much less leaving home. Where our ancestors had to struggle daily to obtain sustenance, or labor manually to earn it, we just drive over to the nearest fast-food place—or we order takeout and have it delivered.

Fast food, in particular, is notoriously fattening. But gourmet restaurants also often rely on high-calorie ingredients and cooking methods. Their stock-in-trade, after all, is a taste experience so memorable you will find it worth the price. All too often, that is achieved at the expense of your waistline. When a simple chicken cutlet can lift you into the realm of the sublime, it's probably because it has been topped with Gorgonzola, layered with Canadian bacon, then wrapped in puff pastry—an absolutely delicious, calorically off-the-charts cardiac killer.

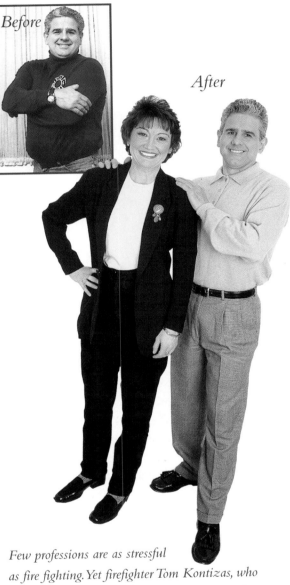

Before

After

Few professions are as stressful as fire fighting. Yet firefighter Tom Kontizas, who was featured on Good Morning America, *lost 40 pounds with Picture-Perfect Weight Loss. "Without even trying," his wife Karen lost 8 pounds just by shopping and cooking for him.*

A Side Effect of Overweight: Sleep Apnea

Sleep apnea is the result of a temporary blockage of the breathing passages. Now research has shown that it is most common in overweight or obese people, predominantly men, with a neck circumference of 17 inches or larger. Apart from the potential consequences of the resultant daytime fatigue, there is evidence that apnea increases the risk of hypertension and heart disease. For the overweight, even a 10 percent weight loss can help.

What's more, we're becoming increasingly accustomed to enormous portions. Huge tubs of buttered popcorn at the movies. Quart-size soft drinks. "Supersized" items that belie the phrase "side dish." It's as if we were proving our prosperity every time we eat.

At the same time that we're eating more, we're exercising less. This, too, flies in the face of human evolution. We evolved as an active species; the human appestat, the part of the brain that regulates appetite and food intake, works best when we're active. Yet we've virtually engineered activity out of daily life—everywhere and every way we can:

- Today's workplace is increasingly automated. Robots do most of the hauling on the factory floor, while computers in the office mean we don't even need to get up to find a file.
- Many neighborhoods lack sidewalks, so a stroll down a country lane is typically more like a slalom on foot in the middle of a Formula 1 race. It's safer to stay home.
- Cleaning chores are less labor-intensive than ever, with telescoping dusters that keep us from having to stretch and powerful vacuums that mean we don't need to bend.

- When we do go someplace, we invariably drive, coming home to the attached garage whose doors open automatically at the touch of a button. Even kids who once walked or cycled to school now get driven—or have their own cars.
- Meanwhile, schools across the country have responded to budget cutbacks by reducing or eliminating physical education activities.
- As for after school, parents in cities, in particular, find their outdoor environments too dangerous for their children to play in without supervision. Instead, they let the kids watch television or play computer games—activities that at best exercise the fingertips and at worst are accompanied by heavy snacking. Even in the suburbs, where kids have a chance to play outdoors, far too many prefer to be couch potatoes.

Yes, there are more gyms than ever before, more fitness videos, more new-fangled pieces of exercise equipment for the home. But we tend to drive to the gym—when we actually get around to going; the videos gather dust on the shelf; and the exercise bike in the bedroom is soon obscured by the clothes we've hung on it. Americans today actually burn 400 fewer calories per day than did our great-grandparents at the turn of the last century. Almost a quarter of us do no leisure-time physical activity at all, while 54 percent of us do less than 30 minutes of moderate activity at a time—usually every other day or so. That's not enough even to maintain weight loss. As for losing weight, a CDC survey of people trying to shed pounds found that less than a quarter of them exercised at least 150 minutes per week, the minimum recommended for weight loss.

All this leaves a lot of people on a virtual treadmill more real than the one they hauled up to the attic years ago. On this virtual treadmill, they're running against metabolism as well as evolution, culture, sociology, and a host of other contributing causes—and they're still overweight.

Sound familiar?

What Doesn't Work

Whatever the causes of your being overweight, in real life—*your* real life—you want to do something about it. Maybe you've tried dieting. You've measured portions and counted calories and eaten only at certain specified times of the day.

Perhaps you've tried one of the fad diets—high-protein or low-carbohydrate or no sugar or zero fat. Maybe you've experimented with one or more of the new weight-loss theories that seem to crop up annually—dieting by blood type, for example, or consciously combining certain foods at certain times.

One thing these decades of changing diet fashions have demonstrated conclusively to both dieters and doctors is that the diets don't work. Sure, you lose weight at first—maybe even a lot of weight. But a diet by definition is time-limited. Unfortunately, once it's over and you return to "real life," the pounds inevitably come back. In fact, all too often, you gain back even more than you lost in the first place. The reason is absolutely physiological: Deprivation backfires. And a diet means deprivation of all kinds as you deprive yourself of certain foods, limit your portion sizes, and eat on a particular schedule rather than when you're hungry. As we'll see, forcing yourself to do what comes *un*naturally eventually has the opposite effect from the one intended: Not only don't you curb your appetite or eat less or lose weight, you actually become increasingly ravenous, eat more, and regain what you've lost and then some.

Where diets are concerned, then, it's time to say, "Been there, done that, got the T-shirt." In fact, one recent study reported that Americans as a whole are fed up with all the diet advice they're getting, especially because so much of it is conflicting advice. They're tired of being told what to eat, when to eat it, and how much of it to eat. And they're showing their anger in a backlash, eating all the foods the diet gurus and nutrition police say they shouldn't eat. It's further evidence of why diets don't work and why Picture-Perfect Weight Loss *does* work: Picture-Perfect Weight Loss doesn't give orders about what you should or should not eat. Instead, it provides you with a way of eating a range of foods, including the foods you love—a way of eating, *not* a diet.

But perhaps you've gone another route to lose weight. Maybe you bought new exercise equipment or joined the gym and began exercising to beat the band. Good for you! A consistent program of moderate exercise is great for your fitness and sense of well-being. Keep it up—forever. It's very, very good for you in every way.

Or did you turn to the most recent behavior-modification guru, the one whose calm, soothing voice on audio tapes was going to "cure" you forever of your appetite? Or maybe you swallowed the drugs or supplements that you hoped would be the ultimate "magic bullet" leading to permanent weight loss. Neither worked. Neither *can* work.

As a new wave of scientific research has confirmed time and again, there is no magic bullet with which to hit the weight-loss bull's-eye. There is no "cure" for an individual's appetite. There is no diet regimen that works for everybody—or that lasts forever.

The reason that diets and pills and voices on a tape don't work is that they simply don't address the problem—that metabolic hand of cards you've been dealt. As Americans, we pride ourselves on being able to fix anything, but you can't fix the metabolism you were born with. When you're told what to eat, when to eat it, and how much of it to eat, you're simply going against all the chemical interactions in your body. When you close your ears to the messages your chemicals are transmitting, when you refuse to respond to your body's demands, when you fight your own metabolism, guess what? Your metabolism wins. Appetite is not a disease to be "cured"; hunger is not a whim you can repress. What we're talking about is a chemically driven message from your metabolism. If

you deny it, defy it, or try to silence it, chances are good you simply won't be able to lose weight—or maintain the weight loss you've achieved.

What Does Work: Picture-Perfect Weight Loss

There's only one way to lose weight and keep it off, and that is to change your relationship with food. What do I mean by that? I mean that you will eat when hungry, that you will eat till satisfied, that you will not exclude from your life the foods you love. But you will eat with awareness of the consequences of what you're eating. You'll bring a big-picture approach to your eating, so that you enjoy the great variety of foods available to you while you lose weight and maintain your weight loss for life.

It's a question of choices, and the choices are all in your hands. After all, who decides what you're going to eat? Who's in charge of what you put in your mouth? Who determines how much exercise you're getting today? You do. Chances are that a lot of the choices you've been making up to now have led to the weight gain you're determined to reverse. You will reverse it—when you change the choices.

The 30-Day Plan in this book gives you the tools for change; it will empower you. My proven method of Food Awareness Training (FAT) will show you the difference between food choices and make you aware of what each choice can mean. What's more, this book will show you these things in vivid demonstrations you'll see in your mind's eye every time you cook a meal or look at a menu or fill out your shopping

Test Your Picture-Perfect Weight-Loss IQ

Which food is lower in calories? Quiz yourself and imprint some memorable images on your brain.

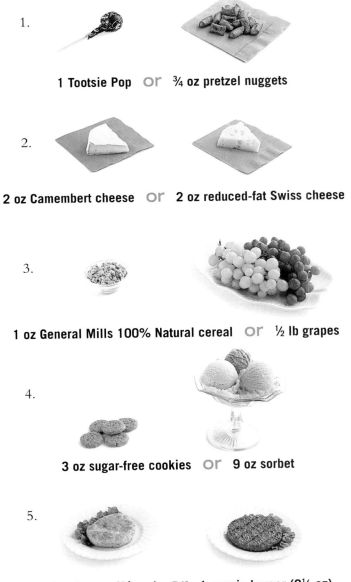

1.

1 Tootsie Pop   or   **¾ oz pretzel nuggets**

2.

2 oz Camembert cheese   or   **2 oz reduced-fat Swiss cheese**

3.

1 oz General Mills 100% Natural cereal   or   **½ lb grapes**

4.

3 oz sugar-free cookies   or   **9 oz sorbet**

5.

1 turkey burger (2½ oz)   or   **1 veggie burger (2½ oz)**

Test Your Picture-Perfect Weight-Loss IQ (answers)

1.

1 Tootsie Pop 50 calories
¾ oz pretzel nuggets 80 calories

Both foods are examples of refined carbohydrates, which aren't the healthiest way to take in calories, nor the most effective for weight loss. But if you assumed that the sweet Tootsie Pop was higher in calories, you can see how wrong you were. Consider also how much more satisfying the Tootsie Pop is than the pretzel nuggets, which are far too easy to ingest mindlessly. Bottom line? If you're going to eat refined carbohydrates, get the most bang for your caloric buck: Stick to hard candy.

2.

2 oz Camembert cheese 170 calories
2 oz reduced-fat Swiss cheese 180 calories

We all love cheese, and we all know that it's high in fat—the kind of saturated fat we should all try to limit. The weight-conscious, however, might automatically go for the reduced-fat cheese; after all, there's something sinfully delicious about real Camembert, so we assume that it must be the high-calorie choice. Not only is it *not* the high-calorie choice, it's also no more packed with fat: Both these cheeses carry 12 grams of largely saturated fat.

3.

1 oz General Mills
100% Natural cereal 130 calories
½ lb grapes 100 calories

Fiber is an essential component of the diet, particularly for the weight-conscious. It takes the edge off the appetite, helps fill you up for the better part of the day, and even helps to fight disease. The goal for Picture-Perfect Weight Loss is to get as much fiber as possible for as few calories as possible. The best way to do that is to get your fiber in fruits and vegetables. The cereal shown here exacts a high calorie price for 1 gram of fiber, while this generous quantity of grapes offers 3 grams of fiber for fewer calories.

4.

3 oz sugar-free cookies 360 calories
9 oz sorbet 180 calories

Three times the amount of food for half the calories: That's the simple equation here. This puny portion of cookies presents a classic food saboteur. The cookies are sugar-free, so eating them makes you feel virtuous. Sorbet, by contrast, is pure sugar, so we assume it must add pounds. Yet a generous helping of the sorbet is far lower in calories. The sum of the equation? While both foods are high in refined carbohydrates, you'll take in far fewer calories with far more satisfaction with the sorbet.

5.

1 turkey burger (2½ oz) 140 calories
1 veggie burger (2½ oz) 90 calories

If you thought poultry was the healthful, low-calorie alternative to beef, you should know that there's an even better alternative. Soy-based products are far lower in calories and add the value of positive health benefits, decreasing your risk for cancer, heart disease, osteoporosis, and other degenerative diseases. What's more, soy products are increasingly numerous, varied, and tasty.

list. That's Picture-Perfect Weight Loss.

It's based on a few simple principles, and it uses a simple approach. Let's start with the three basic principles of Food Awareness Training.

1. Calorie reduction is the key to weight loss. Calories measure the energy value of food. They're one of the key determinants of whether you lose weight, stay the same, or gain weight. Watching out for the fat content in foods may be an interesting exercise, but it is a useless one from the point of view of weight gain or loss. Why? Many low-fat foods are calorically costly. *Picture-Perfect Weight Loss happens when you are comfortable choosing low-calorie foods instead of high-calorie ones.* This book will show you how.

2. Choice is not deprivation. Deprivation doesn't work; in fact, it typically has the opposite effect. Starved for what you love to eat by the rules of a "strict diet," you tend to eat voraciously once the diet is over. That's why there are no forbidden foods in Picture-Perfect Weight Loss, no "correct" portions, and

no specified times to eat. It's also why any reason for eating is okay. Food is not your enemy. It is a necessity that should also be a pleasure. Enjoy it!

3. You can achieve Picture-Perfect Weight Loss while living your life. Maybe your life requires frequent business travel. Maybe you're home all day, taking breaks from housework by peeking into the refrigerator or pantry. Do you take clients to lunch? Eat breakfast on the run? Entertain a lot? Whatever your lifestyle, tastes, needs, or desires, you can still make the choices that will lead to Picture-Perfect Weight Loss.

The approach to implementing these simple principles is equally simple. In Picture-Perfect Weight Loss, you *see* your food choices. What do I mean by that?

They say a picture is worth a thousand words. Turn the page to see one that certainly is. On the left, there's a small amount of a high-calorie food. On the right, a huge amount of delicious low-calorie food. Get the picture?

How to "Read" a Picture-Perfect Weight-Loss Food Demonstration

Each demonstration presents at least two related food offerings. On one side is a high-calorie food or foods, on the other a lower-calorie food or foods. Typically, there will be a huge amount of the lower-calorie food. This is not meant to suggest that you should—or could!—eat that amount of low-calorie food. It's not a recommendation; it's a *demonstration*. It's meant to dramatize the point that in eating even a portion of the lower-calorie foods, you will fill up, satisfy your appetite, and take in fewer calories.

Split the Difference

The difference between the two banana splits can be measured in scoops—six. But of course, no one would really eat a nine-scoop banana split. Eat the same number of scoops of the fat-free frozen yogurt version, get the same taste sensation, and save 450 calories.

3 scoops super-premium ice cream 750 **calories**
⅓ cup nuts 300 **calories**
1 banana 90 **calories**
4 Tbsp chocolate sauce 160 **calories**
4 Tbsp whipped topping 40 **calories**

TOTAL 1,340 **calories**

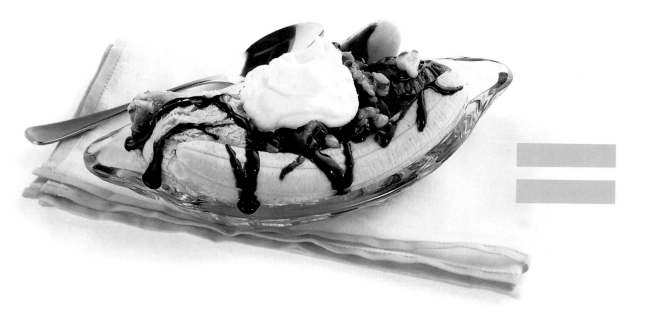

9 scoops fat-free frozen yogurt 900 calories
1 cup diced fruit 60 calories
2 bananas 180 calories
4 Tbsp chocolate sauce 160 calories
4 Tbsp whipped topping 40 calories

TOTAL 1,340 calories

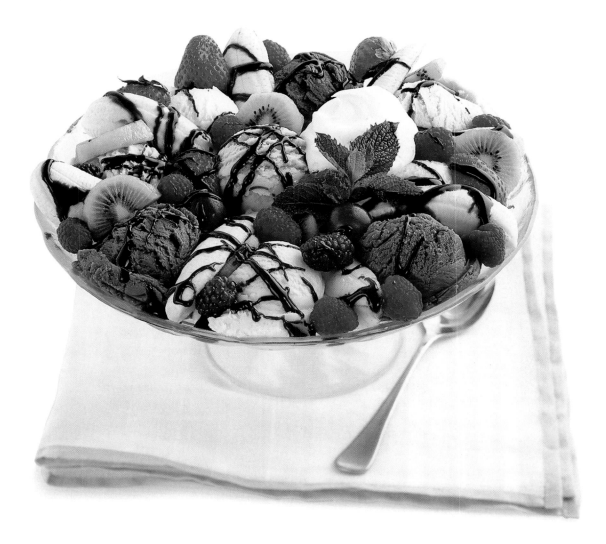

See, two very different sundaes—with the same number of calories. What have you learned from this demo? Four important facts:

1. Eat the food pictured on the left if you want to. No food is forbidden.
2. Eat *all* the food pictured on the right if you want to—or if you can. Yes, you would be eating the same number of calories as the food shown on the left, but you would still be ahead. Why? Because you would be fuller— and more satisfied—than if you had eaten the high-calorie food on the left, and you'll have eaten healthier food.
3. If you eat only some of the food on the right, you're still eating more food than what's pictured on the left, but you're saving a significant number of calories.
4. Anytime you are hungry or in need of food, any food on the right is a good choice.

Above all, here is graphic evidence of the real caloric cost of the food shown on the left. The disparity in the amounts of food shown makes it clear. Obviously, the food pictured on the right is not a suggested alternative for the food on the left; it's a demonstration of caloric equivalents—an exercise in awareness. The bottom line? Eat as much of the food on the right as makes you comfortable—and you will still end up saving calories.*

This book will train you in this kind of food awareness for 30 days, focusing on a different meal and/or food issue each of the 4 weeks. You'll see 115 of these demonstrations, 115 instances of graphic caloric evidence. By the end of the month, you'll have gotten the picture so perfectly you won't even need to think about your choices. Your appetite and your tastebuds will be satisfied; you won't be obsessing about food; you won't need to avoid parties or restaurants— and you will *lose weight.*

And chances are you'll be saying to yourself what patients have been saying to me in the 3rd or 4th week of their Picture-Perfect Weight-Loss programs for close to 25 years: "But Doctor Shapiro, I don't even feel like I'm dieting!"

In fact, so far from feeling as though they're on a diet, patients report that they do not feel deprived, are eating as much as ever (often even more than ever), are comfortable with their food choices, and are losing weight. What has happened? In 4 weeks—30 days—they have simply become empowered. It's what makes Picture-Perfect Weight Loss work.

The Exercise Factor

Exercise is essential to Picture-Perfect Weight Loss for reasons that are both physiological and psychological.

Physiologically, the more weight you lose, the harder it can be to lose more weight. That's because the body reacts to weight loss the same way it reacts to true starvation: It actually reduces the number of calories it burns. That means that you'd have to reduce your calorie intake even further to continue to lose weight.

Burning calories through exercise helps. Exercise actually changes the way the body processes food, making it easier for the body to

---

*Note: Not all brands mentioned in the food demonstrations will be available in every store. Consult with your local supermarket manager about the products that interest you. Also, the number of calories per ounce can be a range; the calories in our demos are accurate within the range for the product.

Exercise Arithmetic

Like ice cream? Then you had better learn to like exercise, too. Here's why.

If you ate just 3 tablespoons of ice cream a day for a year—and did not exercise sufficiently to burn off the extra calories in the ice cream—you would gain 10 pounds. How does it work out?

Given that 3 tablespoons of ice cream equals 100 calories and that 1 pound of fat equals 3,500 calories, calculate as follows: 100 calories of intake over expenditure per day multiplied by 365 days per year divided by 3,500 calories in a pound of fat equals approximately 10 pounds.

The bottom line? If you increase your ice cream intake, you had better increase your compensatory physical activity as well.

use calories for energy rather than storing them as fat.

Perhaps just as significant is the fact that exercise helps preserve metabolically active muscle tissue. Why is this important? Metabolically active muscle tissue uses far more calories than an equivalent weight of fat, so the more metabolically active muscle tissue you have, the higher your resting metabolic rate—that is, the number of calories your body uses when you're inactive. A body that uses more calories at rest is a body that can lose weight more easily and can maintain the weight loss with only moderate calorie restriction. As if these reasons weren't good enough, exercise also acts as a temporary appetite suppressant.

Exercise has a psychological impact, too. Regular physical activity helps lessen the anxiety, stress, and depression that seem to prompt overeating in many people. It "clears the cobwebs" from the brain, lightens the mood, and lifts the spirit.

Best of all, the effect of exercise is both cumulative and pervasive. As your body becomes stronger through one form of exercise, you tend to become more physically active in other ways. You'll find yourself climbing stairs when you grow impatient with the elevator, or you'll discover how much easier it has become to lift and carry those heavy bags of groceries. It's like the old adage: The more you do, the more you *can* do. Your weight loss and your newly fit body are mutually "encouraging," leading to a healthier, trimmer, more active you, ready to take on more of life—and to enjoy it more.

Exercise doesn't necessarily mean jogging 5 miles or getting in three sets of tennis before breakfast. Yes, high-intensity exercise burns the most calories per minute, but the idea is to sustain the calorie-burning over time; that's what burns the most calories over all. For that, your best bet is probably moderate- or even low-intensity exercise that you can keep doing, rather than a quick burst of all-out effort that leaves you exhausted and spent. In addition, recent research recommends breaking up exercise sessions into shorter bouts that you can repeat several times during the day. One study showed that weight loss was greater among those who did four short stints on a treadmill than among those assigned to one long session a day.

Taking the Picture-Perfect Weight-Loss Journey

Picture-Perfect Weight Loss works. It worked for 26 New York City firefighters who lost between 22 and 45 pounds over a 10-week period. You may have seen them on ABC's *Good Morning America*, and you'll meet a lot of them in this book. Another group of New York firefighters was tracked by the CBS news-magazine show *48 Hours*; the most weight lost in the 12-week period was 45 pounds by one individual—with a number of firefighters close to that record—and all kept on losing after the 12 weeks. You'll meet them as well.

You'll also meet members of the group I call the Chicago 7, who were also featured on *Good Morning America*. In the segment called "Lock the Door, Lose the Weight," a group including housewives, professionals, couples, parents, and singles were "locked" into a house for a week of re-education—a kind of intensive cram course in Picture-Perfect Weight Loss—then returned to their normal lives. In 4 weeks, the Chicago 7 lost between 9 and 21 pounds per person, for a total of 91 pounds. And they're still going strong as I write this book.

Also still going strong are 250 citizens of the city of Stamford, Connecticut, who undertook a 7-week program of Picture-Perfect Weight Loss called "Lighten Up, Stamford!" At the end of the program, the leading results were a loss of 19 pounds for a woman and 23 for a man.

In fact, go back to 1995. That's when I read a news article asserting that "7,000 policemen are overweight and out of shape." It's also when I initiated the first program for New York's uniformed officers—with a group of 15 of New York's Finest. In all, they lost 684 pounds as a result of their participation in the program. The least amount lost was 18 pounds; the most was 42—over the course of 12 weeks!

The Picture-Perfect Weight-Loss plan has also worked for thousands of patients I've treated in my New York practice, and you'll meet many of them in this book as well—executives and office workers, homemakers and career women, celebrities conscious of their image and ordinary folks upset about their appearance, young people worried about their health and older people trying to get trim and fit to enjoy a better and longer life.

Maybe you're allergic to certain foods—not a problem. Perhaps you're a senior citizen, and your doctor has restricted your sodium intake or recommended that you ingest more calcium or focus on foods with certain vitamins. You'll do fine with Picture-Perfect Weight Loss. Maybe, like all of us, you have a particular ethnic heritage that you're proud of—or a combination of ethnic heritages—and you love the ethnic foods you grew up on. With Picture-Perfect Weight Loss, nobody will suggest that you give up those foods. On the contrary, it will lead you to a whole new range of food choices. It will expand your awareness of foods from many origins, foods of many types, foods of varying tastes.

Just ask the Picture-Perfect Weight-Loss patients you'll meet in this book. As they'll tell you, not one of them has gone hungry achieving Picture-Perfect Weight Loss. They haven't given up the foods they love. They haven't stopped cooking creatively or shopping in bulk. They dine in restaurants with friends; they go to lunch with clients and colleagues; they enjoy power breakfasts with the boss. You'll learn from them what they do about the urge for a midnight snack, how they satisfy their irresistible sweet tooth, how they "handle" the holidays, how they deal with different kinds of cuisine. They'll tell you how they do all of this with increased awareness about food and food choices—and how you can, too.

There's no secret involved. It's simply a question of empowerment—*your* empowerment. Remember the old proverb that teaches "if you give a man a fish, you feed him a meal; if you teach a man how to fish, you feed him for life"? Picture-Perfect Weight Loss teaches you to "fish"; it's a way you can feed yourself for life. Yes, you will have to change your relationship with food; that goes without saying. But you'll do so comfortably, without changing your lifestyle or your tastes, and without beating your head against a wall trying to undo the metabolic hand of cards you were dealt.

Awareness is the key—awareness of the cards in your hand and awareness of a vast universe of healthy, low-calorie food alternatives. These are all the tools you need to change your relationship with food and lose weight once and for all.

After that, the choice is yours.

Chapter 2

IT STARTS IN CHILDHOOD

Peter is 10 years old and already a computer whiz. Every afternoon, he races home from school and heads directly for his room and the stash of electronic equipment lodged there. His computer is equipped with four joysticks so Peter and his pals can smash four high-speed, piercingly noisy virtual cars into virtual walls all at once. If the other kids are doing something else—maybe playing outdoors—Peter can still play a single-player game, or he can watch a movie on DVD, or he can log on to the Internet and browse, enter one of the chat rooms that passes his parents' security muster, or download new game software.

Peter's mother is happy to offer snacks to her growing boy and his friends. The kitchen is reliably stocked with gallon bottles of soda, cakes and cookies, and all the chips and nachos a boy could want.

Height and weight are entirely individual, but the *average* height for a boy Peter's age is 55 inches with an average weight of 80 pounds. Peter is right-on for the height measurement, but he's already carrying 92 pounds on that average frame.

Sound familiar?

How about Alison? She's 6, cute as a button, a first-grader who is learning to read and loving it! She also loves to eat—with a special fondness for anything fried. Her lunch box favorite is cold fried chicken legs and a bag of potato chips. At home, Alison's mother knows that French fries will keep her little girl happy at the dinner table. As for the fact that Alison is gaining about a pound a month, her loving parents are certain it is "just baby fat" that will somehow disappear in time.

Peter and Alison have a lot in common. Both are setting themselves up for potentially serious health problems when they are adults. Both are headed for increasing isolation—and unhappiness—as their weight sets them apart from their peers. And in both cases, most of the foods they eat, and certainly their eating habits, are in the control of their parents.

Sure, 10-year-old boys want to snack after school. But Peter's mother could stock the pantry with Fruit Roll-Ups, low-calorie beverages, and Tootsie Pops, and she could load the freezer with low-calorie Fudgsicles and Creamsicles.

It's Alison's dad who fixes her lunch box in

Picture This: Food Advertising

The U.S. food industry is the nation's second largest advertiser. In the period from 1988 through 1999, advertising expenditure for soft drinks rose 28 percent, for candy and snacks 40 percent, for restaurants 86 percent. The national advertising budget to promote snacks and nuts alone matches the entire Department of Agriculture budget for nutrition research and education. And the advertisers—pushing mostly highly processed high-calorie foods—are beating the nutrition message hands down.

They're especially successful with their prime target, children. They're getting them young—sometimes even in schools that subscribe to commercial "learning" channels—and turning them on to the very foods that can lead to overweight and health problems down the line.

---

the morning—a father-daughter ritual both cherish—and he could just as easily choose fish sticks instead of fried chicken, could just as easily offer a few pretzel rods and a box of raisins instead of potato chips.

It's up to the parents to establish their children's relationship with food. After all, an awful lot depends on it. And it must start with parents understanding the issues of childhood overweight—and knowing what's at stake. Obviously, young children aren't in charge of shopping for the food they eat, or of preparing it. Over time, they will increasingly take control of their own eating habits, but at this stage, it's the parents who are really in charge. That's why the pattern that parents set now is so important, and it's why their parental actions can really make a difference.

How can parents ensure that the pattern they establish is a good one? According to New York–based clinical psychologist Lynn Vinnick Kaller, Ph.D., a specialist in child and family therapy, parents should take care to make their kids' eating a shared issue. They should offer choices, negotiate, supervise, and monitor. Dictating what kids should eat or nagging them about food is bound to turn food into "a control issue," says Dr. Kaller. On the other hand, making meal choices a shared issue creates a sensible, healthy attitude toward eating and weight—and lets kids turn to other areas, like what they wear, to exercise control.

The Deadly Reality behind the "Cuteness" of Childhood Overweight

Everybody loves a roly-poly baby, a chubby toddler, a "pleasingly plump" schoolboy or girl. In all those slick Hollywood movies, it's the pudgy, freckle-faced little tyke—the one puffing hard as he tries to keep up with his slimmer pals—who wins the affection of the star and the audience's hearts as well.

Unfortunately, behind the cute cuddliness of childhood overweight are some very uncute, unpleasing realities.

Body Mass Indexing for Children

The Body Mass Index (BMI) is determined by dividing body weight in kilograms by height as expressed in meters squared. It doesn't measure body fat per se, but higher BMIs usually point to an increase in body fat and excess weight. A BMI of 27 or higher correlates with increased risk of disease.

Now BMI has been incorporated into new federal growth charts for children as young as 2 years of age, giving physicians an important tool for identifying children with the potential to become overweight. Replacing or supplementing the old weight-for-height charts, the BMI gives pediatricians and doctors treating patients up to age 20 the chance to "intervene when necessary to prevent significant medical problems in adulthood and deal with more immediate self-esteem problems," says Susan Baker, M.D., Ph.D., chairman of the Committee on Nutrition of the American Academy of Pediatrics.

Childhood overweight is as much an epidemic as is adult overweight, and as with the grown-up version, the problem among children is widespread and growing. Back in 1967, about 5 percent of U.S. children ages 6 to 11 were overweight. Just a few years later, during the period from 1976 to 1980, the number of overweight children rose to 6.5 percent. A little more than a decade after that, in the period from 1990 to 1994, 11.4 percent of kids in the 6-to-11 age group were overweight. That's nearly a doubling of the problem, and most of the doubling took place in a decade.

What's more, the doubling covers only those children defined as overweight *in comparison to* their age group. Use the more liberal definition we use for adults—10 to 15 percent above the individual's ideal weight—and the numbers climb even higher. In fact, by the adult definition, the number of overweight children in the United States rose from 15 percent to 23 percent, mostly in the last decade of the 20th century. That means that just about one in four American kids is too heavy.

How heavy is too heavy? That's the other part of the story: A growing number of children are "advancing" from the overweight category to the obesity category. The National Center for Health Statistics has found a growing gap between the weights of normal-weight children and overweight children. In other words, fat children are simply becoming fatter. Pediatricians who once treated children who were 40 percent overweight are today treating kids who are 80 percent overweight.

The Nation's Price Tag

Whatever measures you use to define the problem, the reality is clear: As with adults, overweight and obesity in American children have reached epidemic proportions. And the costs of this epidemic are very, very high.

One cost, of course, is the public health. Back in 1998, the then Surgeon General of the United States, David Satcher, M.D., Ph.D., declared that the epidemic of childhood obesity left "a nation of young people seriously at risk of starting out obese and dooming themselves to the difficult task of overcoming a tough illness."

The risks? As with adults, overweight children are more prone to suffer elevated cholesterol levels, high blood pressure, and abnormal blood sugar counts. They are at serious risk for cardiovascular disease, diabetes, and other chronic ailments.

To take just one depressing example, type 2 diabetes, traditionally known as adult-onset diabetes, is increasingly showing up on the pediatric wards of hospitals. This is a disease that almost inevitably leads to blood vessel damage, putting the patient at risk for kidney failure, blindness, heart attack, stroke, and amputation later in life. To be sure, there's a lag between the onset of the damage and the later effects, but when the blood vessel damage begins in childhood, the consequences can be felt as early as adolescence or at best in the individual's twenties or thirties.

Already, say some practicing pediatricians, signs of elevated blood pressure and cholesterol are being seen in overweight kids of 3 and 4. Might those children suffer heart attacks in their teens? We'll know the answer to that question soon enough, as the trend toward childhood overweight accelerates.

It's an expensive trend. Some experts have estimated that the cost of these risks born in childhood overweight will reach hundreds of billions of dollars by the year 2020. Some of those billions will go to defray the costs of lost productivity in our factories and offices and on our farms, while most of the money will comprise the public health budget that will be needed to pay for treatment and care of an ever larger population of sick people. It's a price we'll all pay.

Overweight Child, Overweight Adult

One of the starkest realities about childhood overweight is that it tends to lead to adult overweight. Studies show that while overweight infants and toddlers are no more likely to grow into overweight adults than thin children, after the age of 3, overweight kids tend to settle into being overweight. They become overweight teenagers and then overweight

Learning Disability

A group of 3-year-olds ate only as much macaroni as they were hungry for, no matter how much was put on their plates. A group of 5-year-olds ate more when given larger portions. The conclusion? According to eminent nutrition researcher Barbara Rolls, Ph.D., of Pennsylvania State University, learned behavior overtakes instinct between the ages of 3 and 5. While the body instinctively would stop eating when satisfied, we *learn* to choose the biggest piece of cake or to "clean our plates."

grown-ups. That's why Peter and even little Alison with her "baby fat" are already at risk. For Alison, in fact, the problem is even more acute. Both her parents are overweight, and studies show that the children of overweight parents tend to copy what they see at home. This means that if you're an overweight adult, you may be condemning your children to the same unhappy condition.

While scientists are pretty certain of the main reasons why children today are overweight—the lack of physical activity, thanks to television and computer games, combined with too much of too many high-calorie foods—they don't really know why being overweight in the growing years tends to lead to being overweight as adults. Part of the reason may be as much psychological as physiological. Perhaps overweight children simply accept their weight as a normal condition—especially if excess weight is something they see in a beloved parent or role model. Or maybe overweight kids simply get into the "habit" of being overweight.

An unhealthy cycle develops. Because the child is overweight, it's harder for him or her to exercise or to enjoy sports. So the child stays on the sidelines while the other kids are burning up calories. That adds even more weight—and makes it that much harder to exercise. And so it goes, on and on.

Meet Tia and Jim Chisholm, two of our Chicago 7 volunteers. You've heard of two-career couples? Tia and Jim are a four-career couple. Both work, and both are university students. Tia holds a full-time job in the housing office of DePaul University and is a part-time student, while Jim does just the op-posite: He's a full-time graduate student in physics with a part-time job in a factory. Tia and Jim were both heavy as children, and although both were athletic teenagers, their hectic lifestyles and crammed schedules leave them little time to exercise these days. Mealtimes tend to be hurried affairs as well, and since Tia struggles with a sweet tooth and Jim enjoys large portions, both have reverted to the levels of excess weight they knew as children. It's a situation they're not about to accept. Precisely because Tia and Jim were overweight children, they are determined not to remain overweight adults—and they are determined to learn healthy eating habits they can pass on to *their* children.

The Pain of Being an Overweight Child

There's little doubt that the highest price paid for childhood overweight or obesity is paid by the child. The psychological and emotional toll as well as the physical cost can be enormous—and can have lifelong consequences.

There's no point in tiptoeing around the issue; overweight children know they are overweight. They get the message every day, and at this important stage of their development, the message can produce a long-lasting sense of inferiority and insecurity.

At school, Alison already knows she's "different." She knows that what makes her different is that she is fat, and she senses a certain isolation, as if there is a "territory" she does not share with the other kids.

Peter is almost always the last person picked for the team in games and sports. In class, no matter how hard he waves his hand in the air,

A Young Boy's Pain—And Progress

They came to see me as a family—mother, father, and 10-year-old son, Albert. All three needed and wanted to lose weight, but the catalyst that actually propelled them into my office was Albert. Even in the fifth grade, even for a boy who excelled in his studies, loved sports, and was popular with his friends, weight had become an issue.

The issue? "Just looking at yourself in the mirror," Albert told me, "and being able to keep up with kids when you're running." For an avid baseball fan who doubles as a pitcher and first baseman, athletic adroitness is certainly consequential. As for looking at himself in the mirror and not liking what he saw, it turns out that Albert had help in that: One day, a classmate insulted him by calling him a name. Even for a popular kid with high self-esteem, the impact was devastating.

Albert's parents chose to support his wish to lose weight by going on the Picture-Perfect Weight-Loss program with him. For all three, there has been substantial progress. Albert has made very real changes in his eating habits—and he is proud of himself for having done so. These days, his lunch box usually contains veggie deli with lettuce and tomato on a roll, a piece of fruit for dessert, and a Blow-Pop for an extra snack. When he goes to McDonald's—his favorite restaurant, as it is for most kids his age—he finds he is just as happy with a tossed salad with light dressing and grilled chicken as he used to be with a Big Mac. This young man is changing his relationship with food, doing things differently for himself, losing weight, and feeling very good about himself. He is also getting healthier, and he thinks that's important, too.

the teacher rarely calls on him. Indeed, studies show that teachers call on overweight kids less frequently, as if subconsciously equating overweight with intellectual failure. And fellow students can be particularly cruel. Peter has already heard some of the names—Piggy, Slowpoke, Whale, Fatty—and he's frequently the butt of painful remarks. He appears to take these things in stride, but the truth is that he has often been reduced to tears by the pain they cause. Many children like Peter come to believe the deprecating remarks about themselves, suffering a loss of self-esteem that may affect them for life.

Families sometimes reinforce these negative feelings by kidding the overweight child about his or her weight, or worse, by using sarcasm. Alison's dad calls her his "garbage disposal." It's meant jokingly and lovingly, but can he be sure his little girl gets the joke? As if such remarks aren't toxic enough, the overweight child is sometimes then encouraged to "be a good sport" or to join in "the fun." But being called these names is no fun at all for the child. On the contrary, like sticks and stones, names can be extremely painful and terribly damaging. What's more, the criticism that follows a response to one of these remarks—"Can't you

Picture-Perfect Prescription: Don't Make Food an Issue

When parents bring a child to my office for weight-loss treatment, the first thing I do is insist that this is no longer an issue between parent and child. I break the loop between the two, interposing myself as objective medical professional, and I ask the parent not to say anything else to the child about food or eating. That takes a weapon out of the hands of the child, and it removes a burden from the shoulders of the parent. And that's what makes it possible for both parent and child to bring a fresh perspective to the food issue—and make some changes that can make a difference.

take a joke?" or "You're too sensitive"—may just add to the psychological burden.

Even when these things are said with love, even when family members are "only kidding," even when comments are made obliquely or subtly—a mother telling her overweight little girl that a certain dress "doesn't look all that flattering," or pointing out a particularly slim little girl as being "so pretty"—the impact on the child can be downright deadly.

Beyond school and home, of course, the media bombard all of us with images of how we're supposed to look. Young children are more prone than adults to embrace these images as a standard to admire and emulate, and for overweight children, it's abundantly clear they don't look the way they're "supposed to." One result of this is that younger and younger children are worried about their own body image, particularly their weight—and, tragically, more and more young children are falling victim to eating disorders.

In one school studied by researchers, more than half of both boys and girls in the first through the fifth grades said they had gone on diets. Another study found that nearly half of the boys in the third to sixth grades in a California school district wanted to lose weight; more than half the girls did. Of a group of elementary school girls who had tried to lose weight, 24 percent had skipped meals, 11 percent had taken laxatives or diet pills, and nearly 7 percent had forced themselves to vomit.

No wonder anorexia and bulimia, the serious, occasionally fatal diseases usually associated with adolescence, are now seen in children—especially girls—of 12, 11, 10, even as young as 8 years old. But even short of these dreadfully harmful disorders, dislike of their own bodies can set children on other dangerous paths—fasting, for example, or the kind of dieting that deprives children of the nourishment they need for growth and maturation as well as for all-around good health.

To those who suffer it, and to those who love them, childhood overweight is no abstraction. It's all too real, all too painful, all too consequential. If you are an overweight adult, then maybe, like Tia and Jim Chisholm, you began life as an overweight child. Watching Jim and Tia progress toward Picture-Perfect Weight Loss, as you will later in this book, is a reminder that you need not accept overweight as a necessary legacy of your childhood.

Equally important, if not more so, if you are an overweight adult, you may be the parent of an overweight child. There are few things you can do for your child that will be more important than taking the right actions now to help him or her lose weight—and step into adolescence confident and in control.

Understanding the Issue

What should you do if your child is overweight? That's the heart of the issue—and the issue is multifaceted and complex.

First of all, it's important to note that not every overweight child is an unhealthy child— or fated to become an overweight, unhealthy adult. Weight gain is very much a part of growing up, and a plentiful variety of food is essential to the process of building strong bones and muscles.

Especially in the period just before puberty, and especially in girls, weight gain— even considerable weight gain—is absolutely normal and may be desirable. That is just one reason why all that body-image scrutiny on the part of young girls is so troubling. If a pre-pubescent girl diets her way through this important growth phase, the results can be disastrous. Some young girls have gone so far as to stave off the onset of their menstrual cycles by simply not eating, or by not eating enough healthy foods. Both physiologically and psychologically, this fear of food is worrying.

Food as Support: Emotional Mayhem

Dieting or fasting to stave off the menstrual cycle—and thus, psychologically, to avoid maturity—may be an extreme reaction, but there is little question that food can in many ways be a psychological issue.

Lisa's parents separated 2 weeks after her eighth birthday. She turned to food for comfort, eating everything her mother put in front of her and supplementing meals by eating alone in her room. Doug had a similar response to an even more devastating jolt. When his mother died suddenly of breast cancer, all he could do was eat—anywhere and everywhere.

Similarly, the kind of derision I talked about a moment ago—rejection at school or sarcasm at home—can drive a child to eat more. In a sense, the child is hiding behind food, internalizing the insecurity created by being emotionally isolated, then "filling the hole" by eating. To the child, food becomes the one safe anchor in an unsafe world, the one friend in a lonely life; very often, in fact, a child responding to food in this way will do so secretly, becoming a "closet eater," like Lisa in her room. Unfortunately, this kind of emotional response can actually help unleash metabolic influences that lead to further eating—and further weight gain. And it can establish a pattern that might easily last into adulthood.

Fear of Food

Parents' attitudes about food also influence their children's behavior. For one thing, parents are role models; their food habits tend to be-

Infant Nutrition: Calcium Caveats for Children

Want to know a good way to boost your child's bone growth *without* boosting calories? Avoid milk—and all dairy products.

That sounds like heresy, I know. Milk and other dairy products contain calcium, and calcium, as everybody knows, is the essential ingredient of bone growth. But studies also show that the early introduction of dairy products can increase the risk of juvenile diabetes. Even pregnant mothers who consume dairy products are putting their babies at risk. That's because the protein in dairy products can cross the placenta and can also enter the breast milk. And this dairy protein is capable of sparking the production of antibodies that lead to insulin-dependent diabetes.

For pregnant and lactating mothers, therefore, the healthiest way to get calcium into your children is to embrace a diet that includes plenty of fruits and vegetables, whole grains, and protein from seafood,* beans, and soy in all its forms. What's more, second-best to mother's milk is a soy-based formula—a good way to give your baby calcium without risk, and a good way to teach your children to like the taste of soy, a low-calorie protein source that will serve them well all their lives.

*Note: *The U.S. Food and Drug Administration recommends avoiding shark, swordfish, tilefish, and king mackerel during pregnancy because of their high mercury content.*

come their kids' food habits, and how they approach eating can influence their children for life. So many of the patients who come to my office in New York have vivid memories of their mothers restricting certain foods because they were fattening or pushing certain other foods because they were considered healthy. Food thus instantly became a kind of dividing line, a standard of behavior. In many ways, the use of food became frightening. Patients tell of asking for an after-school snack and being told they could have "a" snack but not the snack they wanted; instead, many bought the forbidden food secretly with allowance money at the candy store.

Others tell of parents who saw themselves as overweight and introduced their children

early to the fear of food. One patient recalls being weighed by her mother every morning before school. If her weight was even an ounce over what her mother thought desirable, she was given celery for dinner that night. Today, this patient is a powerful corporate executive, high-functioning in every way—except that she is never pleased with her own appearance, never satisfied with the way she looks, never confident or at ease in her own body.

Missing in Action

Parents also affect their children by their absence, which is more and more frequent in today's high-powered, two-job families. What happens when a child's role model simply is not there? Jane is a lawyer specializing in intellectual property. She's one of the best in the business, and because her focus is on international copyright, she's often on the road. When she's "home," she tends to work late, and although she faithfully calls her 11-year-old, Cheryl, every evening at 6:00 from wherever she is, she's with her daughter less than she'd like to be.

Cheryl, of course, gets her sense of self from her mother, as young girls do. But it's hard to get a sense of self from someone who isn't there. Through no fault of Jane's own, Cheryl is absorbing little sense of womanhood at a time when she is developing into a woman. The lack of a role model may seem to her to be a form of rejection, and Cheryl has tried to fill that sense of rejection with food, gaining weight steadily. Other young girls with little sense of themselves may try to avoid womanhood altogether by fasting—damaging their health in the process.

A Pint-Size Challenge

Sometimes, of course, children use food as a weapon. What they eat or don't eat is the one thing they can control in their environment, so eating becomes a way of controlling their parents. Subconsciously, therefore, remaining overweight when your parents want you to be thin is a way of asserting authority. So is secretly eating foods that your parents don't want you to eat—or not eating foods they do want you to eat.

To Diet or Not to Diet

What should the parent of an overweight child do? How should you handle the food situation at home? Should you seek "treat-

ment" for your child? Is there a single solution that works? Should you put your child on a diet or not?

Pediatricians, psychologists, and nutritionists come at this issue from varying perspectives, but all are pretty much agreed that while action can be advisable, putting kids on a diet tends to do more harm than good. For one thing, where young children are concerned, restricting foods only makes those foods more attractive, while urging a particular food on a child typically backfires, actually creating an aversion to the food. Even more important, a diet is a treatment program that measures success or failure. Putting your child on a diet, therefore, adds the pressure of "performance" to all the other pressures your child is feeling. And since diets almost always end in failure, forcing a kid to diet holds the danger of simply adding to his or her misery—the last result you want for your child.

As with adults, there's another way to help your overweight child. Simply put: Apply the principles of Picture-Perfect Weight Loss.

Picture-Perfect Weight Loss for Children

Start by determining whether your child's overweight is normal growth or a health risk. Consult with your pediatrician. Putting on pounds before puberty is absolutely routine, and baby fat may be just that—extra pounds that will peel off as soon as your child discovers soccer or sprouts another few inches or starts cycling to school.

But if there is a problem, as there was with Peter and Alison, it's extremely important to understand it—and to present it to your child—as a *health issue*, an issue of nutrition. For one thing, in doing so, you are starting from a position of love. You're saying something nurturing to your child—"This is good for you"—instead of implying that the child weighs too much. The former can be encouraging; the latter only damages your child's self-image and sense of self-worth. In fact, throughout your child's Picture-Perfect Weight-Loss program, it's essential that he or she receive consistent and total acceptance, approval, encouragement—and all the love you can give.

Second, by understanding this as a health issue, not a treatment program, you take away the pressure. With Picture-Perfect Weight Loss, you're not asking the child to lose weight or even to reduce calories. That's just the sort of thing that lends itself to measurement—and to failure. Instead, you're encouraging your child to make changes. It's a life lesson, not a corrective.

Finally, what's particularly important about Picture-Perfect Weight Loss for children is the same thing that sets it apart for adults: Picture-Perfect Weight Loss is an approach that *empowers the child* to make choices that will be comfortable. Yes, it accomplishes the calorie reduction the child needs to lose weight, but it does so without the deprivation that is always a problem for kids—and that invariably backfires.

In Alison's case, the whole family undertook a program of Picture-Perfect Weight Loss, so there was plenty of love and support, and the encouragement was bolstered by example. The family literally emptied their shelves and started over, shopping for Picture-Perfect Weight Loss (see chapter 5) and changing their eating habits entirely.

At first, of course, Alison asked constantly for the fried foods she loved, and her parents sought ways to wean her from this taste without depriving her of her favorites altogether. Even for a 6-year-old, in Picture-Perfect Weight Loss, no food is forbidden. Instead, I suggested to Alison's parents that the fried chicken drumsticks or French fried potatoes be the smaller portion of the meal, with vegetables and salad in profusion so that Alison could fill up on those foods. I also suggested some subtle substitutions to bridge the way to different kinds of foods; for example, I suggested veggie chicken nuggets or veggie Buffalo wings as a first step to replace the fried chicken. Not only are these tasty alternatives, but they're also low in fat as well as in calories and healthier all around. For the French fries, I suggested oven-baked French fries—basically, baked potatoes in the shape of French fries. In due course, other foods were introduced—fish, a wider range of vegetables, bean dishes, and an array of soy products. In time—in fact, sooner than her parents—Alison learned to widen her tastes and to enjoy a greater range of foods. And everybody in the family lost weight as a result of changing their relationship with food.

Peter lost weight, too—not just by eating the lower-calorie foods that his mother now purchased, but also by exchanging a solid regimen of indoor passivity for a greater proportion of outdoor activity. The multiple joysticks and the DVD player have been moved to the monitor in the living room, and while the computer is still in Peter's room, his parents have made it

---

A Guide to Getting Kids Off the Computer: Get Them Moving

Check out the following practical suggestions to get children away from the computer or television—and, in the process, get them excited about doing physical activities.

◆ Go to the real library.

◆ Encourage face-to-face visits, not just e-mails.
◆ Sign your child up for after-school sports, scouting, or community activities.
◆ Use weekends for family activities outdoors.

---

clear it's there for homework purposes only. Now Peter goes to an after-school sports program that has helped him hone his skills, slim down, and buff up. School recess is a lot easier to deal with now; he's being picked earlier when the kids choose up sides for a game.

In addition, running up and down the basketball court after school leaves little time for snacking. And when Peter's mom picks him up after the sports program, she brings a sports bottle of water and some mixed dried fruit or popcorn or hard candies.

Change *is* possible—and it works. The younger people are when they change their relationships with food, the better off they will be. Where kids are concerned, it's up to the parents who love them to get the change under way.

The Don'ts of Picture-Perfect Weight Loss for Children

Don't make food a bargaining chip. "No dessert until you've finished your carrots. . . . Just taste it—it's good for you. . . . One more bite—please!" Not one of these supplications works. All they succeed in doing is making

food into an issue, encouraging closet eating, and producing results opposite from the ones you intend. Don't withhold food, don't restrict certain foods, don't try to impose a liking for a particular food, and don't make food part of a "deal."

Don't judge your child. Either directly or with body language, don't express your opinions about eating habits, tastes in food, weight, or appearance. At mealtimes with your children, keep a poker face and/or avoid the subjects of food and appearance altogether. Don't roll your eyes.

Don't deprecate your own eating habits, tastes in food, weight, or appearance. And that applies to anyone else's as well.

Don't pile pressure on your children. Must they begin preparing for the fast track at age 6? Is it essential that they attend the fanciest nursery school in town? Should they look a certain way to be accepted by certain people? Children sense these pressures—and often flee from them to food.

Don't talk about foods as being "good" or "bad." Rather, talk about foods that help nourish us.

The Do's of Picture-Perfect Weight Loss for Children

Do give your overweight children the same love and approval you give all your kids. Tell them they're the best thing that ever happened to you, that they're smart, that they're beautiful. They *are* beautiful.

Do set boundaries for your children. These might include 1 hour of television per day, limits on computer time, and so on. And once you've made rules, stick to them. This can help encourage other activities, including the physical activity so essential for growing kids.

Do encourage your kids to exercise. If you live in the city, the streets may not be a safe place for children to play unsupervised, but you can investigate after-school sports programs or join with other parents to share play supervision duties. And here's an idea: Play with your children. Let them know what their bodies can do.

Do listen to your child. When she brings up issues of body image or body awareness or complains about being teased, sometimes just listening can solve the problem or prevent the child from turning to food for comfort.

Do make mealtimes fun. Feed the eyes and heart as well as the body. Use enticing place mats, plates, glasses, and flatware. Talk about healthy eating as you demonstrate it—and give it your loving attention. A handful of carrot sticks will be more appealing if it's offered on a plate with your child's favorite character on it, and the carrots will go down more easily with positive attention from you.

Variety Is the *Health* of Life

Of course you want your children to learn to love a range of healthy foods—especially the low-calorie choices that will help them lose weight and maintain weight loss. Unfortunately, however, trying to cajole small children to love leafy green vegetables—or worse, trying to force kids to eat them—is a surefire way to turn your children off these foods for life. Bribery doesn't work, either. Coercion certainly doesn't work. How can you get your kids to love healthy foods? Here are some tips for starting good eating habits early.

Start *really* early. One- and 2-year-olds put everything they touch in their mouths. Make sure that fruits and vegetables are in range of their searching hands. Cut-up vegetables and fruits make great finger food—so long as the pieces fit small fingers. Even if kids reject these foods at a later stage of development, chances are they'll eventually go back to them.

Don't give up. When children resist a healthy food, don't make an issue of it—but don't give up, either. Keep bringing the food back to the table every other week or so for your own enjoyment. Your persistence may eventually pique their curiosity.

Know that availability is half the battle. Make sure nutritious foods are on hand at all times—and avoid stocking your pantry and refrigerator with the sodas, candy, cookies, and chips that can so easily become lifelong habits. Of course, kids can find these foods lots of places outside the home, but make sure lower-calorie treats—Fudgsicles or Tootsie Pops, for example—are available at your house; they may even diminish your child's yearning for the other stuff.

Remember that you're the role model. If your kids see you dieting repeatedly, losing weight and then gaining it back, checking yourself in the mirror every time you pass one, and clucking over how fat you are, that's the pattern they'll pick up. If they see you eating and enjoying fruits, vegetables, fish, grains, and other healthy foods, chances are they will want to eat them, too.

Bridging the Gap to Healthy Nutrition

Familiarity whets the appetite. That's the theory behind a technique for getting your kids to eat healthier, more nutritious foods. The idea is simple: Package the unfamiliar (nutritious) food in a familiar wrapping.

Suppose your children love breaded chicken but claim to hate fish. Try serving them breaded shrimp or breaded sole as a way to start getting them to accept seafood. Sandwiches are another great way to introduce foods. All kids love sandwiches, but instead of your kid's favorite chicken salad on white bread, try tuna salad on whole wheat to ease him or her into something new and nutritious.

Social Forces Favor Childhood Weight Gain

Food manufacturers spend hundreds of millions of dollars a year targeting young children in their advertising and marketing of fast-food meals, sugar-laden cookies and pastries and candies, and high-calorie/low-nutrition beverages and snacks. Fast-food chains have focused particularly on children in minority neighborhoods in their campaign to sell the bigger portions they call supersizing. Children have responded: They love "junk foods," and for today's two-career family, a fast-food family dinner may be all they can afford—or have time for.

Television is another culprit. Studies show that kids watch an enormous amount of television: 67 percent of American children watch at least 2 hours a day, and 26 percent watch 4 or more hours a day, with the highest rate of viewing among 11- to 13-year-olds. Not surprisingly, researchers found a correlation between the number of hours of television watched and a child's body mass index and body fatness. (Body Mass Index, or BMI, is a measure that takes into account a person's weight and height to gauge total body fat; it's a good way to determine when extra pounds translate into health risks.) Kids in the higher viewing brackets—4 hours or more per day—had a greater body mass index than kids who watched less than 2 hours.

At the same time, kids are less active than ever before. Many schools have responded to budget cutbacks by reducing or eliminating physical education—or by closing gym facilities. With two parents working, outdoor play is discouraged because no parent is available to supervise the children's safety. And many kids simply resist sports or outdoor play in favor of Nintendo, Pokémon, and surfing the Internet.

Put all these social and cultural changes together, and it's no wonder childhood obesity has reached epidemic proportions.

Is there a solution? You bet there is. First, kids need to get up and get moving. They also need to turn to alternative, low-calorie food choices. Want some ideas? Turn the page.

Sandwich Half

Treat your child to a PB-and-J—peanut butter and jelly sandwich—to be enjoyed the low-calorie way. Calorically, it comes in at less than half the tally of an ordinary grilled cheese sandwich. What's more, your child gains in health: Peanut butter contains the good kind of fat, whereas the grilled cheese sandwich's high calorie count comes mostly from the saturated fat in the cheese.

Grilled cheese sandwich

2 slices bread	140	calories
3 oz cheese	300	calories
1 Tbsp butter	120	calories
TOTAL	560	calories

VS.

Peanut butter and jelly sandwich

2 slices light bread	80	calories
2 Tbsp peanut butter	160	calories
1 Tbsp all-fruit jam	30	calories
TOTAL	270	calories

Soy: Mixing It Up

I defy your kid to find a taste difference between these two sloppy joes. The real difference, of course, is in the calorie count—and in the health benefits of the veggie sloppy joe.

Sloppy joes represent only one of many ways to use soy products to create new menu ideas. Be creative!

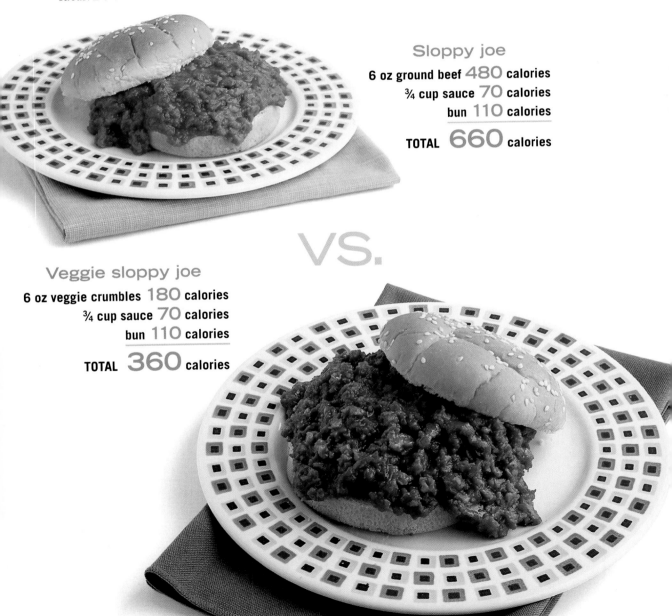

Sloppy joe

6 oz ground beef 480 **calories**
¾ cup sauce 70 **calories**
bun 110 **calories**

TOTAL 660 **calories**

VS.

Veggie sloppy joe

6 oz veggie crumbles 180 **calories**
¾ cup sauce 70 **calories**
bun 110 **calories**

TOTAL 360 **calories**

All-Day Fun

Just because a kid is weight-conscious doesn't mean he or she shouldn't have fun. An all-day sucker is fun all day—whereas a handful of jelly beans is fun for only a minute, and all you want is more.

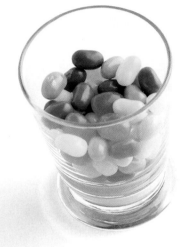

5 oz jelly beans 500 calories

1 all-day sucker (5 oz) 500 calories

After-School Snack

Want to be sure you give your kids a nutritious after-school snack? Study after study confirms that dairy is not the best choice for children, and this cheese, although made with part-skim milk, is still fairly high in calories. Instead, consider treating your kids to bowls of carrot soup and some whole grain crackers. Instead of calories from fat, they'll be taking in nutritious vegetables and whole grain.

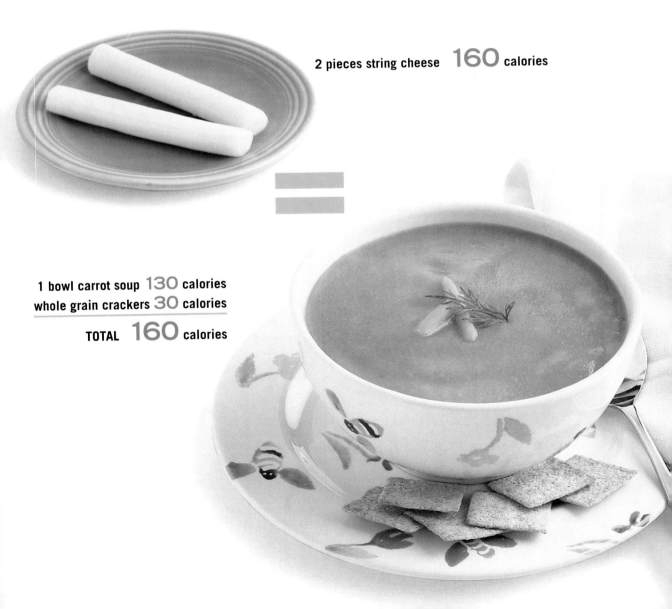

2 pieces string cheese 160 calories

1 bowl carrot soup 130 calories
whole grain crackers 30 calories
TOTAL 160 calories

Red Alert!

Because cranberries are fruit and because they have a tart taste, even the weight-conscious have helped make dried cranberries one of today's trendy snacks. But it's all a bit of a misunderstanding. Yes, the taste is tart, but because cranberries are so very sour, they need a ton of sugar to make them palatable. So when you want your kids to have the nourishment of fruit, think twice before providing it in dried cranberries—and exacting a heavy price in sugar calories.

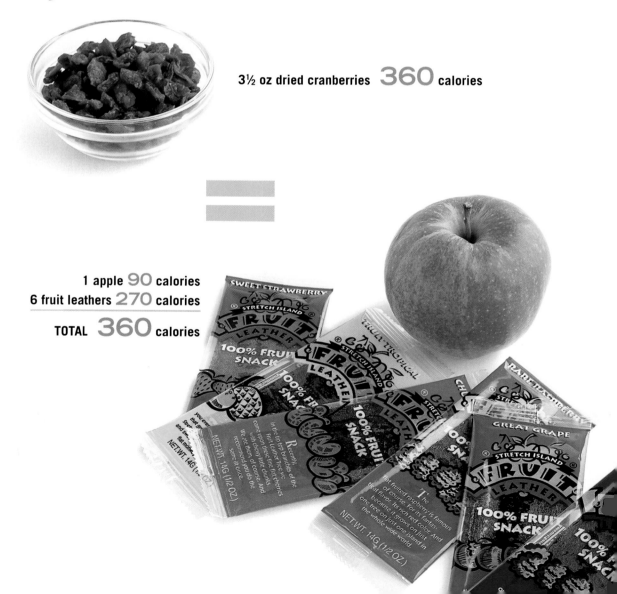

3½ oz dried cranberries 360 calories

1 apple 90 calories
6 fruit leathers 270 calories
TOTAL 360 calories

A Puff of Fluff

Every kid deserves the special treat of cotton candy. If you're worried about the calorie count, compare these puffs of cotton candy to this small handful of jelly beans—and go for the special treat!

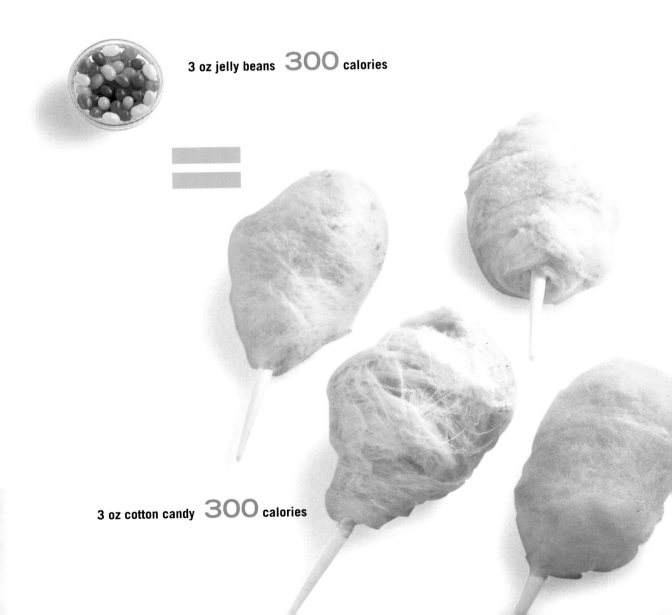

3 oz jelly beans 300 **calories**

3 oz cotton candy 300 **calories**

Lunch Box Fun?

Just how much fun is a small lunch that costs your child 440 calories—much of it from fat and refined carbohydrates? The lunch on the right offers considerably more food and is far healthier. What's more, you're not depriving your child of any of the fun foods kids love—ham and cheese, a sweet beverage, candy for dessert—nor are these foods that set your child apart as "different" or "on a diet." Maybe it's time to redefine "fun."

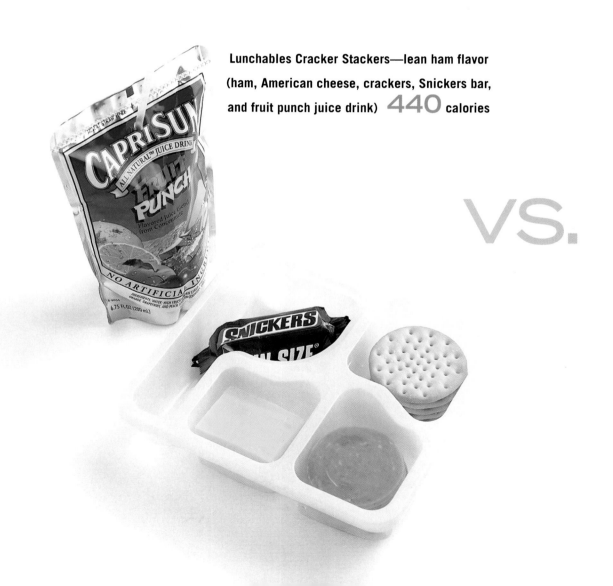

Lunchables Cracker Stackers—lean ham flavor (ham, American cheese, crackers, Snickers bar, and fruit punch juice drink) 440 **calories**

VS.

3 slices veggie ham 60 calories
slice veggie cheese 40 calories
lettuce 0 calories
2 slices light bread 80 calories
pear 50 calories
Tootsie Pop 50 calories
½ oz raisins 45 calories
1 can Diet Rite soda 0 calories

TOTAL 325 calories

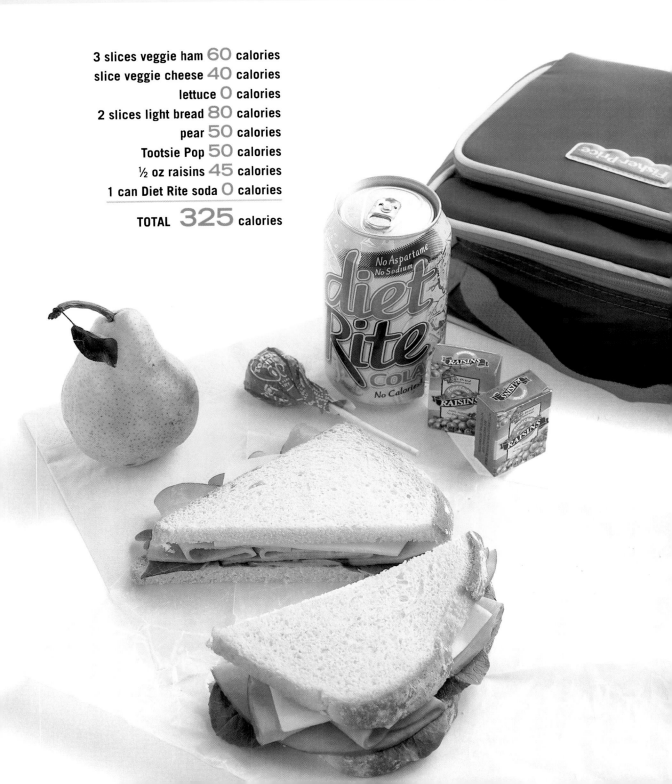

Pack a Snack with Fruit

For your child's lunch box or after-school treat, the low-fat fruit and cereal bar sounds ideal but packs far too many calories. The fruit leather is sweet and chewy, is far more fun, and lasts longer.

1 low-fat fruit and cereal bar 130 calories

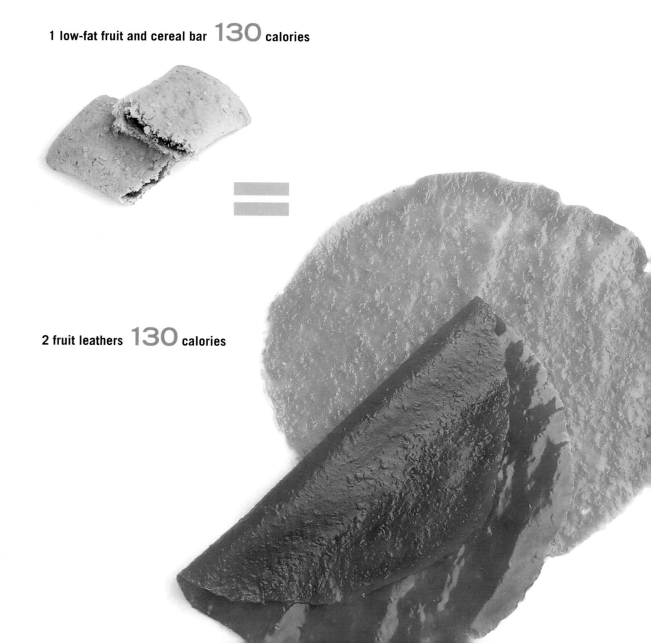

2 fruit leathers 130 calories

Finger Food Snacks

Finger foods lend themselves to after-school snacking, but some choices can carry a high cost in calories. Your kids will have more to munch on—longer—with the snack on the right. And they'll take in some fruit as well!

½ cup **Combos** 200 calories
1 cup **Cheez Doodles** 300 calories
TOTAL 500 calories

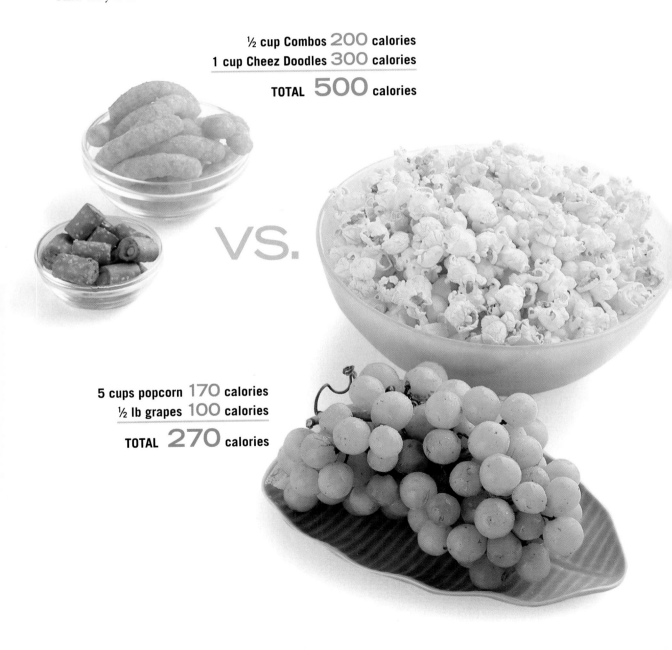

VS.

5 cups **popcorn** 170 calories
½ lb **grapes** 100 calories
TOTAL 270 calories

Chicken Dinner

For the I-don't-like-to-cook crowd, frozen dinners can be a boon. But the veggie chicken dinner on the right is almost as convenient—and far healthier, more filling, more varied, and more appealing than the packaged version on the left. The real bonus, however, is in the veggie chicken dinner's calorie count and far lower fat content.

Swanson Fun Feast fried chicken frozen dinner
(chicken, mashed potatoes, corn, and brownie) 590 calories, 31g fat

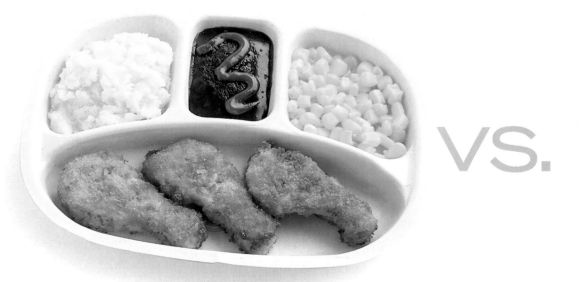

veggie chicken patty 150 calories
baked potato with vegetable topping 80 calories
corn on the cob 90 calories
1 cup baby carrots 50 calories
Popsicle 30 calories

TOTAL 400 calories, 7g fat

Sundae Any Day

Want a sundae? You can spend a lot of calories on the meager portion on the left, or get the same taste—chocolate sauce and whipped topping and all—from the huge sundae on the right. After all, a sundae is for fun and for yumminess; get more of both by going for the frozen yogurt version.

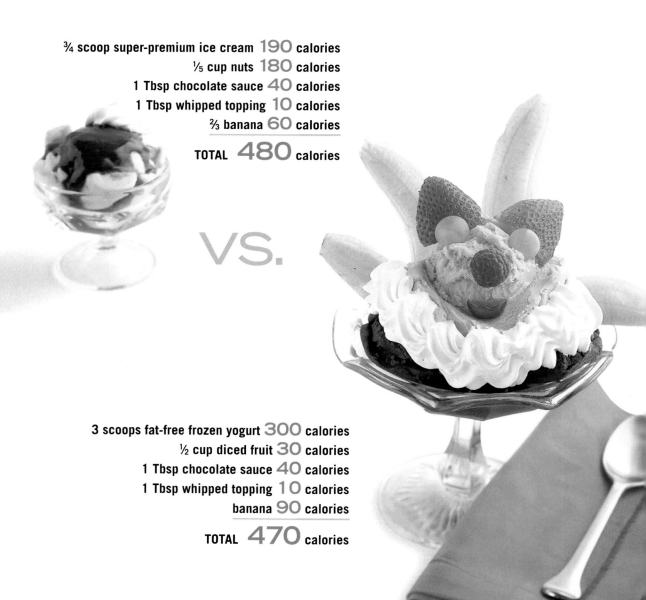

¾ scoop super-premium ice cream 190 calories
⅕ cup nuts 180 calories
1 Tbsp chocolate sauce 40 calories
1 Tbsp whipped topping 10 calories
⅔ banana 60 calories

TOTAL 480 calories

VS.

3 scoops fat-free frozen yogurt 300 calories
½ cup diced fruit 30 calories
1 Tbsp chocolate sauce 40 calories
1 Tbsp whipped topping 10 calories
banana 90 calories

TOTAL 470 calories

The Trick in Treats

There is more than one way to satisfy your child's need for a sweet treat—even a fun, colorful sweet treat. Yes, an M&M cookie is one way, but it's a monster load of calories. So for weight loss and health, consider these other treats.

1 M&M cookie (4 oz) 520 **calories**

3 Popsicles 150 **calories**
2 bananas 180 **calories**
2 licorice sticks 80 **calories**
11 mini–chocolate rice cakes 110 **calories**

TOTAL 520 **calories**

Bite or Burn? The Choice Is Yours

| 1 4-oz M&M cookie | = | 1.1 hours of canoeing |

Child's Play

Looking for a healthy choice for your child's snack? Choosing between these two selections should be as easy as child's play. Despite their "health" reputation—and despite being marketed directly to children—the yogurt snacks and the vegetable chips, which are fried, offer just a little bit of food for a high price in calories. There's another cost as well; its dairy content means that yogurt is not the healthiest choice for children (or adults either, for that matter). You'll do more for your child's health and offer him more to eat for far fewer calories by choosing the fruit and vegetable snacks on the right. And your child will still enjoy cute packaging and foods "styled" for snacks.

2 oz vegetable chips 280 **calories**
Dannon Danimals yogurt 90 **calories**
Yoplait Exprèsse spoon-free yogurt 70 **calories**

TOTAL 440 **calories**

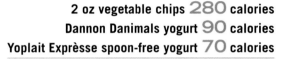

Just Fruit Munchies 70 calories
Just Veggies 70 calories
fruit face 300 calories

TOTAL 440 calories

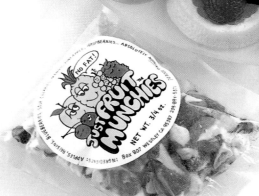

Happy, Healthy Birthday

What's the secret of a child's birthday meal? Fun foods. A variety of foods. And, of course, birthday cake! Yet by playing with the proportions, you can ensure all that and still keep the calorie count low. Check out the two meals shown here. The one on the right offers the same food and the same fun. Nobody is denied anything, and everybody gets the same-sized wedge of all-important cake. But by "flipping the ratio"—a little less pizza and chips in favor of more vegetables and fruits—you cut the total calorie count by more than a third.

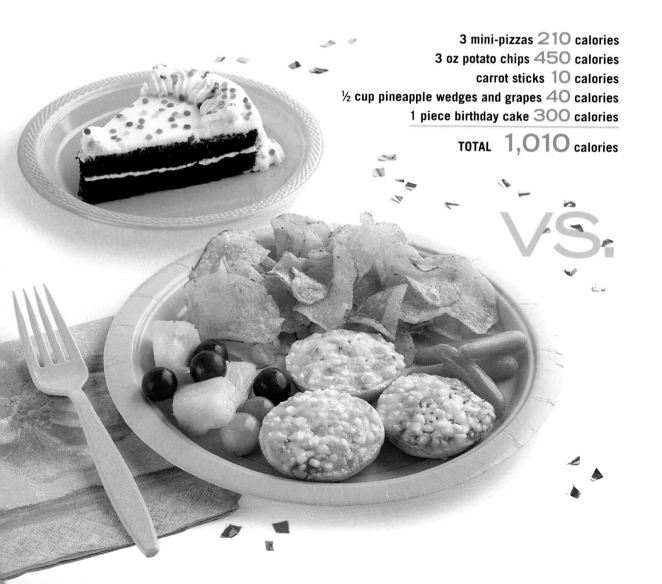

3 mini-pizzas	210	calories
3 oz potato chips	450	calories
carrot sticks	10	calories
½ cup pineapple wedges and grapes	40	calories
1 piece birthday cake	300	calories
TOTAL	**1,010**	calories

VS.

2 mini-pizzas 140 calories
1 oz potato chips 150 calories
carrot sticks 20 calories
1 cup pineapple wedges and grapes 80 calories
1 piece birthday cake 300 calories

TOTAL 690 calories

Chapter 3

THE DANGEROUS TEENS

*I*n this chapter, I want to speak directly to the teenagers in the house.

I know that you're concerned about your appearance—who isn't?—and that the concern often has to do with your weight. I also know that social life has become all-important, and that an awful lot of social life revolves around food. The question is, How can you reconcile the concern about your weight with all that eating? And, just as important, how can you do it without calling attention to yourself?

What do you do at lunch in the cafeteria when everyone is pigging out on cheeseburgers and French fries? What can you eat for an after-school snack that won't instantly add pounds? What do you do at a ball game when everybody is eating chili dogs and fried onion rings? On Saturday at the mall, do you have to detour from the almost obligatory stop for pizza so that you can fit into those hip-hugging jeans you just bought?

Actually, Picture-Perfect Weight Loss provides answers to all these questions. It *shows* you low-calorie choices for all these situations—and for many more—in the food-

comparison demonstrations in this chapter and throughout this book. These low-calorie choices let you satisfy your hunger—which is pretty big at this point in life—fit in with the crowd—also an important goal—and lose weight or stay slim at the same time.

After you've looked at enough of the food demos, you'll get the picture. You'll be able to adjust your relationship with food in such a way that you can feel comfortable in just about any situation involving food—while still doing your best for your appearance and, by the way, for your health.

In my view, though, that's not enough. I think it's also important for you to understand that the eating habits you establish now can affect you for the rest of your life. It's up to you whether the effects are good or bad, healthy or unhealthy, happy or unhappy. For that reason, it's also important for you to understand the pressures that adolescents, in particular, are subject to—and to be aware of some of the real dangers you can face if you mess around with food in unhealthy ways. That's why I ask you to read on.

Do You Want to Be Thin?

It's a silly question. Of course you want to be thin. *Everybody* wants to be thin. Thin is where it's at. Being overweight is uncool. So is drawing attention to your weight by dieting when everyone else is chowing down.

Meet Molly: She was heavier than the other girls—always "on a diet"—and when she went along to the pizza place with the gang, all she ever consumed was diet soda. She never joined in ordering an actual pizza, and she was never counted in when the bill was figured. Eventually, the gang stopped taking her along. After all, if you don't join in, you don't fit in. Molly was overweight, and she was always dieting. Both things put her on the margin.

It's all part of what my staff psychotherapist, Susan Amato, calls "the despotism of slenderness"—and it's everywhere. The despotism of slenderness stares out at us from billboards and television and screams in our ears from radio, movies, and music videos. If you're an adolescent girl, "thin is in" is a message that is drummed into your head loudly and insistently almost around the clock. A study of one teen magazine over 2 decades found that every single article expressed the idea that losing weight would make you prettier—every single article, for 20 years. The fact that weight loss might make you healthy and fit was barely mentioned.

You know what this is all about, of course. It's about money. Companies pay advertisers zillions of dollars a year to capture "the youth market." That's you. All the studies say that you have "disposable" spending money. Either you get an allowance or you work at an after-school job; either way, your pockets are full. It's also assumed that your favorite pastime is to head for the mall and shop till you drop for the latest fashion designed especially for you or for the latest token of what's "cool."

The battleground on which all these companies compete for your money is the media—the magazines you read, the radio stations you listen to, and above all, the television shows you watch. How much time do you really spend watching TV each day? The studies say that teenagers spend an average of 3 to 4 hours a day glued to the tube. (In fact, too much TV-watching is often cited as the main reason that obesity has become epidemic among U.S. teens.) You know what you're watching when you turn on the TV, but do you know what you see? Next time you're plunked down in front of the tube, check out the commercials. See how many of them are about looks. A study of network television commercials found that one out of every 3.8 of them carries an "attractiveness message." That is, they're selling a particular standard of beauty. When you see more than 5,000 such messages, as the study estimates teenagers do each year, you're bound to get the picture.

Getting the Picture

The picture TV commercials are painting—the picture just about everything in our culture is painting—is one in which thinness equates to success and power and everything else admirable and desirable. It's a particular kind of thinness, too. I don't know if you ever read the high-fashion, high-design magazines, but the ads in those magazines feature emaciated-looking women and men. Their bones protrude. Their skin seems tissue-thin. Of course, the stylists who create these ads intensify the look with gray, flat tones that accentuate attenuated bodies. But the point they're trying to make is that this is the look you're supposed to think is the height of fashion, the appearance to strive for.

If you're not looking at those magazines, you're probably looking at magazines aimed right at you, and you're almost certainly looking at MTV. In the pages of these magazines and in the music videos you watch, the movie celebrities and pop stars you admire show off bodies that are "considerably thinner than they've ever been in the past," says Joan Jacobs Brumberg, Ph.D., professor of human development and history at Cornell University in Ithaca, New York. And the supermodels who may be your ideal of how a woman should look are thinner than 98 percent of American women. In fact, where the average fashion model is 5 feet 11 inches tall and weighs 117 pounds, the average American woman is 5 feet 4 inches tall and weighs about 140 pounds. That's quite a discrepancy. One look is fake and contrived, the other real. But you see so much of the artificial that you may have trouble seeing the difference—or you just may not care. You've gotten the message: Thin is where it's at.

Acting on the Message

Maybe you are overweight. If so, of course you want to be thinner.

Maybe your weight is just right. Still, as your mother is always saying about her own figure, you "wouldn't mind losing 5 pounds," just to get ahead of the game.

Maybe you're a guy trying to get on the wrestling team, and you've heard that if you eat just bananas for 4 days—plus maybe take a pill that suppresses appetite—you can probably make the weight and qualify.

Whatever your reason, you've decided to go on a diet. Maybe you go to the bookstore and buy the latest diet fad book—perhaps the most recent version of the high-protein, low-carbohydrate diet that has been around for decades but keeps resurfacing under new names. Or the latest celebrity diet that lets you indulge your fantasy for looking like a Hollywood star.

Maybe you've determined that from now on you will eat nothing with fat in it—not a single food, whether it's a bag of potato chips or a handful of peanuts or a salmon steak.

Perhaps you've found a regimen of fruit and rice that promises to take off 10 pounds in a week.

Or you've bought a scale and a little reference guide and you're going to weigh out portions and count grams to make sure you eat less than before.

Or maybe you decide to eat only one meal a day, or even to eat nothing at all for several days.

Whichever diet you choose, one thing is certain: It won't work.

Oh, you may indeed lose weight—at first. Any rigid eating plan will eventually reduce your total intake of calories, and calories are the main determining factor in weight loss. One reason your calorie intake goes down is the monotony of the diet.

AnneMarie went on a diet that called for fruit and rice three times a day, with juice the only drink allowed. She grew so bored with what she was eating that she almost stopped eating altogether. She lost weight, but she began to dream of the foods she loved; in fact, it seemed food was all she could think about. The minute the diet ended, AnneMarie celebrated with one of her fantasy meals, then went back to her previous eating habits. Within weeks, she had gained back all the weight she had lost—and then some.

That's typical, of course: Weight lost through dieting invariably comes right back. How do I know? I've seen it in literally thousands of patients; they come to me because they're tired of the up-and-down cycle—dieting to lose weight, gaining it back, dieting again, gaining again. They want to get off the roller coaster and find a new way of eating that will get them thin and keep them thin.

As if their experiences weren't enough, every single study ever done on this subject has made it absolutely clear that weight lost through dieting comes back. In fact, what happened to AnneMarie happens in most cases—that is, more than the lost weight comes back. It is estimated that 95 percent of dieters regain their lost weight and more within 5 years of dieting. Not only that, the studies also show that the next time you try to diet, it becomes harder to lose weight . . . and harder still every successive time you try to diet. The reason? Mother Nature tenaciously guards the fat stored within you as a protection against starvation. When you go on a diet and willfully restrict your food intake, she kicks back by slowing down your metabolism. Not only won't you keep off the weight you lose on the diet, you'll actually put more on.

The fact that dieting is doomed to failure isn't the only reason diets are a bad idea. The main reason is that diets are ineffective and can be damaging. That's because dieting is really *inappropriate eating*. Diets tell you when, what, and how much to eat, and that's inappropriate. Why? Because when you follow a restrictive diet, you're not eating for the normal, necessary reasons human beings eat: So we can grow, fuel our energy, help our bodies repair and regenerate themselves, and keep our minds active. And it's inappropriate because when you "diet," you're not eating as a response to hunger; instead, you're actually denying and defying the messages your body chemistry is giving you. The body says it wants to eat now and it wants to eat a full meal—including a salad and dessert. When you're "dieting," you're telling your body, "No! Not now and not a big meal and not the foods you think you feel like eating."

One result of restrictive dieting can be nutritional deficiencies that are downright bad for your health and that can have long-lasting effects. Another result is that you can actually knock your body chemistry out of whack and mess up the mind-body link—no longer even recognizing your own hunger signs. Obviously, that can also have a long-lasting impact.

At this point, you're probably wishing I would mind my own business. But that's exactly what I *am* doing. I'm a doctor, after all. Your health, particularly if you want to lose weight, is the business I'm in. And I know what you're going to say next, too—that "everybody diets." I will agree that dieting has become a national pastime—one that is engaged in by an estimated 40 to 60 percent of American high school girls—but that doesn't mean it's not harmful. And the negative health effects are far more enduring than the ephemeral shedding of pounds.

These negative health effects are harmful in anyone. Among adolescents, though, they can be very serious indeed. Depriving your body of the full, balanced complement of nutrients it needs at this pivotal moment of physical growth and development reduces your ability

Nutrition for Teens:
Meeting the Needs for Calcium and Iron

Any parent of a teenager is familiar with the growth spurt. Occurring somewhere between the ages of 12 and 18, often in increments, almost always noisily, the adolescent growth spurt is a true physiological phenomenon. In fact, it is estimated that 45 percent of an individual's skeletal growth occurs at this time. To fuel the growth of both bone and muscle, the body needs twice the amount of calcium and iron it normally requires.

One consequence of this growth spurt is that teens require adequate amounts of both calcium and iron in their diets. The need for calcium is obvious: It's the essential ingredient of all that skeletal growth. As for the iron, boys need it for the buildup of muscle mass, a process that requires a high volume of blood. Girls need iron, too; their menstrual periods begin, and they need to replenish the iron lost in each monthly flow.

Say "iron" in connection with food, and most people think of a juicy steak or hamburger. Say "calcium," and just about everybody thinks of milk or cheese. But meat and dairy products are not the best or healthiest ways to consume iron and calcium. Both can

VS.

**¾ cup cooked kidney beans plus
¼ cup sauce** 180 **calories,
4 mg iron, virtually no fat**

**1 cooked chuck hamburger
(3½ oz)** 330 **calories,
3 mg iron, 24 g fat
(mainly saturated)**

VS.

1 veggie burger (average size)
100 **calories,
3 mg iron, virtually no fat**

start the ball rolling for a range of conditions later in life, and both can be high-calorie. Instead, teens should aim to get their calcium and iron from soy products, beans, and green vegetables. If those foods don't sound appealing, check out the demos below.

The hamburger contains 330 calories and has 3 milligrams of iron. It also has 24 grams of mainly saturated fat. The chili contains 180 calories and 4 milligrams of iron—with almost no fat. The chili offers an added bonus: It's made with tomatoes and peppers, which are full of vitamin C, and vitamin C actually enhances iron absorption.

Alternatively, consider a veggie burger. It has only 100 calories, 3 milligrams of iron, and minimal fat. Plus, it has all the rich health benefits of soy.

The two grilled cheese sandwiches look alike, but there are major differences between them. The American cheese sandwich on the left costs 460 calories. Since a single slice of American cheese contains 7 grams of fat—mainly saturated—this sandwich has 28 grams of fat. Each slice also contains 10 percent of the Recommended Daily Allowance (RDA) for calcium—40 percent for the sandwich. There's no question that cheese is a good source of calcium.

But soy is better. The sandwich on the right contains 240 calories, and the salad contains 20 calories for a total of 260. Since each slice of soy cheese contains only 2 grams of unsaturated fat, the sandwich totals 8 grams of good fat with 80 percent of your RDA for calcium. In fact, the salad and sandwich together give you 100 percent of the RDA for calcium.

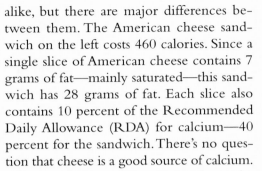

Grilled cheese sandwich

2 slices bread 140 calories
4 slices American cheese 320 calories

TOTAL 460 calories,
40 percent RDA of calcium

VS.

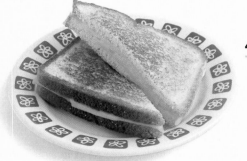

Grilled soy-cheese sandwich

2 slices light bread 80 calories
4 slices veggie American cheese 160 calories
Salad: 1 cup mixed greens with
tomato and 1 Tbsp light dressing 20 calories

TOTAL 260 calories,
100 percent RDA of calcium

Body Image

Take a standard group of white adolescent girls of normal weight, and half of them will tell you they are too fat. That is the finding of a National Health and Nutrition Examination Survey of children and teenagers and the issue of weight. The survey found that black children of both sexes and white boys were far less likely to consider themselves overweight when they were not. It also found that obese kids were concerned about their obesity and wanted to lose weight, but few had access to weight-loss programs that would provide information, individual counseling, and family guidance.

to function well now, and it sets the stage for further health problems in later life—not to mention the fact that it makes it more difficult to maintain a desirable weight.

How to Lose Weight— For Real

You want to lose weight? There's a wrong way to do it and a right way to do it. Inappropriate eating is the wrong way and can lead to results that may haunt you for the rest of your life. Why? Two reasons: One, with inappropriate eating, you fail to take in the proper amounts of nutrients you need; two, inappropriate eating is restrictive eating—that is, you deprive yourself of certain foods and limit your intake of others. This kind of restrictive eating can actually condemn you to weight gain, as we'll learn in more detail later on.

Why is getting the right amount of nutrients so essential? I'm sure you know this answer already: Nutrients are what keep the body working. Protein is the essential body-building nutrient, used to manufacture and repair all the body's cells. Carbohydrates are the primary source of energy. Fats are the fuel for such chemical activities as growth, metabolism,

and the manufacture of sex hormones. Minerals build bones and teeth. Vitamins fight disease. We need them all.

For teenagers, these nutrients are particularly important. Without adequate amounts of all these nutrients, you're shortchanging your body at what is a critical stage in your physical, sexual, and mental growth. This is a time of major bone and muscle growth, and it's the time when the sexual organs are developing to maturity. Inadequate nutrition can affect all of these things. In fact, inadequate amounts of nutrients can adversely impact every body process, your overall physical performance, even your mental acuity.

How? You lose muscle strength, dilute your stamina, and lower your body's use of oxygen. That in turn can result in dehydration and electrolyte imbalances, and it can even make you lose coordination.

Mentally, the mind's reaction times slow. It becomes harder to concentrate. And while some people eat to excess because they're depressed or anxious, dieting inappropriately can cause similar feelings.

In many cases, the adverse impact of inappropriate eating can be permanent. With girls in particular, if the percentage of your body fat goes below a certain critical level, that can interfere with the balance of female hormones. This, in turn, can affect or even eliminate menstruation and may affect your ability to have children later on.

Now you know why nutritionists always advise eating a balanced diet. Obviously, limiting or eliminating any one nutrient—as the high-protein, low-carb diets suggest—is both foolish and scary. A balanced diet is a varied diet, one that gives you all the nutrients your body needs and gives them to you in the amounts you need—as a teenager—for growth and maturation.

As for the second reason, inappropriate eating—restricting certain kinds of food, limiting amounts, and so on—can be dangerous. Here's how it can hurt: Studies show that if you don't respond to your own personal food needs—eating food you like, when you want it, in the amount that satisfies you—you can actually do damage to your body's weight-regulating mechanism. Your metabolism slows, and your body responds as if to starvation, closing down functions in order to save energy. When this "famine response" kicks in, it affects your psyche and causes a pattern of dis-

ordered eating, an obsession with food, and, almost invariably, weight gain.

Scientists know this from having studied real famine victims—people deprived of sufficient food for long periods—who were then restored to food abundance. Even when there was no longer any danger that these people would be deprived of food ever again, they still exhibited the same obsession with food, which is the same starvation psychology that we see in people with eating disorders and/or in chronic dieters. It became a never-ending cycle: Lack of food affected the mind, and the disordered mind then created a pattern of disordered eating, and the disordered eating continued to affect the mind. This link between body chemistry and the mind is real, and the disordering of the link is precisely what happens when you deprive yourself of certain foods or deliberately eat less than your body craves.

In fact, when you feel deprived of food, that's a message from your metabolism. The message is, I'm now going to kick you in the butt and actually make you *gain* weight. Why gain weight? Because you're defying your body's natural hunger, throwing your internal weight-regulating mechanism off-kilter, and in a sense messing with your

Sobering Statistics

The following statistics present a grim view of the diet and eating habits of teenagers.

- Percentage of teenage girls who eat five servings of fruits and vegetables a day: **27**
- Percentage of teenage boys who eat five servings of fruits and vegetables a day: **44**

- Percentage of vegetable servings that are fried potatoes: **33⅓**
- Percentage of high-school girls who vomit, take laxatives, or down diet pills to lose or maintain their weight: **13**
- Percentage of teenagers who do not regularly engage in vigorous physical activity: **50**

Unsafe Speed

A popular drug of choice among teenagers because of its appetite-suppressing capability, amphetamines—also called speed, uppers, bennies, and jollies—stimulate the central nervous system. Under medical supervision, these drugs have been used to treat depression, obesity, and other conditions; in nonmedical or "recreational" use, they keep people awake and may briefly improve athletic performance as breathing, heart rate, and blood pressure shoot up. Eventually, users of these drugs become compulsive, suspicious, and disorganized. Over the long term, they may develop serious mental and physical illnesses.

The abuse of amphetamines to lose weight is entirely discredited. It can lead to malnutrition and dangerous weight loss, and withdrawal can be difficult.

body's intrinsic balance. Your body will fight back; it sets in motion the disordered thinking and eating that lead to weight gain.

Eat Food, Lose Weight

What's the answer? The only way to lose weight and keep it off is to take in fewer calories than you burn up. How can you do that while ensuring you get all the nutrients you need and without depriving yourself? In a way, the answer is easy. When your body tells you to eat, eat a healthy, low-calorie food.

"Sure," I hear you saying, "but what if my body tells me to eat a pint of premium chocolate ice cream?" What my Picture-Perfect Weight-Loss program is all about is showing you that there are alternatives to a pint of premium chocolate ice cream. There are lower-calorie choices that you will find appetizing, and they're pictured throughout this book. For the same number of calories in that pint of premium chocolate ice cream, for example, you could eat 45 Fudgsicles—same chocolate taste, similar creaminess. Or you could have 3 pints of chocolate-flavored fat-free frozen yogurt, or 4 pints of chocolate sorbet.

Of course, you probably can't eat 45 Fudgsicles. Chances are you would eat only one or two—maybe even three. And you would probably want only 1 pint—if that—of frozen yogurt or sorbet. Therefore, by opting for the lower-calorie choice, you are automatically taking in fewer calories. The result? You can get and stay thin by eating food you enjoy. *Picture it: You can lose weight by eating food you like when you're hungry and until you're satisfied. That is the right way to lose weight, and it is at the heart of Picture-Perfect Weight Loss.*

Want to know what to eat at a ball game? How to be part of the crowd at the ice cream store while avoiding the high-calorie choice? Even how to fill the emptiness you feel because you flunked a test or had a fight with your mom or acted like an idiot in front of someone you would much rather have impressed? Check out these food comparison demonstrations.

Basic Blueberry

In a hurry? How much longer does it take to pop frozen waffles in the toaster than fast-food Pop Tarts? Here's another relevant question: Why waste calories on saturated fat just to save a few seconds? Save the calories instead—and enjoy the taste and good nutrition of waffles with real blueberries.

2 blueberry frosted Pop Tarts 420 calories

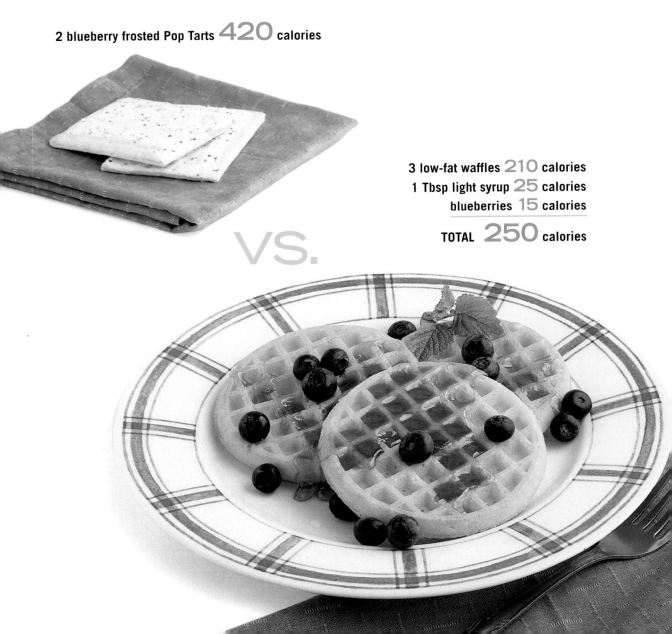

3 low-fat waffles 210 calories
1 Tbsp light syrup 25 calories
blueberries 15 calories

TOTAL 250 calories

VS.

Golden Ouches

Chicken nuggets are a treat, but they can be a calorically costly treat. Veggie nuggets, however, have half the calories of the meat nuggets and are particularly delicious. That's a better treat. What's more, veggie nuggets come in a range of brands. Look for them in the frozen-food department of your supermarket.

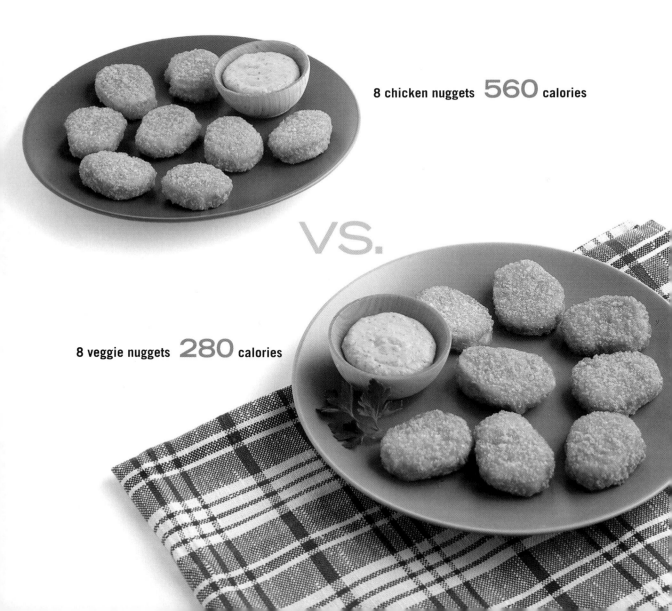

8 chicken nuggets 560 calories

VS.

8 veggie nuggets 280 calories

A Twist on the Pretzel

The fat-free and salt-free designations on a pretzel package are meaningless for weight loss. All they symbolize is a diminished pretzel taste. What's more, the small nuggets go down too quickly, handful after handful—especially since they're not very satisfying. For taste, satisfaction, and weight loss, go for the pretzel rods.

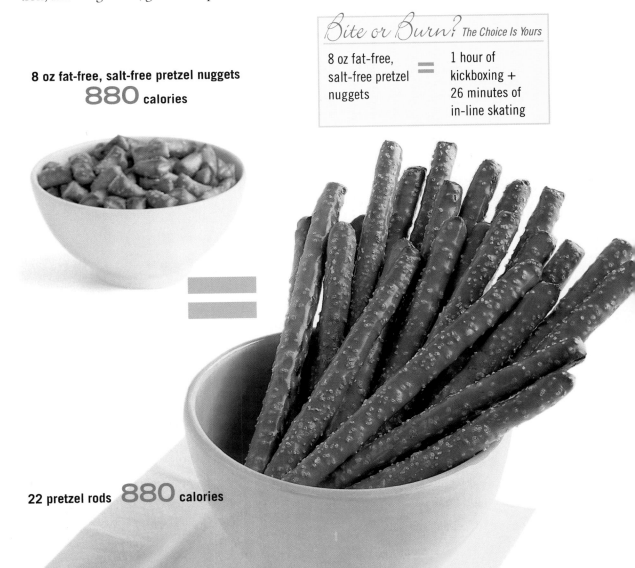

Bite or Burn? The Choice Is Yours

| 8 oz fat-free, salt-free pretzel nuggets | = | 1 hour of kickboxing + 26 minutes of in-line skating |

8 oz fat-free, salt-free pretzel nuggets
880 calories

22 pretzel rods   880 calories

Taking the Edge Off Your Appetite

What's the advantage of a soy product over meat? One advantage is that you get more food for the calories—and, of course, much more in the way of good health. Besides, it's hard to eat just one cocktail frank. You can easily scarf down five, half a dozen, even ten—and that's before you even sit down to dinner!

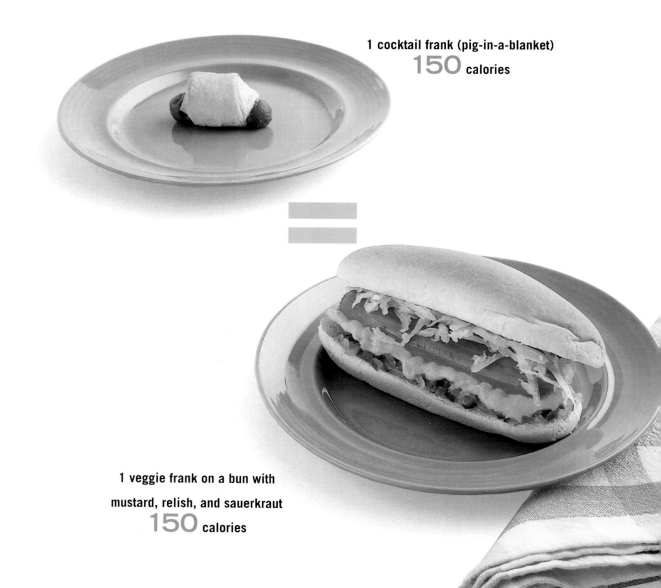

1 cocktail frank (pig-in-a-blanket)
150 calories

1 veggie frank on a bun with
mustard, relish, and sauerkraut
150 calories

Fewer Calories, More Fun

Want something sweet? Want a lot of something sweet? The yogurt raisins may feed your sense of virtue, but they won't satisfy—and they're high in calories. Have the caramel corn. There's more of it, and it's a lot more fun.

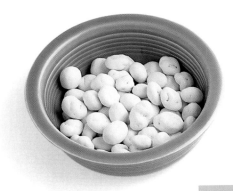

3 oz yogurt raisins
360 calories

3 cups caramel corn
360 calories

One Potato, Two Potato, Three Potato, Four

Where the "side dish" is concerned, think potatoes. In fact, for the weight-conscious, the potato is a powerful secret weapon. Both white and sweet potatoes are satisfying and nutritious, and they lend themselves to a range of culinary possibilities. The ones shown to the right offer just an idea of what can be done with different toppings and condiments. For health, nutrition, and calorie count, any of these side dishes is a far better bet than the standard onion rings pictured below, which are calorically expensive and not all that filling.

Bite or Burn? The Choice Is Yours

9 oz fried onion rings	=	35 minutes of jumping rope + running up and down the infamous 108 steps of the Philadelphia Art Museum—as Sylvester Stallone did in the movie *Rocky*—7 times

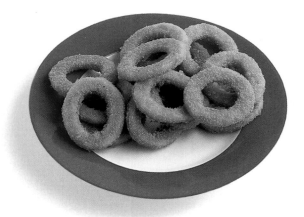 

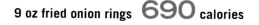

9 oz fried onion rings 690 calories

½ baked potato **80** calories
2 Tbsp bean chili **20** calories

TOTAL 100 calories

VS.

½ baked sweet potato **90** calories
2 Tbsp mandarin oranges **10** calories

TOTAL 100 calories

VS.

½ baked potato **80** calories
1 Tbsp creamy light dressing and chives **100** calories

TOTAL 180 calories

VS.

½ baked sweet potato **90** calories
2 Tbsp pineapple tidbits **15** calories

TOTAL 105 calories

VS.

½ baked sweet potato **90** calories
1 Tbsp light maple syrup and cinnamon **25** calories

TOTAL 115 calories

VS.

½ baked potato **80** calories
2 Tbsp salsa **10** calories

TOTAL 90 calories

6 baked potato halves with toppings 690 calories

Pizza alla Soia

Partial to sausage and pepperoni on your pizza? Try it the soy-based way—with veggie sausage and veggie pepperoni. You'll save calories, gain health, and come out dead-even on the taste!

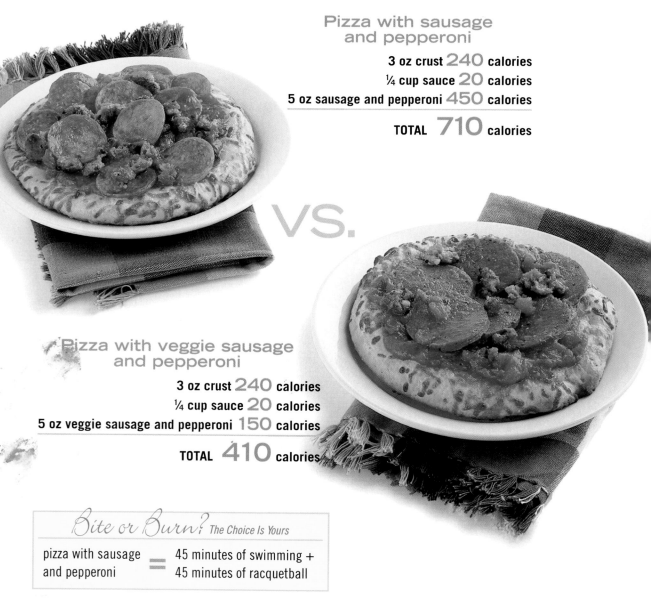

Pizza with sausage and pepperoni

3 oz crust	240 calories
¼ cup sauce	20 calories
5 oz sausage and pepperoni	450 calories
TOTAL	710 calories

VS.

Pizza with veggie sausage and pepperoni

3 oz crust	240 calories
¼ cup sauce	20 calories
5 oz veggie sausage and pepperoni	150 calories
TOTAL	410 calories

Bite or Burn? The Choice Is Yours

pizza with sausage and pepperoni	=	45 minutes of swimming + 45 minutes of racquetball

Ham 'n Cheese

When you yearn for the classic American ham and cheese sandwich taste, go for the version on the right. It is much healthier than the traditional sandwich or the fast-food Hot Pockets on the left—and has about a third as many calories.

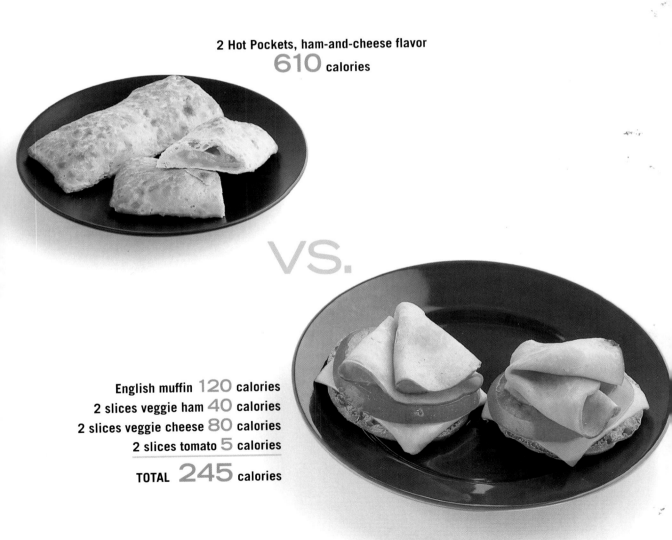

2 Hot Pockets, ham-and-cheese flavor
610 calories

VS.

English muffin 120 calories
2 slices veggie ham 40 calories
2 slices veggie cheese 80 calories
2 slices tomato 5 calories

TOTAL 245 calories

Street Snack

It's easy to rationalize the pretzel; it's a low-fat item that answers to a craving for saltiness and a doughy taste. But if it's a filling snack you're after, think about good old Cracker Jack: A snack-size box weighs in at about a quarter of the calorie count of a single soft pretzel.

1 soft pretzel (6 oz) 480 calories

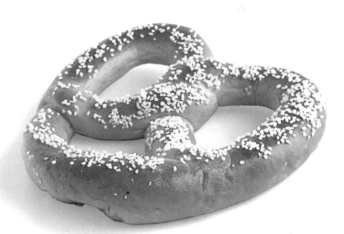 

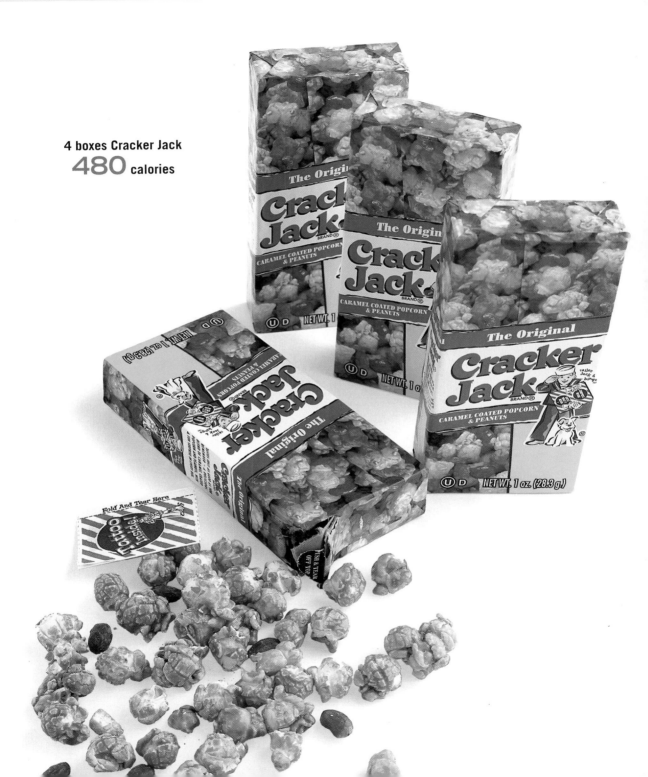

4 boxes Cracker Jack
480 calories

One Little Mini

You'll need a multitude of these mini cookies to feel satisfied, but two scoops of this frozen dessert look and taste indulgent. And even one scoop can certainly satisfy.

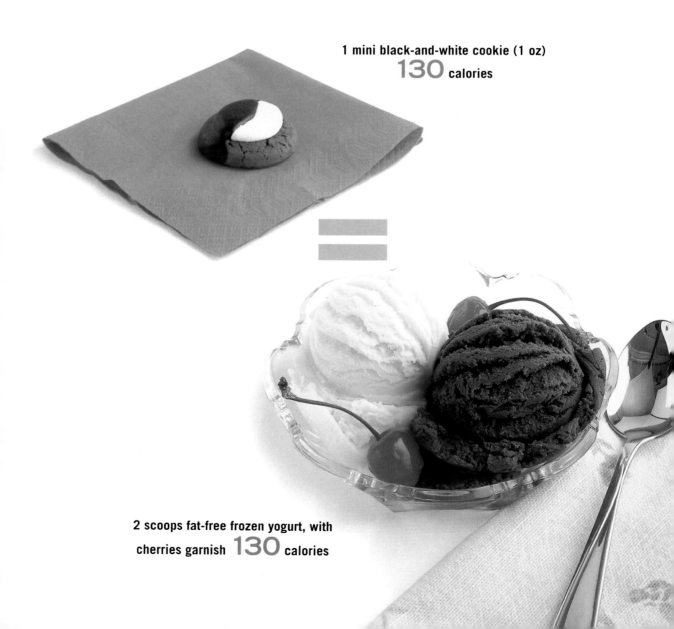

1 mini black-and-white cookie (1 oz)
130 calories

2 scoops fat-free frozen yogurt, with cherries garnish 130 calories

Eating Disorders and Borderline Conditions: Some Statistics

- The number of people with eating disorders and borderline conditions is three times as great as the number of people living with AIDS and the number of people suffering from schizophrenia.
- Five to 10 percent of adolescent girls and women suffer from an eating disorder or borderline condition.
- Forty to 60 percent of high school girls are on diets. On one college campus, 91 percent of the women had dieted; 22 percent dieted "often" or "always."

Danger Zones: A Word to Parents

I've entitled this chapter "The Dangerous Teens" for an important reason: Any kind of inappropriate eating can kick-start a pattern of bad habits that can lead to the next step of disordered eating. And that's the real danger.

What starts as a benign-sounding attempt to lose a few extra pounds can all too easily become a habit. The next step to losing weight will have to be more drastic. That's how inappropriate eating can escalate into an eating disorder—anorexia nervosa, bulimia nervosa, or binge eating. Such disorders can result in long-term physical damage, and can even be fatal.

Eating Disorders and Prevention (EDAP), an organization dedicated to preventing full-syndrome eating disorders, estimates that 35 percent of "normal" dieters eventually turn into abnormal, even pathological dieters, and that a quarter of those eventually progress to full-syndrome eating disorders.

This is why inappropriate eating ought to be a warning signal to parents. It's the first step down the slippery slope to something far worse. Unfortunately, inappropriate eating is on the upswing. More and more boys are falling victim to the body image trap. Making or remaining on the sports team now often carries a weight requirement, and boys who never thought of restricting their food intakes before are looking to starvation or diuretics and laxatives—even drugs—to achieve their weight goals fast.

We also see girls who in no way could be considered heavy deciding they have to lose weight. These girls are simply so influenced by the popularity of the emaciated look that they insist on losing pounds. Their method of choice? Diuretics and laxatives.

And sometimes, your overweight daughter decides that she just has to lose weight—fast—and that means some sort of crash diet that will yield "results."

Parents should intervene whenever they see the signs of inappropriate eating that I'll describe later in this chapter. Work with your teen before it ever has a chance to turn into an eating disorder—and a lifetime disaster.

Diseases Requiring Treatment

With Michelle, it started when she grew into the next bigger clothing size—not an unnatural occurrence in a developing adolescent but upsetting, in some way, to Michelle's sense of herself. While the other girls at the mall were buying tank tops and miniskirts, Michelle opted for baggy pants and flowing tunics. "I need to diet," she announced. "I'll be brown-bagging lunch from now on." In the cafeteria, the other girls could see Michelle out on the lawn, a book propped in front of her and—sure enough—a brown paper bag nearby. No one noticed that she wasn't eating much, that she in fact was eating less and less.

Eventually, Michelle wasn't eating anything; there was nothing in the paper bag at all. At home, she practiced similar subterfuge and evasion, declaring she "wasn't hungry" or "had a big snack after school" or would "eat in her room" because she had homework to do. But the food she took to her room ended up in a plastic bag she surreptitiously carried out of the house and tossed away, and there never was a snack after school. Michelle lived on water and hid her unhealthy thinness in the folds of her new wardrobe. No, she really wasn't hungry; she had stifled all appetite. Michelle was in the midst of the disaster of anorexia.

The full-syndrome eating disorders—anorexia, bulimia, and binge eating disorder—are serious, complex conditions. Anorexia means "without appetite," and it is essentially self-starvation. Bulimia is binge eating followed by purging, typically by inducing vomiting or by abusing laxatives, diuretics, or exercise. In binge eating disorder, the individual consumes large amounts of food while feeling a lack of control over her eating, and she does this again and again. Binge eating disorder differs from bulimia in that binge eaters typically don't purge after a binge episode. Instead, this disorder is characterized by the regular, repeated occurrences of the bingeing—and by the extreme shame and distress felt afterward.

These disorders are extremes—extreme ways of "filling" an emptiness or inadequacy in life, or of compensating for feelings of overwhelming pain, or of taking control of a life that seems out of control.

Almost anything can trigger such an extreme response. Maybe it's an excessive professional pressure, as is often the case with ballerinas or jockeys, whose professional lives depend on maintaining thinness. Perhaps there's a history of physical or sexual abuse, or of anxiety disorders going back to childhood. Some personality types, such as highly compulsive, perfectionist, and self-critical personalities, are more vulnerable than others. And scientists continue to research possible biochemical causes of eating disorders.

Whatever the cause, however, once an eating disorder starts, it can perpetuate itself through cycle after cycle of physical and emotional destruction. Singer Karen Carpenter, dead of anorexia nervosa at 32, and ballerina Heidi Guenther, dead at 22, are perhaps the most famous examples of eating disorder fatalities, but tragically, with 5 to 10 million adolescent girls and women in the United States today struggling with eating disorders and borderline eating disorders, they are undoubtedly not the last.

That is why at the first signs of such a disorder, you must get professional help for the person. Anorexia is not something a person can "get through" on her own. It may take a combination of psychotherapy, nutrition counseling, and medical treatments, and it may require years of recovery, but these disorders can be overcome. As a physician, I believe that in the long run, the best cure for these disorders is prevention, and that may take an overhaul of our popular culture and our ideas of what constitutes beauty. In the meantime, don't dismiss these disorders as "just" calls for attention or habits or addictions. They are severe illnesses and must be treated as such.

Watchful Parents

What can parents do to stop inappropriate eating before it escalates into a full-syndrome disorder? What should you watch for? Of course, each family is different; each family has its own dynamics; and each adolescent who eats inappropriately has his or her own reasons for doing so. But it's important for parents to understand how their own home life and lifestyle may be contributing to their teenager's inappropriate eating, if at all. That's the only way parents can hope to identify and correct the situation before it becomes more serious. In other words, the first step is to see if there's something unhappy and unhealthy at home

Types of Eating Disorders

Each of the three classic full-syndrome eating disorders has unique characteristics.

Anorexia nervosa. The individual literally starves herself to lose weight to an excessive degree. People with anorexia have an intense fear of weight gain and tend to see themselves as fat even though they may have achieved dramatic weight loss and appear to be painfully thin.

Bulimia nervosa. The individual goes through cycles in which she first secretly binges on large amounts of food, then purges herself of the food—and of the calories the food represents. Both phases of the cycle are uncontrolled: In the binge-eating phase, the individual will typically eat beyond the point of comfortable fullness; she will typically purge herself by self-induced vomiting, fasting, or abusive use of laxatives, diuretics, or amphetamines.

Binge eating. The individual eats an abnormally large amount of food during a short period of time and feels that she cannot stop eating. The binge eater tends to eat alone, eat fast, and eat until uncomfortably full. She feels marked distress over these binge-eating episodes, which occur, on average, at least 2 days a week for 6 months.

In all three cases, people with eating disorders evidence an extreme concern with body weight and shape. Anorexics are unnaturally thin; bulimics tend to be of normal weight or slightly overweight; and binge eaters may be of normal weight, overweight, or severely obese. All three types of eating disorders require professional treatment and help.

Warning Signs of Eating Disorders

Following are some questions about your teen's eating patterns and behavior. If you answer yes to several of them, take it as a possible warning sign of anorexia or bulimia and speak to a trained professional immediately.

Anorexia

- Does your child seem overly concerned with losing weight?
- Does she prepare her own food and follow her own diet instead of eating with the family? Have her food habits become bizarre—even ritualistic?
- Does she become overinvolved in preparing food for others, then refuse to eat even one bite, claiming that she is full because she "just ate"?
- Does she hide food?
- Has she lost a lot of weight in a short time? (Weight losses of as much as 35 percent are not uncommon in anorexia.)
- Does she look gaunt?
- Have you found laxatives that you know you did not give her?
- Have her periods stopped?
- Does she toy with her food without actually eating it?
- Does she exercise excessively?

- Has she developed downy hair on her face and arms? (This is a classic physical response to starvation—either imposed starvation or the self-starvation of anorexia.)
- Is she wearing loose, bulky clothing? (People with anorexia may dress in oversize garments either to conceal the weight loss they've sustained or to cover up what they see as their "fat.")

Bulimia

- Check your child's knuckles. Are they scratched or cut? (People with bulimia typically try to induce vomiting by sticking their fingers down their throats; their teeth often lacerate the knuckles.)
- Are you finding laxatives, diuretics, or enemas among your child's things?
- Is there damage to her tooth enamel? (Ask your dentist to check for this.)
- Is her throat irritated?
- Does she spend a lot of time in the bathroom after eating? In fact, does she excuse herself during or immediately after meals? Do you hear excessive flushing of the toilet?
- Has your plumbing been plugged up lately?

that may be damaging the psychological and physical health of your teenagers. If so, you must fix it before the danger gets out of hand.

1. Reevaluate the beauty myth. Perhaps the first thing to take a look at is whether your family life helps perpetuate the idea that

beauty equals appearance and that skinny equals beautiful. Sarah is a young girl who is at least 10 pounds heavier than her ideal weight. She's also bright, a good student, and a fine athlete who loves to ski. Next to most of the other well-dressed skiers in their skin-hugging athletic gear, Sarah looks big. Yet she is so confident in her body and so at peace with her appearance that her weight is not an issue, much less a preoccupation. I attribute it to Sarah's parents—both thin, by the way. They've taught their daughter—they've taught all their children—that true beauty is more than skin-deep and that people come in all shapes and sizes. They love Sarah for who she is; they accept her the way she is. And that's probably why Sarah loves and accepts herself.

2. Reassess your goals. In many families, the stress on achievement starts early. I know families in which children as young as 2 or 3 are already competing for admission to nursery schools. The parents' explanation? They don't want their kids to "miss the boat" in life; to them, that means getting their kids onto the fast track *now*. It also means round-the-clock worrying and working to ensure that their child will be admitted to the right college, will belong to the right set, will have the right appearance. What's the lesson in all of this for the children? That's easy. They're learning early that thin and pretty wins; all others need not apply. In the old days, parents taught their daughters that good girls didn't have sex; today, good girls don't eat. Having a thin, fit, "buff" body has become part of the achievement demanded of children by high-powered perfectionist parents. It's how they define success.

3. Reestablish the proper role model. Of course, children learn not just by being told but also by the behavior of their parent role models. A patient of mine—I'll call her Jan—told me that her mother, who was permanently thin, repeatedly checked herself in the mirror, consistently pushed away certain foods, and constantly fretted aloud over her thighs or waistline or clothes that felt "too tight." Naturally, Jan quickly picked up the idea that appearance is all-important and that food makes appearance. She'd been well taught—to be always "on a diet," always exercising to remain thin, always vigilant to eliminate certain foods. She learned early her mother's preoccupation and, not surprisingly, now found herself passing it along to her own daughter.

By example, children can learn either that eating is a response to hunger or that it is a way of dealing with loneliness, boredom, or anger. When you respond to stress in a mature way, your children will learn to respond to stress the same way—and to save the chowing down for mealtimes.

4. Reassert differences in identity. Many parents change their expectations for their children right around the time of adolescence. Now that the kids are outgrowing their baby fat and baby looks and entering puberty, their parents have new concerns—and appearance and weight can be high on the list. Of course, those concerns are often born of love: No parent wants to see his or her child ostracized, as overweight teenagers very often are. But sometimes, parental concerns have another source—namely, the parents' sense of their own identification.

Be honest: How many times have you seen parents feeling somehow embarrassed about their overweight daughter or son, as if the child's weight were a condemnation of the parents, something that would lower their status among their peers? Sure, they want their child to lose weight: It will reflect better on *them*. To the child, the unspoken but unmistakable message is that the parents will love them better "if only" they lose weight.

A Mother's "Wrong Message"

Marilyn was 8 when her mother dragged her to a nutritionist for help in losing weight. That wasn't the first time she had gotten the maternal message that she was overweight, and it was far from the last time.

The only child of divorced parents, Marilyn lived full-time with her petite, delicately beautiful mother, a woman who, in Marilyn's words, "has her own issues about food and weight." Marilyn's maternal grandmother was heavy, and her father's family tended to be overweight. She now understands that her mother's protective instincts focused on the fear that her daughter, who was born big, would become overweight. The mistake, Marilyn wisely says, was that her mother made her weight an issue—at age 8—"before it was an issue."

Marilyn also understands that her mother is "a controlling kind of person," and while she knows her mother "wanted me to be safe and happy, she sometimes was too controlling." For Marilyn, the one area her mother couldn't control full-time was food, "so I ate and ate for control." Through childhood and adolescence, Marilyn steadily gained weight. Her mother repeatedly decreed diets, even had doctors prescribe medication, "but on my own, I would eat whatever and whenever I wanted."

At college, well out of her mother's control, Marilyn spent "4 incredible years living on bagel sandwiches" and undertaking a rigorous academic program. She also learned a lot about responsibility. She remembers a phone call when her mother asked, as usual, about her weight. For the first time, Marilyn refused to answer. "This is not your problem," she told her mother. "It is my problem, and I will deal with it. It is not your issue, and you may not have this conversation with me anymore." Changing her relationship with her mother in this way was Marilyn's first step toward changing her relationship with food.

But it still took time. After graduation, ambitious for success, Marilyn headed for New York, a new job, and a new life. And she *was* a success—active, engaged, well-regarded. In fact, it was when "things got really, really good that I realized I couldn't live my life as I was. I wasn't happy overweight, and I knew I needed a healthier lifestyle. I was ready to take responsibility."

With the enthusiastic support of her mother, Marilyn came to see me. In the first 7 months under my care, she lost 40 pounds. It was, she says, "remarkably easy." What made it easy for Marilyn was what went on in her mind before anything at all changed in her body. She came to understand her mother's subconscious motivation—"I think her fear about appearance manifested itself in me"—and she and her mother have since discussed it at length, with her mother conceding she had been wrong and regretting it fiercely.

Her mother's regret wasn't what counted, though. What counted was Marilyn's understanding that "I need to take responsibility for my own happiness," and her knowledge that she *could*—that it was in her hands. Once she was empowered in her mind, it's no wonder it was "remarkably easy" for Marilyn to exercise control and change her relationship with food.

5. Reaffirm your connections. A lot of things change when children move into adolescence. Parent-child relationships change—often not for the better. Men in particular seem to have a problem relating to their teenage children. One response is to distance themselves emotionally from their children. "They have to learn to stand on their own," such fathers say of their teenage kids; "they have to learn to work through their own problems." Of course, but is distancing yourself emotionally the way to teach that lesson? Too many fathers suddenly withdraw from their children precisely what the children need at this crucial time in their lives—the support and interest that only a father can give, the sense that their fathers validate their identities. This is no time for fear of intimacy, and buying things for your children is no substitute for giving of yourself. Unfulfilled father hunger, as it has been called, can be the start of a lifetime of disappointing relationships—and a trigger to inappropriate eating.

6. Return to affection. Many fathers also view the onset of adolescence as a signal to cut back on physical demonstrations of affection. Suddenly, they decide that the little boys they used to hug freely are "men" now and no longer need expressions of affection, while their daughters' sexual development makes physical contact both uncomfortable and unseemly—or so many fathers assume. But teenage girls who sense that their fathers no longer want to cuddle them will wonder what they have done wrong. They conclude that whatever it is, it has something to do with the body and its changes. Consciously or not, girls know that eating less can slow the progress of those changes, so many pursue intensive weight-loss efforts.

7. Relieve the stress of unwelcome events. Often, inappropriate eating is triggered by events or situations that neither parents nor children can control. The sickness or even death of a parent, a move to another town, family financial woes, divorce: Any change in family life can change the way

What's Causing Teenage Obesity?

Researchers for the Centers for Disease Control and Prevention have cited a number of factors that contribute to today's epidemic of adolescent obesity. The main culprits, according to William H. Dietz, M.D., Ph.D., director of the division of nutrition and physical activity at the National Center for Chronic Disease Prevention and Health Promotion, are the lack of physical activity and increased television viewing among American teens. Other causes cited by Dr. Dietz include:

- The increased use of microwave ovens, which take control over what kids eat away from parents
- Increased consumption of fast food
- Missed or skipped meals, which cause overeating later in the day
- The increased consumption of soft drinks, which now account for 8 percent of the average daily calorie intake by teenagers
- The number of new food products introduced—12,000 each year

teenagers deal with food. Sometimes, the change in eating habits will be directly related to the change in family life. For example, if a mother becomes ill with cancer and her child suddenly refuses to eat any food that can be considered carcinogenic, that is an obvious cause-and-effect. Or an 18-year-old college freshman, with no parents to tell him to go to bed or eat three squares a day, will let both his sleeping and his eating get out of control. Remember your own first year away from home?

Divorce can be another major precipitant of inappropriate eating, and it is growing more pervasive every day. Today, slightly more than half of all first marriages and 70 percent of all second marriages in the United States end in divorce. The result is that half the children in this country are subjected to divorce at least once, and 35 percent of them are subjected to it twice. It turns their lives upside down. For teenagers aware of the frictions and fractures in the household, eating inappropriately can be the one way they can get attention, attention they think just might hold the family together. Or sometimes children subconsciously see the divorce as their fault, and they begin to eat inappropriately out of guilt. Either way, the change that divorce brings is fertile ground for children to develop eating issues. Strengthening ties with your teens at these stressful times by encouraging them to express their feelings can head off problems later.

Stopping or Preventing Inappropriate Eating in Your Teenager

How can parents protect against inappropriate eating? First, as suggested earlier, examine your family's values and your own goals for your children. Take care that neither your words nor your behavior sends a message that emphasizes body shape, and don't convey an attitude that you will love your kids more if only they lose weight, wear certain clothes, or have a certain appearance.

Second, teach your children that there is a wide-ranging diversity of body shapes and sizes and that finding any one body type "bad" and another "good" is as ugly a prejudice as racism. It's a big world, filled with people of different colors, shapes, and sizes.

Finally, learn, follow, and teach your children a sensible way of eating and exercising for health—and for life. The Picture-Perfect Weight-Loss program in this book *shows* teenagers how they can eat plenty of tasty food and still lose weight.

Picture-Perfect Weight Loss is not a diet; it's an anti-diet. It doesn't demand that teenagers eat certain foods or eliminate certain foods, doesn't disrupt their marathon schedules with special eating times, and won't draw attention to the teenager in a group eating situation or mark the teenager as either "on a diet" or "pigging out."

By learning and applying the basic principles of Picture-Perfect Weight Loss themselves, parents can become role models for their children. By teaching Picture-Perfect Weight Loss to their teenagers, they will help them lose weight and maintain weight loss healthfully and sensibly. With good, low-calorie eating according to Picture-Perfect Weight-Loss principles, you can set an example and offer guidance that will benefit your teenagers for life.

Chapter 4

THE MIDDLE YEARS
AND BEYOND

*D*ick Johnson knew he had to quit smoking. After all, he was in his late thirties now, the father of young children who would one day want to emulate Dad's behavior. What's more, as a reporter and anchor on the early morning news program at WLS-TV, Chicago's ABC affiliate, Dick was something of a public figure—and public figures shouldn't be caught smoking.

Most of all, of course, there was the health issue: not just the long-term danger of deadly disease, but also the more immediate impact on daily life, athletic ability, and energy level. Dick realized that the day was not too distant when he would no longer be able to swat a tennis ball for an hour at a time, or run up and down a basketball court with his kids. For a guy who gets up at 2:45 A.M. 5 days a week, then puts in a 12-hour work day and also tries to live a family life with his wife and children, the handwriting was on the wall. It spelled out: Quit smoking or else.

So Dick quit. Not just once, not just twice, but six or seven times, each time ending in failure. In fact, the only gain Dick realized from trying to quit smoking was in his weight;

with each attempt, he put on anywhere from 5 to 10 pounds. By the time he finally succeeded in freeing himself of the cigarette habit, he was in his early forties and some 60 pounds overweight. Dick is 6 feet 3 inches tall, so he wore the added weight pretty well, and since television anchors are mostly visible from the waist up, his progression from a 46-long suit size to a 52 looked as much like gaining authority as adding weight.

But Dick, of course, could feel the difference. At 47, his middle-age heft was beginning to be almost as much of a health hazard as the smoking had been, and the feeling of low-energy sluggishness was proving just as limiting.

Debbie Davis is another TV professional—a makeup artist at Chicago's Fox television station. Permanently attached to one popular show and on-call to a range of others, Debbie is a woman on the move every hour of the day 7 days a week. Her cellular phone is her most reliable address; otherwise, she's here, there, in an airport, on the road—rarely staying still. No wonder she is a self-described "junk food

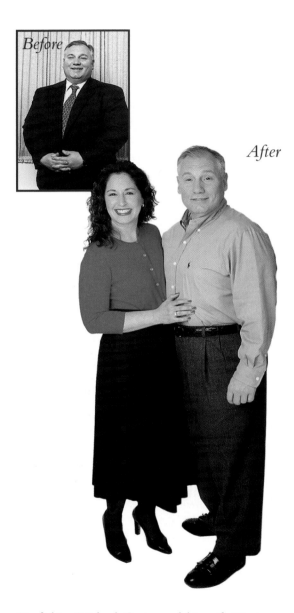

Before

After

Firefighter Michael Carter and his wife Marion together lost 110 pounds on Picture-Perfect Weight Loss. Mike's secret for maintaining his weight: "I can always find an alternative to the high-calorie choice."

junkie." There isn't time for anything else—and, Debbie adds, "it's quick energy." Or so she thought.

The mother of two young daughters, Debbie gained pounds steadily after her pregnancies without being conscious of her weight gain. One day, she woke up to find that she tipped the scale at more than 200 pounds and had gone from a size 12 to a size 18. She's a woman who loves to eat, but she's also a woman in a business based on image. How could she reconcile an erratic schedule, the demands of single parenthood—she is recently divorced—and the responsibilities of a demanding job with what she saw as a failure to lose weight and keep it off?

With a busy career as a corporate auditor, Joanne Rusch was often on the road. In fact, her work and travel kept her too busy even to think about starting a family. If she did get pregnant, she decided, it would be the signal to find a way to work at home. "I saw too many pregnant women hauling computers through airports," Joanne explains. "I didn't want to do that."

Meanwhile, Joanne's biological clock was ticking. It was time. She and her husband decided on a major joint undertaking: to start a financial planning consultancy, working out of their house, and to start a family. Joanne was 39 when she became pregnant, and she was 40 when she gave birth to a beautiful, healthy baby girl. And during the 9 months of her pregnancy, Joanne gained 57 pounds.

For Heidi McInerney, the issue has always been time. With a husband, three small chil-

Who Eats Vegetables?

Apparently, people between the ages of 18 and 34 don't eat their vegetables, at least according to a survey by the Centers for Disease Control and Prevention. It found that most people in that age group ate only one or two servings of vegetables per day, not the five or more recommended by the government. In fact, many in this age group ate no vegetables at all. Only among those 65 and older did more than 40 percent eat three or four servings of vegetables a day.

dren, a household to co-manage, and a part-time job as an optician, time is at a premium.

Call Heidi during the day, and chances are you'll have to shout to be heard above the hum of two washers, two driers, and a dishwasher. By the time she has finished seeing her husband and oldest child off to work and school, feeding the little ones, putting them down for their naps, picking up after everyone, and cleaning the house, "it's all I can do to grab something to eat. Having the time to think about planning and preparing three nutritious meals is out of the question."

And as the only overweight person in a family of thin people, "it's hard to eat differently."

Time is an issue for David Taylor, too. He's 36 and single—which means that when he gets home at the end of a long day, there's no one there to help with all the chores of running a household, cleaning, paying bills, and the like. And David's day is a long one. A media services salesman, he spends 9 hours a day dealing with press and public relations professionals, logging scads of phone time and occasionally heading out of town on a business trip. He's also in a bowling league and is pursuing religious studies in what might be called his spare time.

With a schedule so hectic—and without much interest in cooking for himself—David has always found it most convenient just to pick up his evening meal on the way home. Easiest of all are pizza and fast food—ready-to-eat meals that require no preparation beyond opening the package.

David is a sports enthusiast, especially competitive sports—and particularly tennis. But the Chicago winter, with its subfreezing temperatures and short daylight hours, is hardly conducive to such athletics—unless you invest your life savings in a tennis club membership, which David is disinclined to do. Until the spring and summer bring longer days and the chance to hit a ball outdoors, he tends to participate in sports mostly as a spectator—either in front of the television or surfing the Internet, two situations that typically lend themselves to such high-calorie snacks as David's beloved Salt and Vinegar Pringles. It's a matter of circumstances, and in his mid-thirties, circumstances have brought David Taylor to an uncomfortable and unhealthy level of overweight.

Busy Lives, Stressful Lives

Sound familiar? The lives I've just briefly described belong to five of the Chicago 7—you met the other two, Tia and Jim Chisholm, back in chapter 2. These are the folks we virtually locked into a suburban house in November 2000 for a week-long crash course in Picture-Perfect Weight Loss under the auspices of ABC's *Good Morning America*. I'll bet that elements of their stories sound just like your life.

Same with the scores of firefighters who pour through my office in New York. Given that their jobs are among the most dangerous in the world, you would probably be surprised at the answers they give when asked what really stresses them out. One told me it was his commute into New York City from Long Island—along a highway famously referred to as "the longest parking lot in the world." Another cited the need to take care of five loads of laundry when he gets home at night. A third said it was the fact that he and his working wife pass one another like ships in the night. He told me he couldn't remember the last time they sat down together and talked. In fact, he was planning on asking her out for a date, but first he had to figure out a time when both were free.

These are guys who work 15- or 24-hour shifts, during which they are confined to what is basically a garage, where they wait . . . and wait . . . and wait. If and when an alarm comes, it is always, always tense—quite literally a matter of life and death.

Traditionally, one firefighter is assigned to be in charge of buying, preparing, and cooking the meals for that shift. There's no menu, and there are no options. You eat what that individual puts in front of you—or you don't eat.

And firefighters tend to eat. For one thing, it's a way to alleviate the boredom of all that waiting around. In fact, with all the rich diversity of New York food at their disposal, New York's Bravest, as our firefighters are called, can find themselves munching all day long: bagels for breakfast, doughnuts and cakes with a second cup of coffee, leftovers to nibble on, a hearty lunch, afternoon snacks of chips and candies, and a big dinner at night. Calls typically come at night, so it's not unusual for that big dinner to be interrupted.

While all the firefighters who undertook Picture-Perfect Weight Loss with me are fit enough to carry 75 pounds of weight on their backs up numerous flights of stairs through smoke and fire, many were beginning to feel the effects of the pounds they had been putting on over the years. With minimal access to exercise facilities; plenty of high-calorie food at their fingertips; all the obligations, responsibilities, stresses, and anxieties shared by middle-age folks everywhere; and a high-risk, high-anxiety profession, it's no wonder these guys were weighed down with extra pounds. It's no surprise they were so ready to do something about it that they subjected themselves to the derision—at first, anyway—of a lot of self-styled tough-guy colleagues.

The Weight Gain
You Didn't See Coming

Welcome to the middle years.

Maybe you're not a firefighter, or a media services rep, or a TV anchor, or a corporate auditor, or a mom/part-time professional, or a full-time makeup artist with a cell phone

The "Spare Tire" in Women

Weight gain around the middle is an issue that is front and center for women in midlife, and the "spare tire" that is gained can be dangerous. Why? Doctors think that the particular kind of fat that accumulates at the waistline contributes to high blood pressure and higher blood levels of cholesterol.

What causes the spare tire? One key factor is the decline in levels of growth hormone and estrogen during menopause; a second factor is a possible rise in levels of the stress hormone cortisol, which both increases appetite and sends the extra calories directly to the belly. Confirming this theory, Swedish researchers have found that stressed-out monkeys had high cortisol levels, overate, and developed abdominal obesity.

---

pasted to your ear. But if you're somewhere between the ages of 30 and 55, chances are good that you woke up one morning to find that you had put on a few pounds. Possibly even a lot of pounds.

I'll bet it sneaked up on you. One day, you just happened to notice that your clothes felt snug, or that the person looking back at you from the mirror was unrecognizable, or that you weren't moving with the ease you once took pride in. You suddenly felt uncomfortable in your own body. Once upon a time, you could eat any food in any amount and never gain an ounce. No more.

Slowing Metabolism and the Speeding Approach of Disease

While every individual is different, the middle years in general are a time of small, incremental physiological changes that all too often lead to weight gain. Simply put, your metabolism slows, and it begins to show in your waistline. Your body just isn't burning calories the

way it used to. It's easier to put weight on, harder to take weight off.

Put some of the blame on lifestyle. If you have a job or career, these are your peak earning years. That usually means stress, and stress in turn is typically a good excuse for bad eating habits. Maybe you're on the go, traveling frequently for business, eating as you can when you can, with neither the time to exercise nor access to exercise facilities. Maybe you wolf down lunch at your desk while answering phones that never stop ringing, trying to soothe feelings and keep up with your workload—all of which leaves you feeling simultaneously stuffed and dissatisfied, not to mention suffering from a bad case of heartburn. Or perhaps you dine lavishly with clients, courtesy of a generous expense account, mixing rich food with the need to strike a business deal and close it.

Relationships can become stressed, too, especially because the constant logistical hassles and the separate work lives of husband and wife can leave little time for intimacy or romance. Just ask the firefighter trying to plan a date with his own wife. Or ask Debbie Davis of the Chicago 7; the "negative feelings" she experienced during her divorce were probably directly responsible for her gaining back 10 pounds she had lost earlier.

This is a vulnerable time of life. All too often, it's a time when people form bad eating habits—eating for comfort, eating out of stress, eating what's fast and easy, eating to fill the hole left by the inevitable angst of middle age.

And then one day you hear a siren or see an ambulance go by, and you're surprised to realize it's for the guy down the block or the woman in the apartment upstairs—someone who is the same age as you. You begin to think about the possibility that you, too, could become ill. Suddenly, diseases like diabetes, hypertension and heart disease, cancer, and osteoporosis—all those debilitating, degenerative ailments—don't seem so far-fetched.

How can you decrease your own risk of disease? The studies you read about in the newspapers tell you that what you eat today can directly affect your level of risk for these diseases and ailments. They make it clear that a diet that's based on a wide range of fruits and vegetables and that gets its protein from beans, seafood, and soy rather than from meats and dairy is the best way to lower the risk of degenerative disease. Such a diet is at the heart of Picture-Perfect Weight Loss.

Of course, risk is individual. So is the weight issue, and it is different at different stages of the middle years and for different populations. It's one story for pregnant women and quite another for women at home whose children have gone off to college. The realities the high-powered executive faces are different from those confronted by the artist in her studio. Still, for many people at the midpoint of life, weight gain can cause serious concern. Picture-Perfect Weight Loss offers a healthy, sensible, satisfying solution whatever the circumstances. Here are some examples.

Pregnancy and Weight Gain

Giving birth to your first child in your forties would once have been considered a phenomenon; today, it is almost commonplace. People are marrying later, and—like Joanne Rusch of the Chicago 7—women are putting off preg-

Phytochemicals Fight Lung Cancer

Red, yellow, orange: The colors of fruits and vegetables are not just beautiful, they're beneficial to your lungs as well. Carotenoids and alpha-carotene fill the yellow and orange fruits and vegetables and may help reduce the risk of lung cancer. Red lycopene is beneficial even to those who still smoke. And please note: You won't get the same benefits from pills or supplements; it's the way the phytochemical compounds work together in foods that makes the difference. Of course, these phytochemicals also fight other cancers and heart disease as well.

More Calcium in the Middle Years

It's a fact: Sometime in the middle years, we begin to lose calcium—and thus bone strength as well. Menopausal women are particularly vulnerable. The loss of estrogen makes them prone to osteoporosis, and a simple fall can literally shatter a bone. It's why the shelves of drugstores are packed with calcium pills, capsules, and "candy" bars—all aimed at compensating for our calcium deficiency. And it's why many women in menopause make an effort to drink more milk or eat more dairy products.

It's a mistake.

The animal protein in dairy products may actually undermine bone strength. In the famous Harvard Nurses' Health Study, nurses with the highest dairy calcium intake suffered more hip fractures than those with the lowest intake. And a Japanese study found that soy is better than calcium in preventing bone loss in menopausal women.

In addition to the link between dairy products and weakened bones, it has been shown that a breakdown product of milk sugar, called galactose, is linked to ovarian cancer, while another substance, IGF-1, found in dairy products, can make cancer cells grow rapidly and can thus increase the risk of breast and other cancers. Both galactose and IGF-1 occur in low-fat as well as high-fat dairy products.

The conclusion seems clear: Dairy products are not the way to replenish the calcium we begin to lose in middle age. So what's the solution?

Alternatives like soy, green vegetables, beans, even nuts and seeds—all are great sources of calcium and other important nutrients.

The middle years are a good time to increase your intake of these foods. For menopausal and premenopausal women in particular, the disease-fighting substances in vegetables, known as phytochemicals, can be a boon, for this is a time of life when the risk of cancers, heart disease, and osteoporosis goes way up.

As for soy, using it as a protein replacement for meat, poultry, and dairy products provides the body with important phytoestrogens. These plant estrogens partly replace a woman's dwindling estrogen supply and may help alleviate hot flashes, night sweats, and other symptoms of menopause in many women. What's more, these phytoestrogens actually help protect the calcium in bones.

What's the best way to get these benefits? In tofu, miso, edamame—the straight soy foods—or in the range of soy-based products now available in supermarkets just about everywhere. Accompany your soy dish with a heaping plate of vegetables or a big bowl of salad, and you're adding to the health-promoting benefits of your meal.

As for soy pills, capsules, and "candy" bars, we still don't have sufficient long-term data on their safety or efficacy. My recommendation? Stick to getting your soy in food; centuries of experience in Asian cultures in particular substantiate its safety, and hard data from the laboratory has demonstrated its disease-fighting and bone-protecting goodness—especially when used as a replacement for meat, poultry, and dairy products.

nancy until they have nailed down a career and/or traveled the world and/or done the things they want to do. This gives more urgency to one of the questions every pregnant woman asks: What is a healthy, reasonable amount of weight to gain during pregnancy?

The answer, however, depends on whom you ask—and when you ask it. Thirty-five years ago, doctors told pregnant women to keep their weight gain between 24 and 30 pounds—no matter what their weight when they conceived. A generation later, obstetricians instructed their patients not to count pounds at all; rather, they were told to just "follow their appetites." That's exactly what those patients did, and the odd appetites of pregnancy took many of them to weight gains of 50 pounds or more. While this may not have harmed the developing fetus, it left the new mothers with an enormous weight burden they then had to work hard to take off. Now many of the daughters of these women, worried about potential weight gain, are trying hard to stay thin during pregnancy, and while most doctors agree that restraining your weight gain to perhaps 25 to 30 pounds is probably a sound idea, too much restraint is as bad as too little.

Either extreme can actually be dangerous.

Gaining too little weight can result in low birth weight for your baby—with all the possible attendant problems of slowed physical and mental development and a dysfunctional immune system. Two-thirds of all infant deaths are attributed to low birth weight, so it is a very serious danger indeed. Of course, eating inadequately out of fear of weight gain is not the sole determinant of low birth weight, but it is potentially a contributing factor, and it is one the pregnant woman can control. Many women assume that the fetus will simply absorb the nutrients it requires no matter what the mother's eating habits during pregnancy, but this simply isn't so: Your baby needs you to supply it with nutrients.

On the other hand, gaining too much weight does no one any favors, either. Just as a thin woman gaining too little can set her baby up for problems, so can an overweight woman gaining too much—although in this case, the danger is that the baby may be predisposed to diabetes. In addition, the woman who gains too much can be setting herself up for hypertension, blood clotting, and a range of obstetric complications.

So we're right back to the original question: What's a good number of pounds to gain? Today's answer is that no single number works for all pregnant women.

Fiber May Fight Diabetes

There's new evidence that consuming 50 grams of fiber per day—that's twice the normal recommended intake—can lower blood sugar levels in people with type 2, or adult-onset, diabetes. Lowering your blood sugar levels can delay or prevent such complications as blindness, lower leg amputations, and heart disease.

What's All This about Fatty Fish?

Fatty fish are rich in omega-3 polyunsaturated fatty acids that prevent blood clotting, can reduce triglyceride levels, and may make the heart less susceptible to rhythm abnormalities. The omega-3s are the reason the American Heart Association advises eating at least two servings of fish a week. Take note, though, that they recommend fish—not fish oil capsules, which don't carry the same benefits and do come with potential negative side effects.

Pregnant women should go easy on their fish intake, however, and should abstain entirely from eating shark, swordfish, king mackerel, and tilefish. These may contain high levels of mercury, and mercury can damage the brain and nervous system of a fetus.

For the rest of us, however, fish is an excellent low-calorie way to strengthen the heart by consuming omega-3 fatty acids.

What counts is the adequacy of the nutrition the mother and fetus take in. And there's no reason a woman can't be mindful of calories while she takes in plenty of nutrients. In fact, there's a formula every pregnant woman should probably follow: Take in all the nutrients needed for developing a healthy baby and staying healthy yourself, while keeping weight gain reasonable for both the baby's sake and yours. That means that a pregnant woman should eat adequately, healthfully, and to the point of satisfaction, making the lower-calorie choice when possible. Of course, that parallels exactly the basic formula of Picture-Perfect Weight Loss.

At Home with the Baby

Sandy was a new mother. The event she'd been anticipating with breathless excitement for the last 9 months had finally happened. She had a beautiful baby who was the object of everyone's focus and admiration, she was being assured 24 hours a day that she was the luckiest woman in the world, the house was full of presents and tokens of people's affection, and the fact of the matter was: Sandy was miserable.

There was a huge disconnect between the gauzy, magazine-photo image she had carried in her head for 9 months and the reality she faced every minute of every day. Her world had turned upside down. It now consisted of a baby who just kept crying and making demands on her, while she felt uncomfortable, exhausted, stressed, and not up to the task she confronted.

That was a surprise, because Sandy, who had taken a maternity leave from a high-powered job to have her child, was accustomed to being in control and in charge. Now she was at the beck and call of a tiny baby. Sometimes she would phone the office just to hear the bustle of corporate activity, the click of computer keyboards, the rustle of smartly tailored suits that contrasted so sharply with the sweats and vomit-stained T-shirt that were her current outfit. Not that anyone noticed her at all now that there was a cute baby in the house.

As if all that weren't depressing enough, every time Sandy had a moment to think, she grew terrified that her months away from the office would cost her the career she'd worked so hard to build—that she would "miss out" on an important development opportunity or significant experience, or that some brash new rival would use the opportunity to slide ahead of her.

No wonder Sandy was depressed. She felt utterly isolated. She had barely been out of the house since the baby was born. There didn't seem to be anything to do all day—except eat. And that's exactly what Sandy had begun to do. She ate mindlessly. She ate to pass the time between feedings, to fill the emptiness of postpartum depression, to mask the disconnection between the motherhood fantasy she had pictured in her mind and the reality she was dealing with all day long.

The result? Even before Sandy had lost all the weight gained during her pregnancy, she was putting on more weight—unhealthy weight, for unhealthy reasons, in unhealthy ways.

Combating Postpartum Weight Gain

What happened to Sandy doesn't have to happen at all. There are two ways to combat the weight gain that is all too often a result of suddenly finding yourself at home with a new baby. One way helps your psyche; the other goes directly to the issue of getting back to a healthy weight.

The psyche-soothing approach is fairly simple. First of all, women need to realize before the fact that postpartum depression is both natural and common. This is a subject that has been taboo for far too long; the fact is that almost every new mother feels the letdown, the uncertainty, and the low spirits that typically follow on the heels of giving birth. And it takes some time for your hormones to settle down. (If your depression lingers for more than a few weeks, however, you might want to see a doctor.)

Fortunately, there is a way to break out of the isolation you feel, and that's by networking with other new mothers. I know a number of corporate women on maternity leave who have set up informal telephone sessions in which they discuss what they're doing and what they're feeling—and get to talk to grownups for a change. Expectant mothers meet other expectant mothers at natural childbirth classes, or at preparatory sessions at the local hospital, or in the obstetrician's office; staying in touch with these women after you've given birth is another good way to share with someone who's going through the same thing you're going through—and feeling the same emotions. And of course, in this day and age, one great way to network is via the Internet.

As for the issue of weight gain, it's something women need to be aware of. Some women I know think they can drop the extra weight of pregnancy in no time if they "get a jump start" with a crash diet and intense exercising. Nothing could be further from the truth, of course—and crash diets are an extremely bad idea for new mothers altogether, particularly if you're nursing your baby. The solution, as always, is to eat well—to eat tasty food when you're hungry and until you're satisfied, but to look for the lower-calorie choices. In other words: Picture-Perfect Weight Loss.

The Career Woman at Middle Age

I can't even count the number of women patients of mine who are powerful and successful executives. I applaud their success, and I admire them for having achieved the power positions they hold. But it is also true that with the success and the power have often come the same stresses and strains powerful male execs have felt for years. And as can happen when the stresses and strains pile on, so do the pounds.

In a man, the extra bulk may seem evidence of success—the "paunch of prosperity." In a woman, however, it's too often perceived as failure—a character flaw, a weakness that she hasn't been able to "correct." It's an absurd and offensive and unjust perception, but unfortunately, it's a pervasive view.

Of course, these middle years are pivotal in a career. Now is the moment when you have to vault upward or risk getting stuck at this plateau. That means constant vigilance as you keep an eye out for just the right opportunity; it means being sure that you dot every *i* and cross every *t*. And all of that means pretty constant pressure, the kind of pressure that many people respond to by eating, the kind of pressure that convinces busy people they don't have time to exercise.

My patient Elizabeth would phone in her medical appointments with me if she could; in fact, she'd probably rather transmit them wirelessly from her Palm Pilot. A high-ranking executive in the world of finance, Elizabeth wakes up at 4:30 A.M. in her spacious suburban home, logs on to the Internet to see what the markets are doing overseas, showers, dresses, puts on her makeup, and is picked up by the car service at 5:30. During her ride into the city, she checks out the newspapers, phones her chief of staff on the cellular, and downs a fresh croissant with her travel mug of coffee—a standing order at the local bakery that is picked up daily by her faithful driver.

She's at her desk by 6:15 most mornings and typically holds a 7:30 breakfast meeting with her staff—bacon and eggs with buttered muffins. Then there is a constant series of meetings and presentations until lunch—invariably with a client either in a private corporate dining room or in a New York restaurant—then more meetings and presentations until the car calls for Elizabeth again at 7:00 P.M. If she doesn't have to attend a work-related function—or an event connected with one of the charities on whose boards she sits—she'll head for home. If her husband Jack isn't on the road, the two of them may grab a quick meal together before they head for their separate studies to get some paperwork done. If she's alone, Elizabeth will "just graze," as she describes it, foraging in the refrigerator and pantry—both of which are kept well-stocked by the housekeeper—for whatever appeals to her tastebuds at the time. Facing that 4:30 alarm clock, Elizabeth tries to be in bed by 10:30—11:30 at the latest.

Exercise? Just when, Elizabeth wonders, is she supposed to find time for exercise? As for

Cholesterol Counts

A study of men under the age of 40 showed that those with blood cholesterol levels below 200 had a longer life expectancy than those with cholesterol counts above 240. How much longer? 3.8 to 8.7 years.

watching what she eats, that pretty much comes second to getting the work done, the tasks assigned, the deals closed, the customers soothed. The result is that the higher Elizabeth has risen in the corporate hierarchy, the heavier she has become. For all her success and power, taking care of her health—specifically by losing weight and keeping it off—seems a luxury she is unable or unwilling to indulge.

It's been said many times: The people who need stress management the most are the people who don't give themselves the time to deal with it.

The fact is that there is a way to do business over meals—even lavish meals—and still lose weight and maintain the weight loss. And there are ways to deal with the pressures and stresses of a career at its peak without damaging your health or giving in to the kind of eating patterns that simply add weight without reducing stress or lowering the pressure. You guessed it: It's the Picture-Perfect Weight-Loss formula. It doesn't matter if you're on an expense account or under the gun, stuck in the airport or downing a meal at 37,000 feet: You are presented with food options, and nobody is better equipped than a high-powered executive like yourself to assess your options, make a choice, and then execute the decision that is going to achieve your weight-loss goal.

Working at Home

What about the home office crowd? Their numbers are growing as more and more people commute into the next room to go to work. There are home-based entrepreneurs, corporate telecommuters, artists with a studio in the basement, freelance consultants and writers and journalists who need only a laptop and a phone to get the job done—all are happy to save the commute time and work from some sort of home office.

For wherever the home office is—the basement, kitchen table, garage—you don't have to dress in a suit, don't have to work at a desk if you don't want to, are not on anyone's schedule but your own, and can get up and head for the refrigerator whenever you feel like it.

And that, of course, is the danger. Going into an office, after all, imposes structure: You take a break when it is scheduled, lunch when the cafeteria opens up, and lack ready access to food. At home, however, where *you* make the structure, and where there is food at your fingertips at all times, it's all too easy to eat mindlessly all day.

One patient, a freelance writer, says she finds herself grabbing a snack every time her concentration is broken. The phone rings, or someone knocks on the door, or there's a news bulletin on the easy listening radio station she prefers—and next thing you know, she's up from her desk chair and foraging through the refrigerator. For the home office crowd, in short, every day is Sunday, and all too often it is much too easy to eat anything and everything available.

The remedy? Make sure the kitchen is full of food that can satisfy the appetite at the lowest possible cost in calories. Need some suggestions? You'll find them on the Picture-Perfect Anytime List. These are foods you can reach for at any time and know that you're getting a low-calorie option. You'll find the Anytime List described in full in chapter 5.

The Empty Nest

Lots of stay-at-homes have a different kind of career: They're homemakers and proud of it. If that's you, you know that your job—raising good, healthy, happy kids—was the toughest and most important one in the world. But once you watched your children go off to college or out to work, your work was done; your career was over.

Nina stayed at home to raise her three sons. Her oldest is now in law school, the middle boy is a college junior, and 4 months ago, her baby entered his freshman year at a university a thousand miles away. The house Nina had taken such good care of all these years is empty.

Meanwhile, her husband's career is at its absolute peak, and while he was never around much while the children were growing up, without them to focus on, Nina notices his absence acutely. The emptiness around her has made her realize that her life has been bound up entirely with the lives of her children. Now, suddenly, she feels she has nothing to fall back on.

There are lots of responses to facing an empty nest. Nina's is to eat. She knows a few other women who don't go out to work, and they occasionally meet for lunch and a shop-

Menopause and Weight Gain

That old wives' tale about putting on weight at the change of life turns out to be true. Typically, menopausal women can gain weight and body fat—much of it the result of a slowing metabolism. Some numbers tell the story:

Body weight: Ninety percent of menopausal women gain an average of 12 pounds.

Metabolism: The metabolism of a menopausal woman typically decreases by 10 to 15 percent. (If you typically take in 1,800 calories per day, a slowing metabolism would mean you would gain weight unless you reduced your average daily intake to 1,620 calories per day.)

Percent body fat: This figure may increase 1 to 4 percent.

Upper-body fat: The increased ratio of testosterone to estrogen at menopause typically increases a woman's waist-to-hip ratio from 0.75 to 0.95. (Divide your waistline in inches by your hip measurement in inches to find your waist-to-hip ratio.)

ping trip. Or she finds herself grazing in the pantry or refrigerator each time she finishes a household chore. Truth is, there are fewer chores now—how many times can you make a bed no one sleeps in anymore?—and more time between chores, and that seems to make more opportunity for grazing.

She's only 4 months into life as an empty nester, and Nina has already gained 16 pounds.

For Nina and others like her, as for the work-at-home crowd, the Anytime List is an essential tool as far as eating is concerned. But you'll need to find new activities to fill your life as well: another kind of job, volunteering, going back to school. It's time now to pay attention to *you*—and nutrition and weight are only part of it.

A Word for and about Men

Just about every situation I've described in this chapter—except pregnancy, of course—can apply to men as well. The male metabolism also slows in these years, health troubles can start here, and certainly, at the upper end of middle age, men surely go through something similar to menopause—at least, psychologically.

Men, too, feel the approach of old age, the deceleration of their physical abilities, the emptiness of a house that was once filled with kids. They certainly feel the pressures of work and the demands of a career. Perhaps even more than women, men tend to see their identities bound up with their career success, and the middle years are the time when that success is secured—or when it slips through their fingers.

So men, too, tend to put on weight in these years, ignore nutrition, forget about exercise.

Or, conversely, they try the latest fad diet and turn themselves into weekend warriors trying to "work off" in 2 days of overexertion the overstressed overeating of the work week. Of course, it doesn't work.

Losing Weight—And Keeping It Off—In the Middle Years

Whatever the middle years bring to you—whatever your situation, whatever the crisis of the moment—eating in response can cause weight gain at a time of life when it is harder than ever to shed pounds. If there's one life lesson we all should have learned by middle age, it's that actions have consequences. In the middle years, eating without awareness and failing to exercise adequately bring consequences that are difficult to undo.

There is often a psychological trigger for mindless eating, yet the consequences of the eating only exacerbate the depression. There are often business reasons for eating, but the business can be accomplished just as effectively over a healthful, low-calorie meal. As for the insistence that there is "no time for exercise," there's a simple answer to that: Find the time. Make the time. And at all times, make exercise an integral part of your life. In part 2 of this book, I'll lay out a program of exercise, but no program is sufficient in a culture in which gadgets make it possible to do just about anything without getting up out of your chair. Instead, we must learn to incorporate exercise into our lives—by taking the stairs instead of the elevator, by biking rather than driving to work, by taking a brisk walk on your lunch hour, or by mowing your own lawn or raking your own leaves. Half an hour of vigorous activity a day is recommended—and I do mean *vigorous*—but if you can't do a solid half hour, how about a 10-minute walk back to the office from lunch, a walk up at least a couple of flights of the office building stairs, and another brisk 10-minute walk with your spouse in the evening?

Picture-Perfect Weight Loss works even more powerfully when exercise is an integral part of your life. Of course, that's primarily because exercise burns calories. But there's more to it than that, and as we'll learn in more detail in part 2 of this book, the weight lost through exercise is weight that tends to stay lost as long as the exercise is continued. So think of exercise as an absolutely essential component not just of your Picture-Perfect Weight-Loss program but of your life.

The middle years are crucial. They weigh on the mind—and can weigh on the body. But if you can use these crucial years to make both food awareness and the exercise components of Picture-Perfect Weight Loss daily habits, you'll maintain weight loss—and fitness—forever. And remember: This is *only* the middle. The good habits you get into now can set you up for a whole new lease on life when you are a senior.

Senior Shape-Up

Meet Philip. At 87, he's my oldest current patient. (In fact, if you read my earlier book, *Dr. Shapiro's Picture-Perfect Weight Loss,* you've already met him.) When Philip first came to see me, he had just lost his wife after nursing her through a debilitating and ultimately fatal illness. He was depressed and lonely, ready to

follow his wife to the grave, and his physical condition certainly seemed to be leading him there. Philip was overweight and sluggish, and he suffered from diabetes, gout, and heart disease. All he wanted, he told me, was to take off 20 pounds for what he expected would be the final 2 years of a bleak and empty life.

That was 11 years ago. Today, Philip still starts every day with a brisk walk, volunteers his business expertise to small start-up companies, attends his beloved New York Philharmonic as often as he can, and dines out just about every night—still maintaining his 40-pound weight loss.

The lesson is clear: Old age isn't what it used to be. Today, it can be a whole new time of life, a fresh start. It's a period that can be rich in experience and fulfillment, a true Third Age. Two things in particular can help make it so: your eating habits and the habit of exercise.

In fact, with more time available than in the earlier seasons of life, a great many seniors at last have the leisure to engage in exercise in a relaxed way or to indulge that long-dormant interest in cooking. True, many live on fixed incomes, so gym memberships or gourmet ingredients may be out of the question, but neither is necessary. Walking through the mall in the morning is absolutely free, and if you take along the Picture-Perfect Anytime List as your shopping guide, you can do your marketing at a discount supermarket right there once the walk is over.

Nutrients and No-No's for Seniors

While all nutrients are essential at every stage of life for everyone, for seniors in particular,

When It Comes to Calcium, What's "Enough"—And Where Can You Get It?

How much calcium do you need to consume to ensure that you get its benefits—bone strength, blood coagulation, muscle contraction, blood pressure control, maybe even colon cancer prevention? The National Institutes of Health recommends that a woman in her fifties or sixties gets 1,500 milligrams of calcium a day—1,000 milligrams if she's on estrogen replacement therapy. The National Academy of Sciences advises 1,200 milligrams for all women in their fifties or older. That seems a safe bet, but even 1,200 milligrams per day is about twice as much calcium as most women actually take in.

What's particularly important to remember is that calcium is found not just in dairy foods but also in grains, leafy green vegetables like kale and Swiss chard, fruits, fish, many soy products, beans, and nuts. If you're a woman in your fifties, you should probably shoot for 1,200 milligrams per day, and you should try to get most of that from plant foods, rather than from dairy.

the usual recommendations to eat plenty of fruit and vegetables and to go easy on meat and dairy are especially pertinent.

Both senior men and women should think twice before downing a glass of milk or indulging a passion for cheese or other dairy products. Recent studies have shown that two substances that occur together in many dairy products—estrogen and IGF-1, an insulin-like growth factor—spur the growth of cancer cells, particularly breast and prostate cancer. Researchers found, for example, that men with higher levels of IGF-1 were more likely to develop prostate cancers than men with low levels of IGF-1.

How can you take in needed calcium without using dairy products? You've probably seen the answer in the earlier chapters, but it's worth repeating here: Soy foods, leafy green vegetables, nuts, beans, and fortified cereals give you all the calcium you need more effectively and more healthfully than dairy foods—and at a far lower cost in calories.

Soy products, by the way, can actually decrease a man's risk of developing prostate cancer and even slow the growth of the disease in men who have it. And green vegetables are one of several good sources of a nutrient that is particularly important for the elderly: folate. A B-vitamin that is also found in beans, citrus fruits, tomatoes, almonds, whole wheat bread, bananas, and cantaloupe—as well as in spinach, romaine lettuce, broccoli, and other green vegetables—folate is necessary to regulate your body's level of homocysteine. What is homocysteine and why should it be regulated? It is an amino acid produced in the body, and studies have shown that too much of it in the blood can put you at higher risk of coronary heart disease, stroke, and blood clots. The way people now worry about cholesterol is the way they should worry about homocysteine. According to many experts, homocysteine, which causes fat deposits along the artery walls, may be more dangerous.

Folate—and its supplement form, folic acid—keeps the level of homocysteine down. The amount of folic acid suggested for regulating homocysteine is 400 micrograms per day. This is the amount typically found in most one-a-day multivitamins—and I recommend that everyone take a multivitamin every day.

Still, even with a multivitamin, the best way to get this nutrient is in food, and your best bet is green vegetables or beans. A cup of cooked spinach, for example, has 265 micrograms, and a cup of cooked white beans has 250. Since the FDA's Recommended Daily Allowance (RDA) of folic acid is just 180 micrograms for women and 200 micrograms for men, you can see what a punch a cup of vegetables can provide.

The best idea of all is to cut back on dairy and meat, try soy substitutes and beans, and eat as many vegetables and fruits—cooked, canned, raw, in soup, or any way you like them—as you can.

In fact, the eating principles of Picture-Perfect Weight Loss are absolutely picture-perfect for the needs of seniors. With its emphasis on fruits and vegetables; its focus on beans, seafood, and soy products for protein; and its goal of keeping the calorie count and saturated fat content low and the enjoyment factor high, this plan is just right for an age group that needs lots of nutrients and energy without weight gain.

Of course, seniors should check with their doctors about any food restrictions or food requirements they might have—but then, that's true of anyone at any age.

Exercise!

At the same time that seniors are taking in the nutrients of a balanced, sensible, low-calorie diet, it's also extremely important that they exercise. In fact, the National Institute on Aging says that regular exercise on a permanent basis can actually help prevent disabilities and such diseases as heart ailments, diabetes, and some types of cancer. The questions are obvious: How much exercise and what kind?

Check with your doctor before starting any exercise program, but once you get the go-ahead, it's important to commit to a regular schedule. Every day of the week, if possible—certainly most days of the week—get at least 30 minutes of sustained physical activity, the kind of physical activity that makes you breathe harder. This is called endurance activity; it is sustained, continuous, rhythmic aerobic effort, and it's calculated to build up your stamina. If you can't put in 30 minutes all at once, try three 10-minute sessions. But make sure you do a total of 30 minutes during the day, and make sure that each 10-minute session leaves you a bit breathless.

How breathless? Here's a useful formula: If you can talk without any trouble at all, your exercise activity is too easy. If you can't talk at all, it's too hard. During a brisk walk, you should be able to carry on a conversation with your companion or teammates, but you'll be puffing what you say rather than speaking it.

Walking is one of the best endurance activities there is; it's good for the heart, leg muscles, and overall trimness. It's also an exercise you can do anywhere on Earth, and it doesn't cost a cent.

But walking isn't the only endurance exercise for seniors. Cycling is also excellent. So is dancing. So is doing a sport you've always loved to do—or learning a sport you've always wanted to learn. Swimming, tennis, paddleball: All keep you on the move in a sustained way over time.

In addition to endurance, you'll need to exercise your muscles. The aging process does result in loss of muscle mass—and thus of physical strength. But the main reason for muscle loss over time is that many seniors stop doing everyday activities that require strength. The solution? Don't stop doing such activities. In fact, go out of your way to undertake them. Do the household chores. Mow the grass. Rake the leaves. If you rake the leaves while walking uphill, you'll combine muscle-building exercise with an endurance activity! Begin a more

or less formal program of resistance training focusing on low-impact weight-bearing exercise. Menopausal women in particular can benefit from such exercise, since bone density is a serious concern once they've stopped producing estrogen. Yes, such exercise can certainly include lifting light weights. Just be sure you know the right way to do the lifting. To find out, rent a video or borrow a library book that explains it. The benefits are worth it: Strong leg and hip muscles support you better, making it less likely that you'll fall. And strong muscles may contribute to bone strength as well.

Balance is another thing you can improve through weight-bearing exercise, and also through exercises like tai chi and yoga. Tai chi is based in Chinese Taoist philosophy and focuses on principles of yielding, softness, centeredness, slowness, balance, suppleness, and rootedness. It is graceful, slow, and a boon to

Salt: What's the Story?

Where weight loss is concerned, salt, which contains no calories, is a nonissue. While the amount of salt in your diet might influence the amount of fluid in your body, it will have no effect whatsoever on your losing or gaining fat.

If your doctor has limited your intake of salt, it is probably for reasons of high blood pressure or hypertension. In that case, there are still plenty of alternatives for flavoring your food: a range of canned tomato products for making sauces, for example, and just about anything with a tart or sweet and sour flavor. In addition, as the contents of

your supermarket shelves demonstrate, a lot of soups and sauces are available in low-sodium versions; help out their flavoring with lemon juice, herbs and spices, vinegars, horseradish, or even wine.

But here's an important point to consider: If you've been advised to limit your salt intake because of high blood pressure *and* you're overweight, the Picture-Perfect Weight-Loss program is probably the best eating plan you can follow. Eat the Picture-Perfect Weight-Loss pyramid and exercise routinely; you will lose weight and, in turn, help lower your blood pressure.

Exercise and Ulcers

Data from a study of 11,000 people who work out aerobically shows that the exercise may help reduce the risk of duodenal ulcers in men. Among the 11,000, the most active lowered their risk by 62 percent, and even moderately active men enjoyed a 46 percent risk reduction. Since ulcers are caused by bacteria, a possible explanation may be that the body chemicals related to exercise strengthen the immune system in its fight against the bacteria.

balance. It requires no particular skill, demands no particular proficiency.

Yoga, another ancient and well-proven set of exercise postures—from India this time—helps you shape up even as it teaches you to chill out. Yoga can be particularly helpful for people with arthritis; it also helps relieve or manage stress, improve muscle tone, build up strength and stamina, and improve circulation. Yoga keeps people incredibly limber—and strong—no matter what their age.

In fact, stretches of all types are increasingly important the older we get. The range of motion that stretching increases is extremely important in keeping the body's joints supple and "well-oiled."

So keep moving. One way or another, push your body's limits just a little bit each day. Remember: If you keep on doing it, you find that you *can* keep on doing it. It's half the weight-loss battle—and it will keep you feeling young.

If knowledge is power, the information you learned in Part 1 should prove potent indeed. You've learned a lot about why people are overweight, and you've learned about the consequences of being overweight—not just for your appearance, but for your overall health, well-being, and longevity.

❧

You've also learned the basic principles of Picture-Perfect Weight Loss—principles about awareness and empowerment, about expanding the range of your food options and choosing mindfully.

❧

In Part 2, you'll find the working heart of the Picture-Perfect Weight Loss 30-Day Plan. Here's where you get down to business and begin to change the way you eat—and the way you look, feel, and live. You're about to take 4 weeks to get to Picture-Perfect Weight Loss—1 week at a time.

Are you ready? Yes, you are.

Go.

PART II

THE 30-DAY PLAN
FOR PICTURE-PERFECT
WEIGHT LOSS

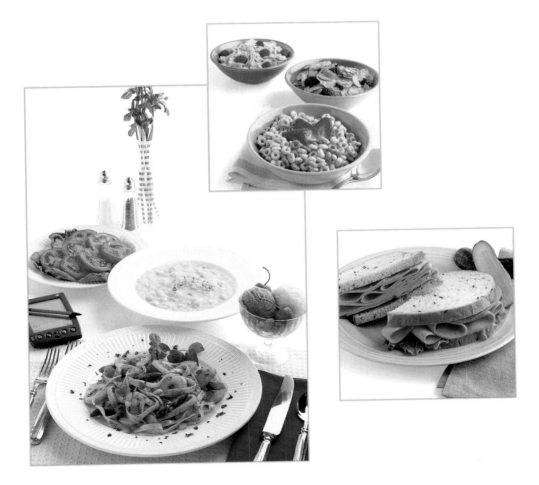

Chapter 5

Day 1: Let's Go Shopping

30-Day Plan

						1
2	3	4	5	6	7	8
9	10	11	12	13	14	15
16	17	18	19	20	21	22
23 / 30	24	25	26	27	28	29

By the end of Day 1, you will have:

- *Really* learned to read nutrition labels
- Understood how supermarkets work
- Changed the food inventory in your refrigerator, freezer, and pantry
- Taken the first, empowering step toward Picture-Perfect Weight Loss

*I*f you do what you did, you get what you got." Today, you'll start *doing* something different from what you've done in the past; that's what it will take to *get* something other than all that extra weight you have now. That makes today Day 1 of changing your relationship with food—the one sure way finally to lose the weight you want to lose and keep it off.

Where do you start to change your relationship with food? The answer is simple. You start in the supermarket. Or the deli. Or the roadside farmer's market. Or the ethnic grocery store. Or wherever you buy the food you and your family will eat.

After all, choosing the food you'll buy is the first step in the process of eating. So to change your eating habits, you must first change your food-shopping choices. Think of the market as your first chance for empowerment, your first opportunity to make the kinds of low-calorie choices pictured throughout this book. Every

food-shopping trip is an occasion for you to assert that you've taken control, and that weight loss is your choice for life.

To that end, this chapter will offer some shopping guidelines. I'll lay out the Anytime List I referred to earlier in this book. Make it your own personal shopping list, and you'll be well on your way toward Picture-Perfect Weight Loss for life. In addition, through the pages of this book, I'll walk the aisles of the supermarket with you to offer some suggestions on what to look for in key categories.

Food Awareness Training: A Review

First, let's review the principles of FAT—Food Awareness Training—that you were first introduced to in chapter 1. Remember?

Principle One states that calorie reduction is the key to weight loss. Picture-Perfect Weight Loss happens when you are comfortable choosing low-calorie foods instead of high-calorie foods. Therefore, when shopping for food, you need to make a conscious effort to look for, find, and buy the lower-calorie options that you like.

Principle Two of Food Awareness Training states that choice doesn't mean deprivation. In fact, deprivation doesn't work. Instead, it can actually cause the opposite effect—that is, weight gain. That's why there are no forbidden foods in Picture-Perfect Weight Loss, and it's why I stress that food is not your enemy. Nor is there any such thing as a "correct" portion or an "incorrect" reason for eating. When you want to eat, do so—and eat till you're satisfied.

This doesn't mean, though, that you can lose weight without making changes in your food choices. On the contrary. I'll repeat what I wrote earlier: "If you do what you did, you get what you got." Picture-Perfect Weight Loss asks you to stop doing what you've done and do something different, to make some fundamental changes. With Picture-Perfect Weight Loss, however, you have the tools to make changes without condemning yourself to a restrictive diet and to the guilt—even the self-loathing—that tends to go along with such limited regimens.

Principle Three says that you can achieve Picture-Perfect Weight Loss while living your life. In fact, I insist on it. Put on a lavish dinner party, head for the refrigerator when you need a break from housework, take your clients to lunch, travel 5 days out of 7—whatever your life is, whatever your tastes are, Picture-Perfect Weight Loss lets you accommodate them comfortably. Through Food Awareness Training, you can make the choices that will lead to Picture-Perfect Weight Loss without causing your own personal world to stop spinning.

Remember: You are not on a diet. Instead, you're involved in a lifelong process of making healthy, low-calorie choices at every meal, in every eating situation, and whenever and wherever you shop for food.

Put these three principles together, and you have a pretty straightforward guide to shopping for Picture-Perfect Weight Loss.

- You'll be shopping for low-calorie choices.
- You'll be embracing a wider range of choices—including some foods you've never tried before.
- You'll be shopping for foods you enjoy—foods that fit your taste and your lifestyle.

More for Less: More Foods for Less Weight

Once inside the doors of your supermarket—or corner grocery or specialty store or deli—remind yourself of this: You're not giving up the foods you love; rather, you're adding to your life more foods that you're going to love just as much. You're seeking alternatives, not necessarily replacements. You're trying to extend your options, not narrow them. You're going to lose weight, and in doing so you're going to gain health, well-being, a better appearance, and a way of eating you can live with and enjoy for a lifetime.

To a chocolate lover, for example, there's no such thing as a substitute for chocolate—but there may be new ways to get your chocolate that mitigate the calorie impact, and there are certainly other options for satisfying that sweet tooth.

Or maybe you're a meat-and-potatoes guy. Strange as it may sound, there really are a whole bunch of low-calorie alternatives that

Ground Out

Half the beef consumed by the beef-loving American public each year is ground beef, which the Center for Science in the Public Interest tells us is probably the single most damaging food we eat. How is it damaging to our health? Let me count the ways:

- After cheese and whole milk, it's our third biggest source of saturated fat.
- Unlike with whole cuts, the fat in ground beef can't be trimmed away.

- Even if it's labeled "80 percent lean," that refers to fat by weight; at only 20 percent fat by weight, the fat is still contributing 70 percent of the total calories.
- Ground beef is more likely than any other food to contain potentially harmful *E. coli* bacteria.

At 27 pounds per person per year, that's a lot of danger in a little hamburger . . .

---

are just as tasty as meat and potatoes and that will more than satisfy your palate. You just haven't found them yet.

Your weekly or daily shopping trip is your chance to be both thoughtful and creative about changing your relationship with food. The chapters that follow will expand your thinking and stir your creativity with ideas and suggestions that focus on specific meals, one week at a time. And the food demonstrations that you will see throughout this book will serve as an encyclopedia of possible choices— and a reference tool you can go back to again and again. But it's *your* tastes, *your* preferences, and *your* imagination that will really make the difference. As I've said before in this book and will say again: Your Picture-Perfect Weight Loss is in your hands.

With that in mind, let's go shopping.

Look and Learn

I call my weight-loss program *Picture-Perfect Weight Loss* for a reason. Choosing begins in awareness, and awareness begins with seeing.

In any supermarket—not to mention hyper-market or megamarket—and even in the corner deli, you will see an almost dizzying array of choices.

Fortunately, today's foods offer a key aware-ness tool: the nutrition label. Once you know how to read it, it can be a useful guide to making the low-calorie choice. New York City policewoman Dorothy Mellone recalls that the first time she went shopping using the principles of Picture-Perfect Weight Loss, she spent 4 hours in the supermarket reading every word of every label of every food she was thinking about buying—and making choices based on what the labels told her. Dorothy's husband gave up and went to wait in the car, but Dorothy pressed on. That was 6 years ago, before she lost the 50-plus pounds she shed in 6 months of Picture-Perfect Weight-Loss eating, the 50-plus pounds Dorothy has kept off ever since. Now, she doesn't have to read labels; she has been a Pic-ture-Perfect shopper for so long that she knows exactly what she's doing, and shopping for low-calorie, healthful, nutritious foods is second nature to her.

Dorothy's experience is instructive: Becoming a savvy label-reader is important, but it's also a skill that will improve with time. Right now, it's essential to remember that it's calories we're looking out for—specifically, calories from saturated fat and refined carbohydrates—and that it's the lowest-calorie choice we're aiming for. A product that claims to be fat-free or cholesterol-free or sugar-free is all well and good, but only if it meets the basic criterion of being low in calories.

To see this for yourself, check out the calorie count in a fat-free muffin. It's high, considering that the calories come mainly from refined carbohydrates. Or have a look at "cholesterol-free" potato chips. They are cholesterol-free all right—but they cost about 150 calories for perhaps a dozen or so chips. What's more, the calories in potato chips often come mostly from hydrogenated fat, one of the bad fats where heart health is concerned.

Sugar-free "candy" bars tend to have only slightly fewer calories than regular candy bars. But since the label says "sugar-free," chances are you'll eat more of the sugar-free bars—and that's not a desirable consequence at all.

Be careful not to be influenced by a range of advertising claims about things that have little or nothing to do with real weight loss. Healthful calorie reduction is your aim, and the Nutrition Facts label, required by law on just about every commercially packaged food, is a key weapon in identifying what the healthy, low-calorie choices are among all those dizzying possibilities confronting you. The label can quickly clue you in on the calorie count of a food—as well as tell you

where the calories come from and what kinds of nutrients the food provides.

Grab a jar or can of something from your pantry or refrigerator to see what I mean.

The first thing to check on the nutrition label is the serving size. The reason is obvious: Calories are measured per serving, so the size of the serving matters. If a serving of beans clocks in at half a cup and costs 120 calories, and if the recipe you're preparing calls for 3 cups of beans, that adds up to 720 calories. On the other hand, if you're throwing together a tuna sandwich, using half a can only, and a can contains two and a half servings, with each serving costing only 70 calories, chances are you're taking in only about 88 calories (half of 2.5 servings)—exclusive of the bread and mayo, that is.

All the nutritional values on the label pertain to a single serving—or if not, the label will clearly state what measurement is being used. Nutritional values for total fat, saturated fat, cholesterol, sodium, total carbohydrate, fiber, sugars, protein, and vitamins and minerals will typically be expressed both as a plain-number measurement and a percentage. The plain-number measurement tells you the actual amount of the nutrient in the food—usually measured in grams or milligrams. The percentage number is the proportion of the Daily Value (DV).

And just what is a Daily Value? It is a reference number, set by the FDA and based on current nutrition recommendations, that gives a general idea of a food's nutrient contribution to the total daily diet—specifically, to a total daily diet of 2,000 calories, which is the reference intake on which Daily Values are based.

The DV is not a recommendation. It is not

an allowance. It's a descriptive indicator. Because it is based on a 2,000-calories-per-day diet, you can use the Daily Value percentage to compare foods and to see how the amount of a nutrient in a serving of food fits in a 2,000-calorie reference diet. For example, compare fiber percentages from food to food, or compare protein from product to product. If you're taking in more or less than 2,000 calories per day, simply adjust the figures to gauge the percentage of DV you're getting for the calories you're eating.

Keep in mind, though, that you eat a variety of foods in the course of a day. At least, that's what Picture-Perfect Weight Loss recommends. So you don't need to try to get in 100 percent of the DV of any one nutrient in a single food. Even 20 percent of a nutrient's DV is a good contribution to your nutritional needs, depending on what else you're eating.

The bottom line? Use the nutrition label as you shop for food. It offers you key information: the calorie count of a food and its relative nutritional content. That makes it a useful tool, a guidepost through the supermarket wilderness.

Three Key Shopping Tips

I want to offer three other thoughts on shopping for Picture-Perfect Weight Loss. Simply put, think variety, taste-enhancers—spices, garnishes, herbs, sauces, condiments of every sort—and soup. All are powerful tools in your weight-loss program.

Avoid Boredom

Why is variety important to weight loss? Because boredom is tantamount to deprivation, and deprivation, as we know, is extremely detrimental to losing weight and keeping it off.

Is there any such thing as a diet that isn't boring? Fad diets often restrict people to one food—for example, nothing but pineapple, or only protein for breakfast and dinner and only carbohydrates for lunch. Other diets set up a daily, weekly, or even monthly menu. Your entire eating future is laid out for you. There are no surprises, there's no wiggle room to add the foods you find appetizing—or even the food you just suddenly "feel like" eating right this minute for no apparent reason. Boredom denies your natural appetite, and restrictive diets eventually fail for just that reason.

In fact, the boredom doesn't just prompt people to go off the fad diet or violate the daily menu; it can actually cause weight gain. Why? Because boring eating is work; it's drudgery. And if you've put up with drudgery for a few days, or for a week, or for more, then you deserve something delicious as compensation. Or so you tell yourself—in what easily becomes a convincing argument. The consequence, however, is that you end up eating a rich, high-calorie meal or meals as a "reward" for the work of eating all that bland, tasteless food.

How to avoid boredom? Never was there a better time to try new foods and expand your tastes than when you are undertaking the Picture-Perfect Weight-Loss program. Let's face it: Far too many of us are stuck with a limited food vocabulary. We know what we like, and we tend not to stray too far from what we know. So protein means meat or dairy, a salad consists of iceberg lettuce, vegetables equal potatoes, and dessert is chocolate cake. Period. End of discussion.

The truth is that there is a vast universe of foods out there, and it likely includes foods you will come to enjoy; in fact, there might be something out there you'll like even more than what you're eating now. Without exception, every one of my patients has told me how Picture-Perfect Weight Loss opened him or her to new taste sensations. From the firefighters who found they love veggie burgers . . . to the priest who once thought seafood meant fish sticks and now knows it includes salmon, tuna, mahi mahi, and lobster . . . to the lawyer who "discovered" beans at age 45—whole new worlds of taste, texture, and nourishment can open up to you, if you let them.

Try something you've never tried before. If you don't like it, you never have to eat it again—but at least try it. It will make your weight-loss program easier—and a lot more fun.

In fact, we Americans have a leg up on the rest of the world when it comes to the available variety of food. There are two reasons for that. One is that the rest of the world is represented in our nation of immigrants—along with all the culinary arts and favorite foods each immigrant group brought with it—and more and more of these "ethnic" options are available in more and more markets. Reason two is that we're blessed with widely divergent regional differences. Our varied climates and soils are capable of producing a range of foods, and modern technology makes it possible for chilly New England to enjoy what comes from the hot, dry plains, and for desert-dwellers to feast on beans and seeds from the cool, wet north.

So as you push your cart through the produce section, reach beyond the iceberg lettuce and string beans to try broccoli rabe from Italy, plantains from the rain forests of the Caribbean, calabaza squash from south of the border, or Chinese bok choy. Closer to home, try the mustard and dandelion greens of our own deep South. Farther afield, Pacific islanders have built an entire way of life around taro roots; try some.

Beans and other legumes are *the* staple food in many parts of the world. Have you tried dal from India, hummus (made from chickpeas and tahini) from the Mediterranean and the Middle East, black-eyed peas from our Native American tribal lands, fava beans from Africa, adzuki beans from Japan? They lend themselves to a range of recipes—from sharp to sweet, hot vegetable stews to cold beans in salads.

In addition to the fish you've been used to since childhood, how about trying some variations on the theme—smoked salmon, for instance . . . or canned sardines or kippers or smoked mackerel or smoked oysters . . . gefilte fish from a jar, topped by hot horseradish . . . pickled herring . . . maybe smoked trout or whitefish? Your eyes have probably just passed over these items on the store shelves in the past. Now's the time to try them.

If your idea of condiments stops at bright red ketchup, bright yellow mustard, and dark brown steak sauce, it's time to move on—to Caribbean jerk sauce, sweet-and-sour sauce, mint sauce, cocktail sauce, an endless range of barbecue and grilling marinades, and such pepper-hot sauces as Tabasco, pukka, jalfrezi, and jalapeño, to name just a few. There are also mustards that are stone-ground, flavored with horseradish or honey, or imported from faraway places like Dijon.

Even fruits, of which we have an abundance

Undiscovered Vegetables: Make New Friends

Picture yourself in your supermarket's produce section. The apples are on your left, right next to the oranges. On your right are the celery, cucumbers, and carrots. In the middle, as though they can't quite decide if they're fruits or vegetables, reside the tomatoes. Next time you're at the store, take a closer look. I bet that interspersed among the green lettuce, yellow peppers, and red tomatoes are vegetables you've never noticed. Just as strangers are friends you haven't met yet, some of those unfamiliar vegetables could be your new favorites, just waiting to be discovered.

Here are a few ideas:

- Artichokes aren't nearly as difficult to eat as their spiny shapes suggest. Members of the sunflower family, artichokes originated in Sicily and were brought by the French to Louisiana and by Spaniards to California. The tender bases of the petals and the fleshy heart to which the petals are connected are the parts you can eat. You can boil, steam, or microwave them and serve them in stews, salads, and casseroles.
- Bok choy's crunchy white stalks and tender, dark green leaves have a mild taste. Bok choy can be eaten raw, but many people prefer to cook it. It's often used as an ingredient in stir-fries and Oriental-style soups.
- Broccoli rabe is related to both the cabbage and turnip. Italians cook this leafy green vegetable in a variety of ways, including frying, steaming, and braising. They also mix it into soups and salads.
- Calabaza is another unique selection in the produce section. This squash is popular in Central and South America as well as in the Caribbean. Peel it first and remove the seeds and spongy fibers, then welcome it into your soups and stews.
- A staple of soul food, collard greens are a variety of cabbage. Unlike cabbage, collard doesn't form a head but instead grows in a loose rosette at the top of a tall stem. It tastes like a cross between cabbage and kale. If you like your collard greens Southern style—that is, boiled with a hunk of bacon or salt pork—try substituting veggie bacon or other veggie deli meats so you'll still get the taste you like. These greens are also good in stir-fries or omelettes.
- Escarole is a variety of endive. With its broad, slightly curved pale green leaves,

in this country, have recently enjoyed a culinary franchise expansion. It isn't just pears and apples anymore. In fact, it isn't just Bartlett pears and Macintosh apples; now you can find scores of varieties of the common fruits. In addition, there are the relatively uncommon fruits: mango, papaya, apricots, a range of melons in every color—from golden watermelon to Persian melon to Crenshaw and casaba melon to Galia melon from Israel and carillon melon from France, green and escarole has a milder flavor than the other endives, Belgian and curly endive. Enjoy escarole chopped and combined with other types of greens in a salad. Or cook it briefly for a tasty side dish or as an addition to soups.

- Jicama, also called Mexican potato, is common in Caribbean cooking. Peel it first, then serve it raw or cooked. It has a sweet, nutty flavor and crunchy white flesh. Jicama can also be used as a substitute for water chestnuts, a wise choice because it is an excellent source of vitamin C.

- Kabocha squash, also known as chestnut squash or Japanese pumpkin or Sweet Mama, is a winter squash with deep-orange flesh and a dense, almost starchy texture. The flavor is sweet and very satisfying; in fact, I find kabocha to be the "squashiest" of the winter squashes—a real winner. Cook it any way you like—boiled, baked, steamed. It's a great source of fiber and beta-carotene, which means that it's good for you as well as good-tasting.

- Plantains are actually fruits, but they're prepared like vegetables. They resemble bananas, but unlike bananas, plantains' starchy flesh must be cooked. Green plantains taste like potatoes or squash; they're sweeter when ripe. Plantains are an excellent source of beta-carotene, which the body turns into vitamin A.

- Radicchio leaves are easily spotted with their dark maroon-red color threaded with white veins. They're most often used as a salad green, but they can also be grilled, sautéed, or baked.

- Taro root is a starchy, potato-like tuber that is cooked, pounded into a paste, and then fermented to make the Hawaiian dish poi, but you can simply add it to soups and stews or boil, fry, or bake it like a potato. It's native to Asia and grown in tropical areas. Taro root is a staple food in West Africa, the Caribbean, and throughout the Polynesian islands.

- Watercress is a vegetable with a long history. Persian, Greek, and Roman soldiers ate this leafy vegetable to prevent scurvy during their battle campaigns. This member of the mustard family grows in cool running water. Its pungent flavor is slightly bitter, with a peppery snap. You'll likely find it in your grocery in small bouquets. Try it cooked, tossed in salads, or as a great way to add crunch on sandwiches.

red and white and black grapes, figs, kumquats, kiwifruit, jicama, nectarines, clementines, persimmons and pomegranates, berries of every shape and hue, and such tropical fruits as passion fruit, pomelo, and custard apple. Try them all.

The bottom-line message? Broaden your culinary horizon and widen your vision. There's a world of food out there. You have a better shot at Picture-Perfect Weight Loss when you experience the richness of the world's

Supermarket Seaweed

Sea vegetables, once found only in Asian or specialty grocery stores, are beginning to appear in upscale supermarkets. Call them weeds if you like, but people all over the globe have been harvesting these sea foods for centuries and gaining the benefits of their nutrients—calcium, beta-carotene, manganese, iron, copper, vitamin E, iodine, and protein.

Sea vegetables are useful in a great range of dishes. What's exotic to us—for example, rice rolled in nori—is as common in Japan as a lunchtime sandwich is here. Common varieties, besides nori, are kombu (kelp), hijiki, and wakame, all of which are great in salads, vegetable platters, and soups.

foods in all their diverse colors, textures, and tastes—available today in your local market.

Try Out the Spices of Life

Variety is essential to Picture-Perfect Weight Loss. After all, variety is the spice of life. And spicing up your meals is important to Picture-Perfect Weight Loss and to shopping for Picture-Perfect Weight Loss.

Buy a vast array of taste-enhancers, such as spices, garnishes, herbs, sauces, and condiments. Why? Because they add taste, flavor, excitement, and the potential for unbridled creativity to your cooking and eating. Add some dried basil to a salad dressing . . . slather an exotic imported mustard on a sandwich of vegetarian salami . . . enliven a soup with fresh pepper . . . season your vegetable dip with Thai curry paste. Especially because you're about to extend the range of your food choices, the time is right to experiment with recipes. A well-stocked shelf of flavorings will help your trial-and-error process and give you more options. And options, in a very real sense, are what Picture-Perfect Weight Loss is all about.

Soup Up Your Weight Loss

Soups are another powerful tool of weight loss. The groups of firefighters I've worked with are particularly big soup fans, and many have become highly creative soup chefs. First of all, for you as for burly firefighters, a bowl of hearty soup can be an entire meal. Second, it's a great way to get your vegetables—even if you're someone who tends not to like vegetables. Finally, you can use soups in other recipes—as a marinade, for example, or to create a sauce.

I recommend shopping for a variety of low-calorie soups, then spicing them up with condiments, herbs, and spices to taste. Enjoy the result—either as a soup or to soup up some other food.

Package Deal

One more word as you prepare to head out the door for the supermarket: Don't reject canned, packaged, or frozen foods. I know that in some quarters, there's a tendency to think that fruit and vegetables must be fresh to be good. It ain't necessarily so.

Now don't get me wrong. I think fresh fruits and vegetables are the best foods on Earth—for health, weight loss, and sheer goodness. But the fact is that the goodness, the weight-loss potential, and the health benefits of fruits and vegetables are often just as powerful in packaged form as in the fruits and vegetables that were fresh-picked this morning.

Did you know that fruits and vegetables intended for packaging are typically harvested at their absolute peak of freshness? That freshness is preserved by the packaging, whatever its form. And while it is true that the processing required to preserve a food can cause the loss of some nutrients, it is also true that the loss is tiny—almost infinitesimal.

Besides, the loss is more than offset by the benefits that packaging provides. What are those benefits? For one thing, the technologies of preservation mean that you can enjoy fruits and vegetables out of season, even all year long. Summer fruits throughout the winter . . . autumn squash in the spring. These anomalies are not only a health benefit but also a luxury that would have astonished preceding generations.

The convenience of canned, packaged, and frozen fruits and vegetables is another luxury. Think of it: Any time of year, any time of day or night, just cut open a can or pull open a package, and with minimal preparation, you are ready to serve and eat pineapple from the tropics, beans from the Mediterranean, potatoes from the Great Plains—all without leaving home.

Fruits and vegetables are the heart of Picture-Perfect Weight Loss. Technology makes it possible to enjoy them in all their variety all the time—without limit. That's a boon to anyone trying to lose weight and keep it off for life.

Dr. Shapiro's Anytime List

You first heard about the Anytime List in the previous chapter, and you can guess how it got its name: Where Picture-Perfect Weight Loss is concerned, anything on the list is good to eat anytime, in any amount, for any purpose, driven by any motivation.

The Anytime List contains soups, sauces and condiments and marinades, dressings and dips, candy, desserts, and beverages—plus any and all fresh fruits and vegetables. Think of the list as your menu of staples for your pantry, refrigerator, and freezer. Reach for any of these foods anytime to make a meal or grab a snack.

On their own, the foods on the list provide a banquet of varying tastes. Supplement them with low-calorie choices from among the foods you

Salty Snack

If you're craving a salty snack but are concerned about the high calorie count of peanuts, try roasted soybeans. Dry-roasted or oil-roasted—and available in a range of flavors—an ounce of soy nuts has half the fat content of peanuts (although it's the healthier unsaturated fat in both cases) and considerably fewer calories. Soy nuts also provide folate and fiber, iron and other minerals, and disease-fighting isoflavones.

Shopping for Your Kids

At just about your waist level as you push your cart along the supermarket aisle—at eye level for your kids—are the products made especially to appeal to children. Be watchful of these foods pitched to kids. While many are good choices, in terms of both calorie count and nutrition, others are high-calorie products with little nutritional value, if any.

The latter point up my key recommendation about shopping for children who may be overweight. It's this: Shopping for kids is like shopping for yourself. The same principles that guide you in buying supplies for *your* Picture-Perfect Weight Loss should guide you in buying the foods for your children's Picture-Perfect Weight Loss.

Be particularly mindful of snack foods. Growing children do snack, of course, and snack food manufacturers make no secret of the fact that they are going after the kid market. If your child is overweight, be especially careful about snack foods that *sound like* they're weight-conscious choices—dietetic candies, for example, or all-natural chips. As the demonstrations show, some of these can be what I call saboteur foods—you buy into the advertising claim that this is a weight- or health-conscious choice, so you eat even more of the snack than you might have if it were not "dietetic," only to find out that the calorie savings isn't that great, if it exists at all, and the nutritional value is low.

For your children as for yourself, expand the scope of food options. Remember: No child should feel deprived of the tastes he or she enjoys, but by expanding options, you can also expand the range of your child's enjoyment. I know it sounds bizarre, but weight loss really can be fun!

---

love, and you should have no trouble creating wonderful recipes that satisfy your tastebuds, boost your nutritional health, and contribute to your weight loss. My physician's prescription for the Anytime List? Take as needed.

The Anytime List

Fruits and vegetables: All fruits and vegetables—raw, cooked, fresh, frozen, canned, in soups. For the best flavor, try to buy fresh fruits and vegetables in season. Avoid any packaged fruits that have added sugar.

Soups: Satisfying, easy, and versatile, soup can be a snack, a meal, or a cooking ingredient. And soups with vegetables and/or beans offer a nutritional bonus. Just be sure to avoid cream soups.

Sauces, condiments, and marinades: Use these to add flavor, moisture, texture, and versatility to every food at every meal.

- Oil-free and/or low-calorie salad dressings
- Fat-free or light mayonnaise, fat-free sour cream, fat-free yogurt (plain) or light yogurt with NutraSweet
- Mustards: Dijon, Pommery, and others
- Tomato purée, tomato paste, tomato sauce
- Clam juice, lemon or lime juice, tomato juice, V-8 vegetable cocktail

- Butter Buds, Molly McButter
- Nonstick cooking sprays such as Pam, in flavors such as butter, olive oil, garlic, and lemon
- Vinegars: balsamic, tarragon, wine, and others
- Horseradish: red, white
- Sauces: A-1, barbecue, chutney, cocktail, duck sauce, ketchup, relish, salsa, soy, tamari, Worcestershire, and others
- Onions: fresh, juice, flakes, or powder
- Garlic: fresh, jarred, juice, flakes, or powder
- Herbs: all, including basil, bay leaves, chives, dill, marjoram, oregano, rosemary, sage, tarragon, thyme, and others
- Spices: all, including allspice, cinnamon, cloves, coriander, cumin, curry, ginger, nutmeg, paprika, and others
- Extracts: almond, coconut, maple, peppermint, vanilla, and others
- Cocoa powder
- Soups as seasoning

Dressings and dips: Fat-free or light versions are recommended. The light version may be called low-fat, reduced-fat, or low-calorie, and it's often tastier than the fat-free version. Use as toppings or even cooking liquids as well as for dipping and dressing. I recommend keeping several variations of dressings and dips on hand—including at least one creamy version.

Candy: Avoid the "dietetic" variety; it contains almost as many calories as the real thing but is far less satisfying. The upshot? You'll tend to eat more—for more calories. I do recommend:

- Any chewing gum or gumballs
- Any hard candy: sourballs, candy canes, lollipops such as Tootsie Pops or Blow Pops, Jolly Ranchers, Werther's Original Butterscotch, Hershey's TasteTations, and others

Desserts (frozen): Any fat-free frozen yogurt—or nondairy substitute—or sorbet is a fine addition to the freezer. Try for the lower-calorie choices among them.

- In soft-serve, stick to varieties that contain up to 25 calories per ounce, as in Skimpy Treat, TCBY or ICBY, Columbo fat-free frozen yogurt, and low-fat Tofutti
- In hard-pack, choose items with up to 400 calories per pint, as in Sharon's Sorbet, low-fat Tofutti, all Italian ices, and Sweet Nothings
- In Creamsicles, Fudgsicles, Popsicles, and other frozen bars, opt for those with up to 45 calories per bar, as in Welch's Fruit Juice Bars, Weight Watchers Smart Ones Orange Vanilla Treats, Tofutti Chocolate Fudge Treats, Weight Watchers Smart Ones Chocolate Mousse, Dolly Madison

Avocados? Absolutely!

High in calories? Sort of. High in fat? Just the unsaturated kind, the kind you *want* to have. Further, avocados are packed with potassium, beta-carotene, vitamin C, and folate—and they're also a source of cholesterol-lowering sterols. A rich, tasty meal in itself, a single avocado offers about 6 ounces of edible fruit. Like all fruits and vegetables, it's the best kind of food you can eat for healthy weight loss.

Impulse Buy?

Truth be told, you didn't buy that bag of chips or that package of cookies or that candy bar by accident but by design—the supermarket's design. Marketing managers have spent millions of dollars to research what we buy and why we buy it, and they design their stores and their marketing campaigns in response. It's why high-calorie treats are densely packed in the inner aisles while staples are along the outer walls of the store, so that you have to pass through stacks of starches and cookies to find a head of lettuce. It's why candies are right at the checkout counter, where we have time to talk ourselves into buying them while we wait. It's also why you can often get two of something you probably didn't want in the first place for the price of one. And so on. Everything about supermarket design, including the music played and the smell of bread baking, is meticulously planned to capture your mind and bend it to choose certain foods.

Slender Treat Chocolate Mousse, and Yoplait
- In individually packaged frozen bars, choose ones with about 70 to 120 calories each, as in FrozFruit, Häagen-Dazs Orange and Vanilla sorbet bars, and Starbucks Coffee Frappuccino and Mocha Frappuccino bars

Beverages: Low-calorie beverages are good to keep on hand to supplement water, but avoid beverages labeled "naturally sweetened" or "fruit-juice sweetened."

- Coffees and teas
- Crystal Light, Diet Snapple, Diet Natural Lemon Nestea, Diet Mistic, and others
- Diet sodas: orange, chocolate, cherry chocolate, cream, root beer, colas, and more
- Seltzer: plain or flavored (check the calorie count if the product is labeled "naturally sweetened")
- Hot cocoa mixes: Stick with ones with 20 to 50 calories per serving, as in Swiss Miss Diet and Nestlé Carnation Diet (avoid cocoa mixes with 60 calories or more)

- Milk shake mixes: Choose varieties with no more than 80 calories per serving, as in Weight Watchers chocolate fudge and Alba Fit 'n Frosty

More Essential Ingredients

Okay. Let's assume you've stocked your shelves and cupboards with the items on the Anytime List. Let's assume further that your refrigerator, freezer, and pantry are stuffed with fresh and frozen and canned fruits and vegetables. In other words, you have the core of Picture-Perfect Weight Loss on hand right now. But you probably still want to shop for a few more essential items. Here are some tips and recommendations on how to look at the choices with which you'll be presented.

Cereals

Let's start with breakfast cereals. The choices here are staggering, so let me offer a general rule: Go for whole grain or high-fiber cereal, and if possible, look for cereals that contain bran. After that, the array of flavors and textures is your choice as you look for the lowest-calorie option. Be very careful to check the serving size when you're perusing the nutrition labels on cereal boxes. These vary dramatically from manufacturer to manufacturer, product to product. Be an aware cereal shopper!

Breads and Spreads

Is a peanut butter and jelly sandwich your standard lunch? Afraid you'll have to give it up for Picture-Perfect Weight Loss? Not necessarily.

Light breads at 40 to 45 calories per slice, made by just about every manufacturer, are my recommendation for the weight-conscious, but if you do choose regular bread, look for whole grain, which is the preferable nutritional choice. To be sure it's whole grain, make sure the nutrition label says "100 percent whole."

As you climb the baked goods ladder, the calorie count also rises. Have a look:

- 2 slices of light-bread toast: 80 calories
- 1 English muffin, plain: 120 calories
- 2 slices of regular toast: 140 calories
- 1 average roll (2 ounces): 160 calories
- 1 bagel, plain (5 ounces): 400 calories

Where jams and jellies are concerned, the lower-sugar versions are best—10 to 40 calories per tablespoon versus the 50 to 60 in "regular" jams. And don't be misled by honey, a wonderfully "natural" food that is actually more concentrated in sugar than sugar itself. With no particular health benefits and weighing in at 60 calories per tablespoon, honey is best avoided if weight loss is your aim.

As for peanut butter, yes, it's a high-calorie item. But it is also amazingly good for you. Peanut butter contains lots of nutrients that are important for heart health—niacin, folate, phosphorus, vitamin E, and phytosterols.

Oils and Dressings

Everyone knows that vegetable oils are good for you, but their 120 calories per tablespoon are a high price to pay for the goodness. For the weight-conscious in particular, I recommend substituting ready-made light dressings or dressing mixes.

In addition to serving as a substitute for oil or butter, the ready-mades are a great food preparation ingredient—and that makes them a highly useful tool in Picture-Perfect Weight Loss. Brush a low-calorie ranch dressing on a baked potato, for example, or daub shrimp with low-calorie Italian dressing in preparation for the grill. Or mix up a ready-made dressing with some low-calorie salsa to create a healthful vegetable dip. The results are delicious.

The recommended ready-made dressings come in two categories:

The "Whole" in the Label

Among breads, the prize for the most nutritious goes to those that contain whole grains. Unless the ingredients list *starts* with the "whole" designation, you're getting refined wheat flour, which is not nearly as nutritious as the whole grain ingredient.

- Light or reduced-fat dressings—15 to 50 calories per tablespoon
- Fat-free dressings—2 to 15 calories per tablespoon

Another tip for salad lovers trying to shed pounds: Use a flavored vinegar as a salad dressing (or as a cooking ingredient) and forget the oil altogether.

Frozen Meals

When convenience is an issue, frozen meals are an excellent option. For breakfast, lunch, or dinner, they offer a range of choices—including a variety of ethnic tastes and textures. Of course, you should shop for the lower-calorie choices; in general, they provide excellent nutritional value for the calories.

My one reservation concerns the small portion sizes of vegetables in most of the lunch and dinner frozen meals. Of course, there's a simple solution to this: Just add a vegetable side dish or a salad to your frozen meal, or start off with a cup or bowl of vegetable-rich soup.

Beverages

The rule of thumb here is to eat your calories rather than drink them. All juices, regular sodas, and flavored drinks are full of calories. Yet the soft drink you guzzle with a meal and the glass of juice you down for an afternoon pick-me-up are almost afterthoughts. Why spend calories on afterthoughts? Besides, if you're just dying for the taste of orange, you are far better off eating an orange: You'll get lots of vitamins and minerals, lots of fiber to fill you up, and about 45 calories—versus a glass of orange juice at about 120 calories.

Stick with water or diet drinks—and check out the recommendations on the Anytime List.

Rice, Pasta, and Other Starchy Grains

Look for whole grain varieties, which are more nutritious. While brown rice, kasha, and whole wheat pastas are probably available in your supermarket, you may have to head for a specialty store to find such exotic entries as

Fortified Waters

Just when you thought it was safe to go back to plain old tap water, food manufacturers have come out with cranked-up "fitness" waters. Marketed to slake the thirst for better athletic performance and greater endurance, these new drinks, including Propel and Glaceau Soy Water, Vitamin Water, and Smart Water, to name a few, of course do nothing of the kind. They're fortified with caffeine, sweeteners, herbs, vitamins and minerals, or soy, but their extra strength is a dubious proposition, and their "fortifiers" are better taken in elsewhere. After all, if you need more soy in your diet, you should be eating more soy products.

On the other hand, some of the vitamin-stuffed waters are stuffed with too much vitamin; Glaceau Vitamin Water has twice the RDA for vitamin A and can be harmful for pregnant women.

Best bet? Get your fluids in diet beverages, foods, and good, clear H_2O.

Energy Defined

The "energy" promised in nutrition bars—and now in gels, the latest explosive food trend—might say "better performance" to you, but its real meaning is calories, and that's about all these bars provide, although at an inflated price. There are the high-carbohydrate bars with high calorie counts, the low-carbohydrate bars that are high in both calories and fat, and the 40-30-30 bars that are only slightly less caloric than your average candy bar. The bottom line? There is no magic to the nutrition bars. They're a marketing phenomenon that may be an alternative to a Hershey's with almonds, but they certainly don't live up to the claims of boosting your athletic, mental, or nutritional performance.

quinoa, whole wheat couscous, bulgur wheat, barley, and millet.

In general, as you stand in the supermarket aisle planning your meals in your mind, think about relegating the starchy grains to side-dish status. Fill up on vegetables and protein, and put rice, pasta, couscous, and polenta in third place in your Picture-Perfect Weight-Loss program.

Frozen Desserts

Look for low-fat, low-calorie fudge bars, fruit bars, and other treats. But be certain to check the calorie counts; some products advertised as "light" are nearly as high in calories as the real thing.

If you're shopping by the pint, look for frozen yogurt, nondairy dessert, sorbet, Italian ices, or other frozen desserts with calorie counts under 400 per pint, sometimes as low as 240 per pint.

If you absolutely cannot stomach fat-free frozen desserts, another option is low-fat desserts. These have the advantage of coming in a range of flavors to satisfy your dessert yearnings, but go for the products with 2 grams or fewer of fat per serving.

Head for the Market . . .

Enough shopping tips for one day? Check out the demos that follow. Then get to the market and start buying!

Day 1 goals:
- [ ] Shop with the Anytime List.
- [ ] Buy four food items you don't normally eat and try them. You may just be pleasantly surprised, and you'll certainly be on your way to Picture-Perfect Weight Loss.
- [ ] Buy a notebook. The next chapter will tell you why. Make sure it's small enough to go with you during the day, but big enough for you to write in comfortably.
- [ ] Prepare to make changes. Remember that if you do what you did, you get what you got.

Somewhere over the Rainbow

Somewhere over the rainbow, bluebirds sing, and this one small rainbow cookie will give you just about a bird-sized bite of sweetness. For the same number of calories, you could eat a multi-flavored rainbow of sweet, cooling sorbets, enough to fill this towering parfait glass. And chances are good that half of the tower would satisfy . . .

4 3-oz scoops of sorbet
200 calories

1½ oz rainbow cookie
200 calories

=

Consumption Assumptions

We assume that anything with chocolate and nuts must be high-calorie; we assume the low-fat caramel is the weight-conscious choice. But check the numbers—you can actually eat more of the chocolate kisses for the same calorie count as the low-fat caramels. Plus this: When you know you're dealing with a high-calorie food, you tend to exercise caution, so chances are you won't eat all nine kisses. On the other hand, the "low-fat" label on the caramels may lull you into throwing caution to the wind.

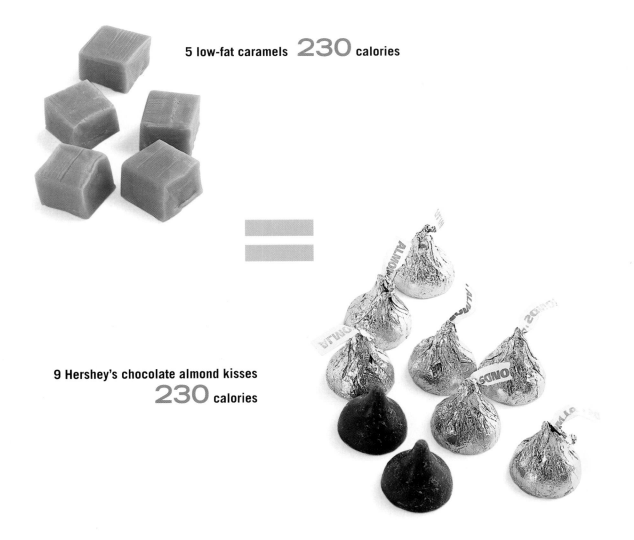

5 low-fat caramels 230 calories

**9 Hershey's chocolate almond kisses
230 calories**

Breakfast Treat

A whole box of these delicious Belgian waffles is the caloric equivalent of not quite one whole bagel. The lesson is clear: Consider light pancakes or waffles as a breakfast choice. They constitute a real calorie bargain and—topped with fruit—make a special breakfast treat.

¾ of a 5-oz bagel 300 **calories**

4 waffles (an entire box of Van's 7-grain Belgian waffles) 300 **calories**

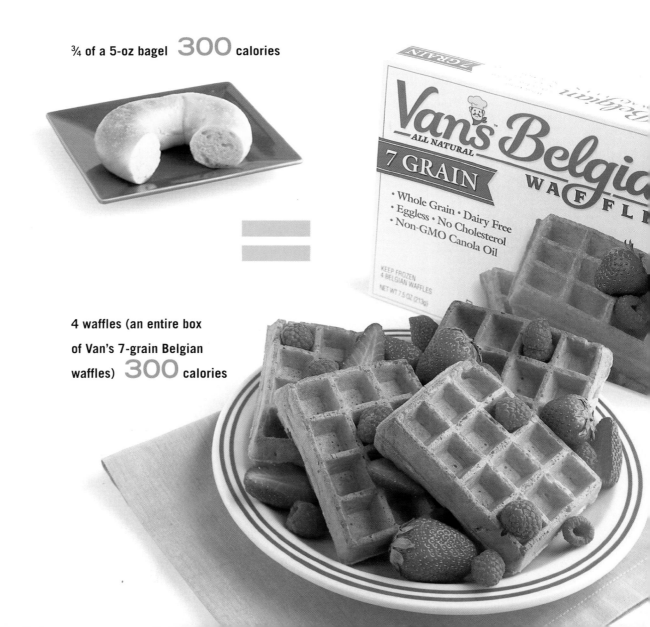

"Let Them Eat Muffins"

Want to have your muffin and eat it, too? You can breakfast on English muffins 4 days in a row for the cost of a single corn muffin breakfast. Stick to the English muffins for a real bargain in breads.

1 corn muffin (4½ oz)
480 calories

1 box English muffins
(4 muffins)
480 calories

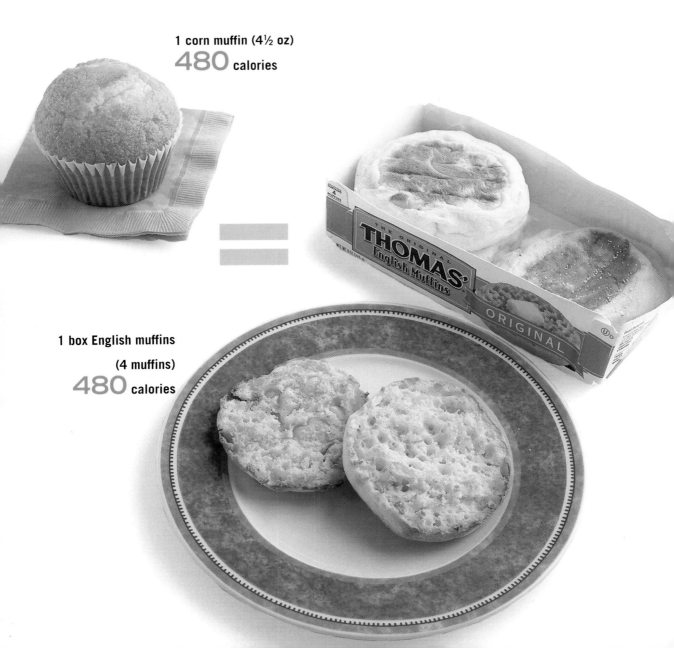

An Expensive Breakfast

A highly concentrated source of calories, granola makes for a breakfast that's costly in terms of weight loss—and is all too easy to snack on right out of the box. Box for box, you'll get much more nutrition for far fewer calories with the wheat flakes.

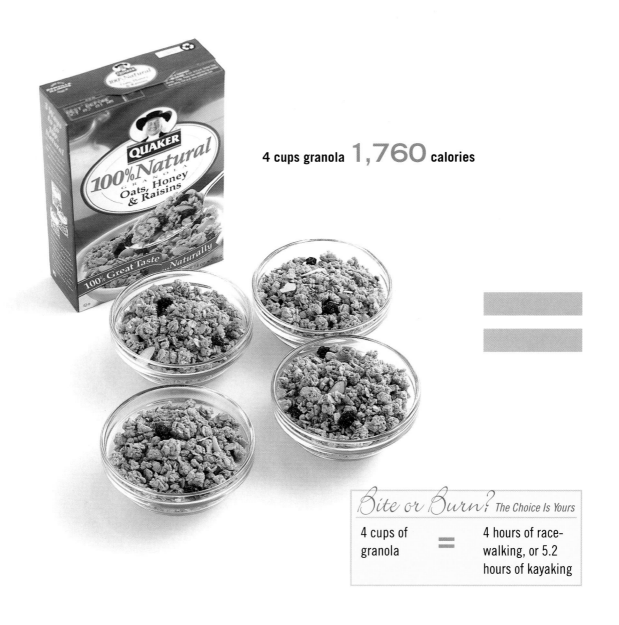

4 cups granola 1,760 calories

Bite or Burn? The Choice Is Yours

| 4 cups of granola | = | 4 hours of race-walking, or 5.2 hours of kayaking |

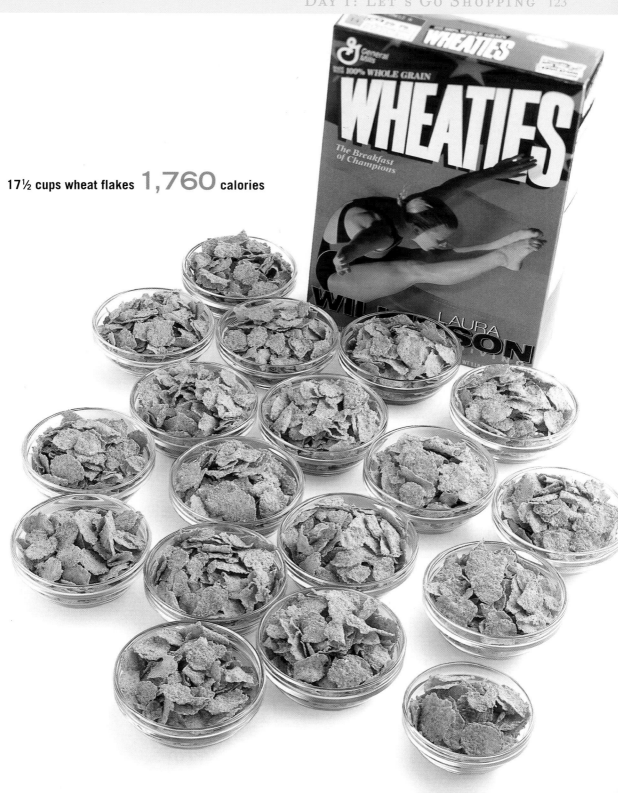

17½ cups wheat flakes 1,760 calories

Is It Clear?

The bottled beverage looks absolutely clear and is "naturally flavored." The flavor comes from the sugar: Every teaspoon pictured on the right is in the beverage. Lesson? Read the nutrition label; even on something as simple as a bottle of water, it pays to be clear about what you're getting.

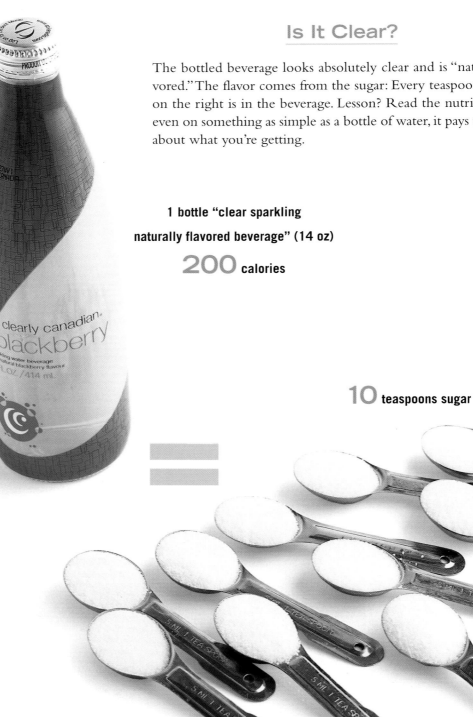

1 bottle "clear sparkling naturally flavored beverage" (14 oz)

200 calories

10 teaspoons sugar

Saboteur!

The reduced-calorie sweet saves you little, but because it is reduced-calorie, you may rationalize taking in more of it than you normally would. This makes it a classic saboteur. Stick to lollipops when you want the taste of chocolate.

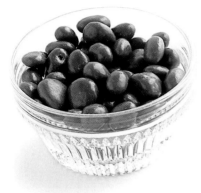

3 oz reduced-calorie

chocolate-covered raisins

300 calories

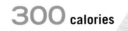

6 chocolate lollipops

300 calories

Deluxe Dessert

When you crave something rich for a deluxe dessert, think about getting it in a low-calorie frozen bar—for one-tenth the calories of a super-premium bar.

1 super-premium ice cream bar 330 calories

10 assorted low-calorie frozen bars 330 calories

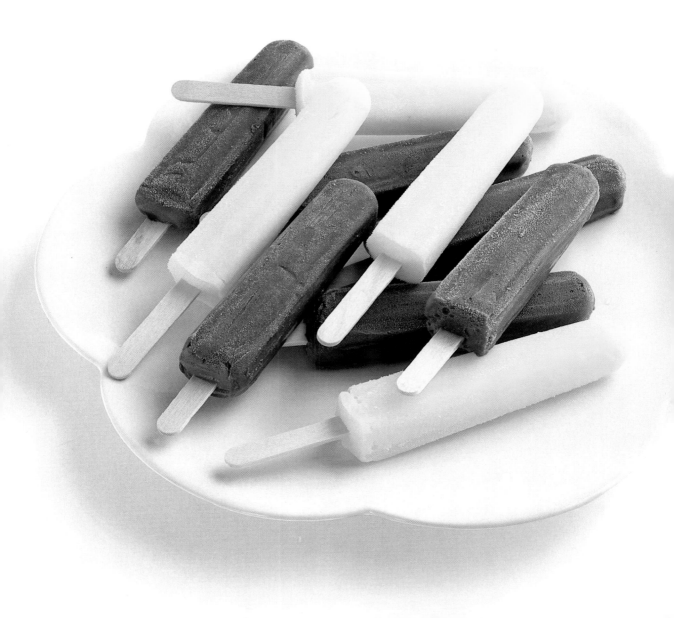

Frozen Desserts

Shopping for a frozen dessert? Here's a graphic illustration of the relative calorie costs. Notice what a good bargain the sorbet is. Best of all, though, are the individual chocolate mousse bars; you can eat even several of them and not come close to the calorie count of the other options. And both the sorbet and the mousse bars are on the Anytime List, so enjoy them at any time.

1 pint super-premium ice cream **1,280** calories

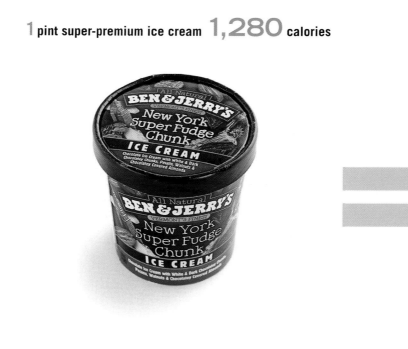

Bite or Burn? The Choice Is Yours

| 1 pint premium ice cream | = | 5.4 hours of skydiving |

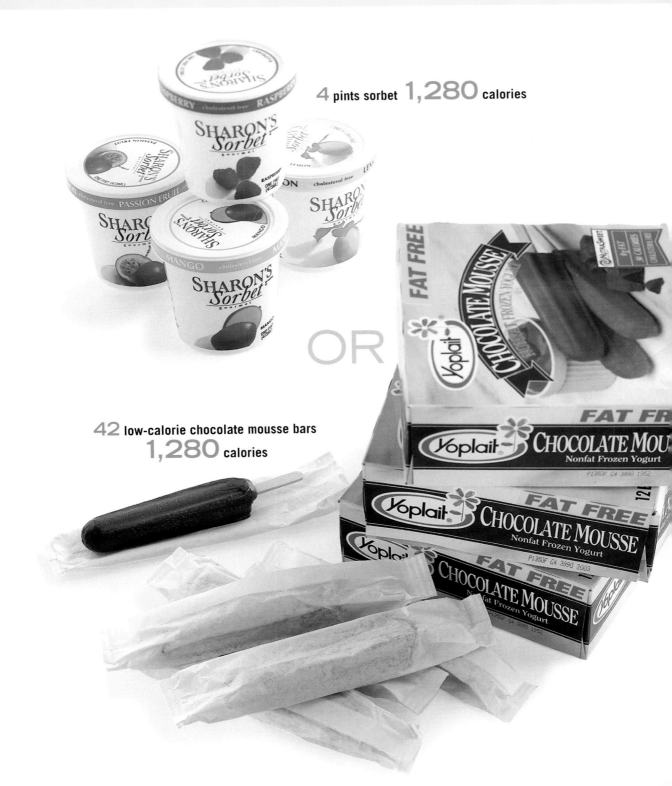

4 pints sorbet 1,280 calories

OR

42 low-calorie chocolate mousse bars
1,280 calories

Dr. Shapiro's Picture-Perfect Weight Loss Food Pyramid

The Picture-Perfect Weight-Loss Food Pyramid is a guide to healthy, low-calorie choices. It maps the proportionate amounts of foods in an overall eating plan. Here's what it tells you:

Make fruits and vegetables the foundation of your eating. Just as the pyramid is necessarily widest at the base, let fruits and vegetables be the foods you eat most—most often, most regularly, and most of.

Next, go for protein. But as often as possible, get your protein in beans and other legumes, seafood, and soy products rather than in meats, poultry, and dairy. (*Note:* The FDA recommends avoiding shark, swordfish, tilefish, and king mackerel during pregnancy because of their high mercury content.)

When you take in grain products, choose whole grain or light versions if possible.

Where fats and oils are concerned, choose nuts, seeds, olives, avocados, and either olive or canola oil wherever possible.

For sweet treats, stick with hard candies and fat-free frozen desserts.

If you don't see your favorite food category on my pyramid, keep in mind that no food is forbidden with Picture-Perfect Weight Loss. The pyramid presents my recommendations for a healthy way of eating that will provide all the nutrients you need as you lose weight and maintain your weight loss.

Make the pyramid your guide, and you will be thin for life.

Hard candies, fat-free frozen desserts
SWEETS

Nuts, seeds, olives, avocados, and olive and canola oil
FATS AND OILS

Preferably whole grains or light versions
GRAIN PRODUCTS

Soy products, beans, legumes, seafood
PROTEIN FOODS

Any and all—fresh, frozen, canned, packaged—as much as possible, as often as possible
FRUITS AND VEGETABLES

Chapter 6

WEEK 1: FOCUS ON BREAKFAST, ON CHANGE, AND ON *You*

30-Day Plan

By the end of Week 1, you will have:

- Committed to change
- Learned the basic principles of Picture-Perfect Weight Loss
- Started a food diary/personal journal
- Begun to exercise
- Changed your thinking about breakfast and your breakfast choices
- Begun to lose weight

In just about every firehouse in New York City—perhaps in every firehouse in the country—there's a steady supply of breads and pastries on hand for munching during the day. Somebody is bound to bring in a dozen bagels—and maybe some cream cheese for good measure—and there's invariably one guy who passes Dunkin' Donuts on the way to work and can't resist stocking up on doughnuts, crullers, and Munchkins for his fire-fighting brethren. That's why it was always easy for Lieutenant Larry Quinn Jr. of New York's Bravest to down a couple of bagels along with his breakfast coffee and orange juice, and maybe grab a sugar-coated doughnut or two for a midmorning snack.

What's more, since the firefighters responsible for cooking aim for quantity as much as for quality, there's generally food left over from the previous evening meal, despite the hearty appetites on which firefighters pride themselves. So if you ask firefighter Billy Quick what his usual breakfast used to be, he's likely to answer: "A meatball sandwich" or "leftover breaded veal cutlets."

For fire department chaplain Father John Delendick, the breakfast issue was slightly different. Father John typically began each morning with a healthy bowl of cereal. But as he went about his morning routine, he would add a jelly doughnut at this firehouse, a bagel at that firehouse, or "whatever was around." On Sundays, as a special treat, the organist at Father John's church always used to leave two jelly dough-nuts—Father's favorites—as an after-mass treat.

These days, Lieutenant Quinn typically breakfasts on an English muffin, maybe a ba-nana, an orange or two, and coffee. Billy Quick might whip up an egg-white-and-spinach omelette for himself. And Father John's Sunday treat is a generous helping of French toast made with light bread and Egg Beaters, doused with light syrup, and accompanied by veggie bacon or sausages. During the week, if his daily bowl of cereal isn't enough, Father John sup-plements it with a couple of oranges.

Yet Father John will tell you, calmly but forcefully, that he has "not given up anything" since he began his Picture-Perfect Weight-Loss program and changed his eating habits at break-fast, lunch, and dinner—although he managed to lose 52 pounds in 5 months. Billy Quick, fea-tured on the CBS newsmagazine *48 Hours* in a show about weight loss and health, shed 30 pounds in 4 months. Lieutenant Quinn lost 29 pounds in 12 weeks—12 weeks, he points out, that included the Thanksgiving, Christmas, and New Year's holidays.

Then there's Tracy, another patient of mine. As the marketing director for a well-known fi-nancial services firm, Tracy's life seems a world away from the firefighters' routines. There's *no* downtime on Tracy's job. Almost from the mo-ment she gets up in the morning until she re-turns home at night, she's in meetings and conferences, on the phone, at working lunches or client dinners. Breakfast always used to be a muffin Tracy could pick up on her way into the office—preferably a corn muffin, which appealed to her sweet tooth as well as to her understanding of nutrition. And, because weight was a problem, Tracy made sure it was

a fat-free muffin. Just one muffin, she used to think to herself. Nothing to it.

Actually, as Tracy learned when she began her Picture-Perfect Weight-Loss program, there is something to the fat-free muffin: some 600 to 700 calories every morning. Three months later and 27 pounds lighter, Tracy breakfasts on maple-flavored oatmeal with fruit. Her sweet tooth is satisfied, her nutrition need is more than satisfied, and the calorie count comes to some 130 calories for the oat-meal and 50 or so for the fruit, depending on how much fruit she eats. What's more, the fruit is an excellent source of nutrients, and it also gives her a good portion of fiber, which is a wonderful way to take the edge off her ap-petite for the day by filling her up early.

No wonder all these people—from dedi-cated public servants to priest to fast-track ex-ecutive—are convinced of the efficacy of their Picture-Perfect Weight-Loss programs. No wonder they all continue to lose weight. No wonder they're all committed to their changed relationship with food for life.

And for all of them, breakfast is the first time in the day that they evidence that com-mitment. It's their opening shot in a day of empowered choices for Picture-Perfect Weight Loss, and it sets the tone for their changed re-lationship with food first thing in the morning—day after day after day.

Five Steps to Changing Your Breakfast—And Your Life

Week 1 of the 30-Day Plan for Picture-Perfect Weight Loss is about more than just changing the way you think about your first meal of the day. It's actually about changing your life—by starting to change your relationship with food.

This is the moment when you begin forging the principles of Picture-Perfect Weight Loss, putting them in place so that they eventually become routine. That's an ambitious agenda, but I make it doable by breaking it down into manageable steps. You're not going to change your relationship with food all at once but rather one step at a time. Actually, for Week 1, I want you to undertake five specific steps.

To get started, go get that notebook I advised you to buy when you went shopping. It starts coming in handy right now.

Step 1: Focus on Motivation

Why are you doing this? Why are you starting today to undertake a program of Picture-Perfect Weight Loss—a program that asks you to make a long-term, even lifetime commitment to change?

Of course, everybody knows the answer to this: You're doing it to lose weight. You want to look better, feel better, live longer. Everybody knows *all* the reasons why people try to lose weight.

But you're not "people." You're you. And the first step you should take toward Picture-Perfect Weight Loss is to know the desire or need that is triggering you to undertake the program—your personal motivation for changing your relationship with food.

Maybe the trigger for you, as for so many of the firefighters I've worked with, is suddenly feeling "weighed down" by the extra weight you've accumulated—so much so, in the firefighters' case, that they wondered about their ability to do the job.

Maybe, like Joanne Rusch or Tia and Jim Chisholm of the Chicago 7, your motivation

is to be the kind of role model of health you want your children to emulate.

Maybe it's something as "simple" as that upcoming college reunion . . . or looking good in a bathing suit, not just this summer, but every summer to come . . . or being tired of feeling different, left out, set apart from the world of thin people.

Whatever your personal motivation is, discover it, articulate it clearly, even say it out loud. Then write it down on its own page in your notebook—set apart so you can revisit it from time to time and be refreshed by it.

Why is this important? Because if you don't understand clearly what motivates you, it's all too easy to lose focus. Especially at the very beginning of the program, when everything is new and different, when Food Awareness has not yet become automatic and the principles of Picture-Perfect Weight Loss have not yet become second nature, you will need to hold on tight to your motivating reason. You'll have to think in ways you haven't thought before, try foods you haven't tried before. You may feel uncomfortable in certain situations—change is often uncomfortable. Remembering exactly what weight loss can mean to you is just about the most powerful weapon you can have to keep you focused.

Make the notebook your workbook, your personal journal of the change you're going through, including any feelings of discomfort. Studies show that writing things down is a "focusing device," as the behaviorists call it, and what you're focusing on is your own power to make change, the importance of the change you're making, and the very personal need or desire that motivates you.

One more point about motivation. You've

Presentation

We eat with our eyes. Even the simplest of foods can become special when presented attractively. A touch of garnish, a unique serving dish with a flower next to it, or a colorful arrangement makes food look so good you really want to eat it. Try focusing on presentation when you serve your next big plate of vegetables.

failed before? You've lost weight in the past, then regained it? Forget about it. Failure is an old and worn-out recording. Don't replay it. Think of your past failures as rehearsals that didn't really count. Instead, fast-forward to today. Today is when change starts. From this moment forward, you're on the Picture-Perfect Weight-Loss program, and all the signs are positive.

In fact, I recommend marking the moment in some way. When Tia and Jim Chisholm returned to "real life" from the house in which the Chicago 7 had lived for a week of Picture-Perfect Weight-Loss total immersion, they cleaned out their refrigerator and pantry, getting rid of all the foods they decided should no longer be a part of their lives. Another patient of mine canceled her newspaper delivery and decided instead to bike or walk into town for the paper each morning. *Because any kind of change can break a cycle, these gestures, while symbolic, mark the moment. They draw a line between one phase of your life, the one in which you were overweight, and the new you to come.*

Step 2: Honor Thyself

A patient told me about the day she tried to begin her Picture-Perfect Weight-Loss program. She was determined to start the day by getting on the exercise bike in the basement and doing 10 minutes before breakfast. She had just climbed aboard when her husband's voice boomed out from the bedroom, asking if he had any clean socks. She got off the bike, got the clean socks from the laundry room, and took them up to him. Then she climbed up on the bike again.

Next it was her daughter who interrupted. She popped into the basement, urgently announced her after-school plans, and demanded her mother's undivided attention. My patient climbed down off the bike and entered the pertinent information in her calendar.

Back on the bike. This time it was her son. He couldn't remember where he had put his hockey stick. Her husband again: Was she going to cook breakfast? Daughter: Just wondering if the dog had been fed. And so on. Later that morning, a friend called needing a ride to the market because her car was in the shop—could my patient please drive her where she needed to go?

The upshot? My patient never did any exercise at all that day. She never found—never *took*—the 10 minutes she had promised herself.

You have to. You have to do Picture-Perfect Weight Loss for *you*. Sure, mothers are typically the pivotal point in a family. They're the caregivers, the hub around which the family moves. But everyone—even a small child—can wait 10 minutes while you do your exercise . . . or prepare a special meal . . . or take a relaxing bath . . . or go for a brisk walk. You deserve it. You're worth it.

Even if your motivating trigger is to be an example for your children—in fact, *especially* if your motivating trigger is to be an example for your children—set that example by caring for yourself as you want them to care for themselves.

Hang a sign that says "Honor Thyself" on your refrigerator or on the mirror in your bedroom—or both. It's a reminder that where Picture-Perfect Weight Loss is concerned, this one is for you. And don't get off the exercise bike until you've finished your routine. Your family will quickly get the idea that they need to request things from you before or after your exercise session.

To help you remember the importance of your weight-loss program, try to line up your own support system. It might be a family member; it might be a friend—someone who can help you hold on to your motivation, someone who will be comfortable with a different you. New York psychologist Adele Fink, Ph.D., whose practice is "75 percent" focused on people with weight issues, talks about how unsettling a person's weight loss can be to family and friends. They're comfortable with the old you, says Dr. Fink; they "want you to stay the same, and your weight loss—your change—can be threatening to them."

One patient told me about lunching with two friends. When she pulled her own bottle of low-calorie salad dressing out of her bag, one friend was appalled, the other applauded. Obviously, it was the one who applauded who became a reliable source of encouragement when it was needed. My patient knew that this friend wanted her to be her best, and that made the friend a prime candidate for serving as a support "system."

Now suppose you're the parent of a child or teenager starting the Picture-Perfect Weight-Loss program. Remember that your son or daughter must do this by and for himself or herself. Set the example. Be the role model. Serve as a support system. But don't interfere—no comments, no negative remarks. Let your children do their own thing; it's the only way they'll succeed. The best help you can give and the most powerful influence you can provide is to live the program yourself.

Step 3: Start Your Food Diary/Personal Journal

Somewhere in your notebook—first page, last page, or right next to your motivational analysis—write down your current weight. Call it your starting weight. Months from now, even weeks from now, you'll be thrilled with how far you've traveled from this number.

Now turn to the first blank page and start your Week 1 food diary. (The diary worksheet will change in the weeks to come.)

The food diary is one of the most important tools of the Picture-Perfect Weight-Loss program. It's the best way I know for understanding your eating behavior, and that understanding, in turn, is the best spur to changing your behavior. For that reason, accuracy and attention to detail in keeping the food diary are absolutely essential.

Use the template shown on page 136 as a guide to creating your own food diary.

It's pretty straightforward. Every time you eat anything—meal or snack or "bite" of anything at all—write it down in the diary immediately. The "immediately" part is important. It's important first because we really do forget what we've eaten—and it's the forgotten bite that can make the difference, so "catching up" on the diary later is never as effective as making your entries the minute you eat. And it's important also because keeping the diary faithfully is evidence of your commitment to the important mission you've undertaken—the mission of losing weight by changing your relationship with food.

Record the exact time and exactly what you ate. It's not enough to write "soup and sandwich." A cup of soup or a bowl? What kind of soup? And what kind of sandwich? On what kind of bread? Anything "on" it? With what

beverage? Same for a quick snack: Don't just write "crackers"; write "four cheese crackers."

Next, rank your desire to eat—at the time you ate the food—on a scale from 0 to 4, with 0 for no hunger at all and 4 for ravenous.

Then fill in the entries that describe the circumstances in which you were eating.

Were you alone or with others? If you were with other people, who were they? How many other people? What's their relationship to you—friend, spouse, coworker? Were you at home or out? If you were at home, note which room. If you were out, note if the location was a restaurant, a friend's home, or some other place. What was your mood just before you ate? Were you bored, tense, happy, content, angry,

Week 1 Food Diary

Date/Time	Food (Preparation, Serving Size)	Degree of Hunger (0–4)	People/ Place	Mood	Activity

tired, depressed? Write it down. Finally, set down what else, if anything, you were doing at the time. Were you watching television, or perhaps reading in your easy chair, or maybe being a spectator at a sporting event or movie or show? Whatever it was, write it down.

The importance of keeping the food diary—and doing so faithfully—cannot be overestimated. One patient, himself a physician, says that "the diary confronts you with exactly what and when and what mental state you were in when you ate." He claims that he began losing weight as soon as he started keeping the food diary. And he stresses the "keeping" part. "In a stressful life, I tended to eat without thinking. I knew better, but knowing and doing are two different things. Until I started keeping the food diary. The diary was the incentive for constant and consistent awareness, and awareness was the incentive for consistently better choices."

Step 4: Get Moving

We've talked about it throughout part 1. We've discussed its importance for young people, the elderly, and those in the middle. Every health professional you speak with, every new piece of research, every health column in every newspaper will confirm what you already know so well: Exercise is good for you, and it's particularly good for you if you're trying to lose weight. Make up your mind that this week, you will get moving—and you will continue to move for the rest of your life. And understand that 30 days from now, you are going to feel better and look better because you have begun to move.

For Week 1 of Picture-Perfect Weight Loss, I ask that you start walking. That's an exercise you can do anytime, anywhere, in almost any weather. It doesn't require special equipment or a specially laid-out track in a gym or fancy sports gear—although I recommend sturdy, worn-in shoes and comfortable, loose-fitting slacks or shorts and a top. You don't even have to think of it as an exercise program. Just go for a walk. Take the first steps to enjoying a healthy life.

If you're a city dweller, I recommend what I tell my New York patients: Walk a few extra blocks before getting on the bus or heading down into the subway or hailing a taxi. If you live in an apartment building, exit the elevator a few floors before your stop and take the stairs the rest of the way. Head for the nearest city park: Walk across it or around it—or both.

If you live in a house with stairs, walk up and down them a few times in succession. Stride back and forth across your yard. Take a walk around the block; explore your neighborhood. Walk to the corner store to buy that item you forgot to get yesterday . . . or to the library to return a book . . . or to a neighbor's house for a visit.

Walk briskly. Swing your arms. Move those legs. Breathe deeply. You don't have to run, or get out of breath, or sweat. All you have to do is *move*.

Walk any time of the day. Many people like to get up out of bed and get moving. For them, a morning walk jump-starts the day; it gets the juices flowing and the mind working. Others like to break up the day with a brisk lunchtime walk that clears the cobwebs from the brain. My own recommendation is to take a walk after work. It's a way of losing the day's stress without resorting to cocktails and hors d'oeuvres; it's the perfect appetizer for a healthy, Picture-Perfect Weight-Loss dinner to come.

Whenever and wherever you walk this first week, do it with a sense of mindfulness. Be aware of the need to move, and be on the lookout for opportunities to move: by parking as far as possible from the supermarket, or by giving up the elevator for the stairs, or by raking the lawn yourself—right now—instead of waiting for the weekend and your husband to do it. As with food awareness, exercise awareness will eventually become second nature to you, and exercise itself will become a part of everything you do. It won't be "exercise" anymore; it will be lifestyle physical activity—and it starts right now in Week 1.

Step 5: Discover New Choices for Breakfast

"Breakfast is the most important meal of the day." That's the standard cliché, and Americans sometimes feel guilty if they don't sit down to a real meal for breakfast, or if their morning appetite ends at a cup of coffee or a mug of tea. In my view, that guilt is misplaced. If you're not hungry, you don't really need to have breakfast at all.

Except for children. They really do benefit from a nutritious morning meal. Study after study shows that kids who eat a nourishing breakfast do better in school and develop more healthfully than children who do not have breakfast.

While adults might also benefit from having breakfast, if you simply don't feel like eating, breakfast isn't a necessity. So your first breakfast choice—your first Picture-Perfect Weight-Loss eating option—is to decide whether you want breakfast at all. If it's a meal you'd just as soon skip, do so without guilt and without worry.

Don't make the mistake of denying yourself

breakfast to "save" calories, though. The denial will only come back to haunt you during the day. Biology will take over and prompt you to eat more—and to eat higher-calorie foods. As always, deprivation backfires. Skip breakfast if you're not hungry for it, but not because you think fasting in the morning will help you lose weight. It won't.

If you do have an appetite for breakfast, think of it as the daily kickoff of your Picture-Perfect Weight-Loss program, the meal that sets the tone for your changed relationship with food. In that sense, for you, breakfast really may be the most important meal of the day.

What's New?

Your goal for Week 1 should be to try something new for breakfast, to branch out from the usual and experience options you simply hadn't thought of before for breakfast. In fact, I'm going to recommend that three of the week's seven breakfasts include foods you've never eaten before. The reason? Ask the Chicago 7. We introduced them to a range of new choices for every meal of the day. The more new foods they were exposed to, the more they liked. Their tastes expanded, and so did the eating possibilities available to them.

Never had a reduced-fat egg product? This is the week to try one. Been eating the same cereal for the past 20 years? Find something new this week. Always wondered what those bialys in the bagel shop tasted like? This is the week to find out. Adding new tastes to your palate is a boon to your state of mind as well. As psychotherapist Susan Amato puts it, it's a "reminder that you're adding good things to your life—and to your kitchen—not subtracting."

Getting a Start on the Day's Nutrition

I want to offer two overall guidelines for thinking in a fresh way about your first meal of the day. You'll find these guidelines amply reflected in both the breakfast demonstrations shown in this chapter and in the breakfast choices I'm about to suggest. Both will give you an excellent start on obtaining the nutrition you need.

Include fruits (and/or vegetables) in your breakfast. Remember Dr. Shapiro's Picture-Perfect Weight-Loss Food Pyramid? You want fruit and vegetables to play a dominant role in your eating from now on. Adding fruit to your breakfast choices is a great way to start—a banana in your cereal, melon with berries, an apple to supplement a bialy. And as the suggestions that follow demonstrate, you can also use breakfast to get a leg up on the day's vegetable intake by going for a watercress omelette, or maybe eggs Florentine (with spinach)—made using reduced-fat egg products like Egg Beaters or Scramblers.

Introduce soy into your life. Soy products are so good for us in so many ways that it's no wonder they're becoming increasingly available everywhere. I predict, however, that this is just the beginning. More and more manufacturers are catching on to the soy idea; they're creating more soy products, and they're making them more tasty. Breakfast is a great way to experiment with these products—by trying soy milk with cereal, or by popping a soy sausage patty on your English muffin, or by having soy bacon with your Egg Beaters.

Some Picture-Perfect Weight Loss Breakfast Ideas

Now, let's put it all together in some breakfast suggestions. Remember: These ideas are just a starting point. Expand your breakfast repertoire with the food demonstrations pictured in this chapter. They offer a range of ideas—from cereal with fruit to a soy-based breakfast sandwich. But as you become increasingly aware of what you eat, let your own imagination and newly expanding palate guide you to more and more breakfast choices.

Cereal for Breakfast

Go for a low-calorie, whole grain or high-fiber cereal. Accompany it with low-fat soy milk in any of a range of flavor choices, or, second-best, with fat-free milk. Finally, add fresh and/or dried fruit to the bowl.

Coffee and . . .

If your idea of a good breakfast is a piece of toast or a roll or a muffin or a bagel with coffee, make it light toast or a whole grain roll or an English muffin or a bialy. Spread it with jam. And by all means, add a piece of fruit or even a plate of fruit. Remember: Fiber is your friend!

Eggs and Bacon

This week is a good time to try Egg Beaters or Scramblers or any of the other reduced-fat egg products. Check out vegetarian bacon or sausage as well. These products are typically soy-based, so they're a good way to start getting your soy. As always, include fruit with the meal.

Waffles and Pancakes

You'll be surprised at how tasty light waffles and pancakes are. I recommend Van's whole

Notes on Oats

Oats are high in protein, rich in soluble fiber, and an excellent source of thiamin, or vitamin B_1. The particular kind of fiber they contain is called beta glucan, and it is particularly effective in lowering the "bad" LDL cholesterol that can endanger coronary arteries. Oat fiber may also lower high blood pressure and help control blood sugar. As a plant food, oats contain disease-fighting phytochemicals that may reduce heart disease risk, relax blood vessels, and maintain bloodflow.

Get your oats in any form of oatmeal, fiber-rich oat bran, and a number of breakfast cereals and breads. Make sure the label says "whole grain oats," and look for products with at least 2 grams of fiber per serving.

grain, dairy-free waffles and pancakes; they're healthful and delicious. Pour on light syrup, and smother with blueberries or any other fruit. Add some soy-based bacon or sausage, and you've covered all your bases.

Breakfast Sandwich

Perhaps you only have time to "grab a sandwich" for breakfast. No problem. Try a vegetable sausage patty and soy cheese on an English muffin. Grill it up, then garnish with fruit.

For Kids

Many of the breakfast foods geared to kids make great Picture-Perfect Weight-Loss breakfasts. A good number of the kids' cereals are low-calorie and whole grain, so all you need to do is introduce flavored soy milks or fat-free milk to give your child a weight-loss boost. Be aware that the calorie counts of some of the special varieties of Pop-Tarts can be high. A good alternative is the mini-version of light waffles—especially if the mini-waffle is accompanied by fruit.

All of the suggestions above also work for children, of course. In fact, why not introduce your kids to them this week? It's a good way to expand their palates toward a more healthful, nutritious, low-calorie breakfast habit.

Week 1 goals:

- [ ] Weigh yourself—and note your starting weight in writing.
- [ ] Start your food diary. Make it a personal journal as well.
- [ ] Commit to 10 minutes of exercise per day. Get moving.
- [ ] Begin to change your eating habits by making every breakfast you eat a Picture-Perfect Weight-Loss breakfast.
- [ ] Eat a food you've never had before at three of the week's seven breakfasts.

Going Bananas for Bagels

For one overwhelming reason—taste—the bagel has become a national pastime. But alas, it offers almost no nutritional benefit at all. So while it's worth having a bagel from time to time, you should also consider a number of alternatives.

Bananas are one of those alternatives. Actually, five bananas are one alternative to a single bagel. As good for you as only fruit can be, bananas also serve as a partial replacement for starchy foods. They're a good bet nutritionally—and a good bet calorically, five times over.

1 bagel (5 oz) 400 **calories**

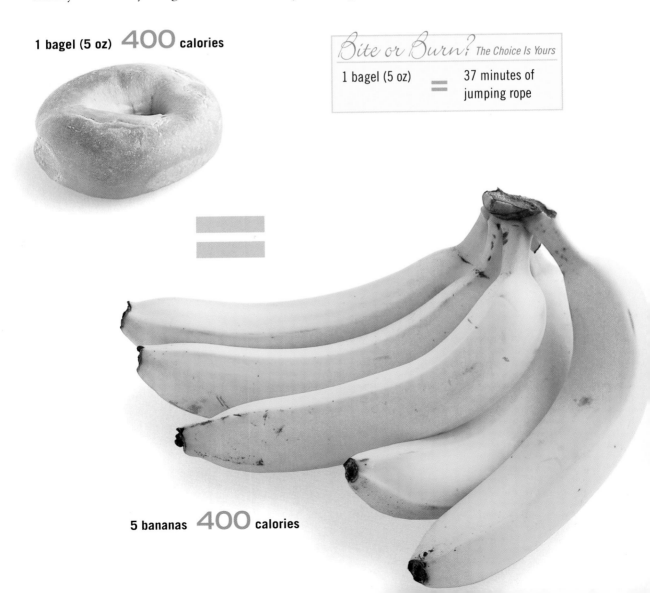

Bite or Burn? The Choice Is Yours

| 1 bagel (5 oz) | = | 37 minutes of jumping rope |

5 bananas 400 **calories**

Cereal Killer

Beware the cereal with the oh-so-healthy-sounding name. It may be dense with taste, but it can also mean a high-calorie start to the day. For the same calorie count as the single bowl of granola on the left, you can enjoy all three bowls of cereal on the right—with fruit. And almost certainly, just one of the bowls of cereal on the right will be more than enough and more than satisfying.

One other caution about the granola types of cereal: They're so much like cookies that they're all too easy to snack on right out of the box—adding even more calories than their nutritional benefit is worth.

4 oz granola cereal 480 calories

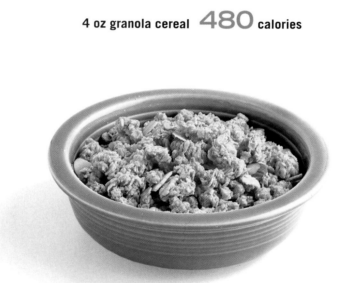

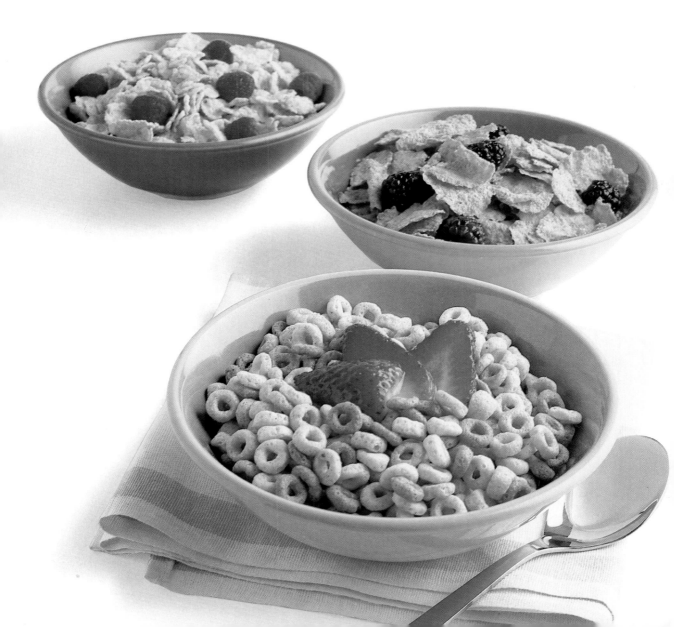

4½ oz total of cereal (1½ oz in each of three bowls)—
multigrain Cheerios, Special K, Wheaties 450 calories
fruit garnish 30 calories

TOTAL 480 calories

Bread and Biscuits

For the weight-conscious, light bread can serve an important function—and it's a lot tastier than people suppose. It would take these 11 slices of light-bread toast, each spread with a fruit topping, to equal just one buttered biscuit. What's more, both the butter and the biscuit contain the bad kind of fat, thus giving the buttered biscuit a health demerit, while the light bread is a good source of fiber—a nutritional plus.

1 biscuit (4½ oz) 450 calories
1 Tbsp butter or margarine 120 calories
TOTAL 570 calories

11 slices light toast 440 calories
11 Tbsp fruit spread 130 calories
TOTAL 570 calories

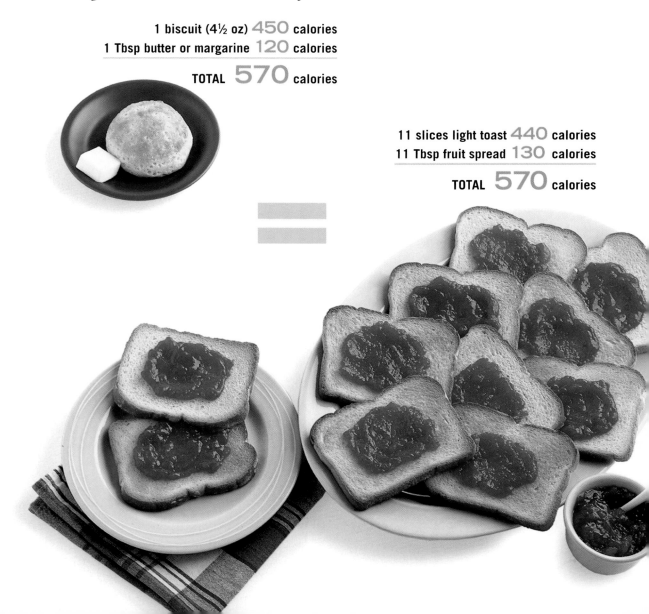

Getting Your Fiber Fix

Yes, fiber is good for us, and yes, a fiber-filled breakfast is a great way to start the day. This bran muffin looks "healthy," and eating it makes us feel virtuous. But for the weight-conscious, that virtue exacts a high price in calories. You'll get the same fiber fix with any of these other bread choices—even better, with this low-calorie assortment of melons and berries.

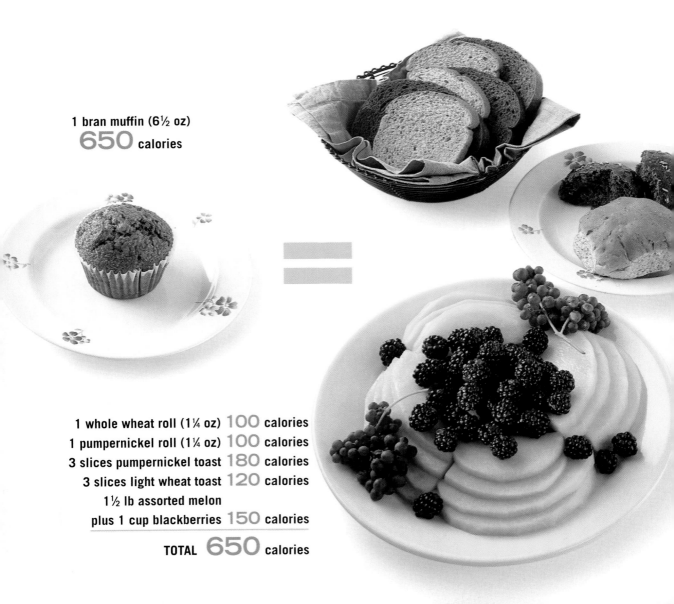

1 bran muffin (6½ oz)
650 calories

=

1 whole wheat roll (1¼ oz) 100 calories
1 pumpernickel roll (1¼ oz) 100 calories
3 slices pumpernickel toast 180 calories
3 slices light wheat toast 120 calories
1½ lb assorted melon
plus 1 cup blackberries 150 calories

TOTAL 650 calories

Starter Sandwich

When you're hungry and in a hurry, the packaged breakfast sandwich looks like a good bet. Look again. The soy-based sandwich gives you twice the portion size and much more healthfulness.

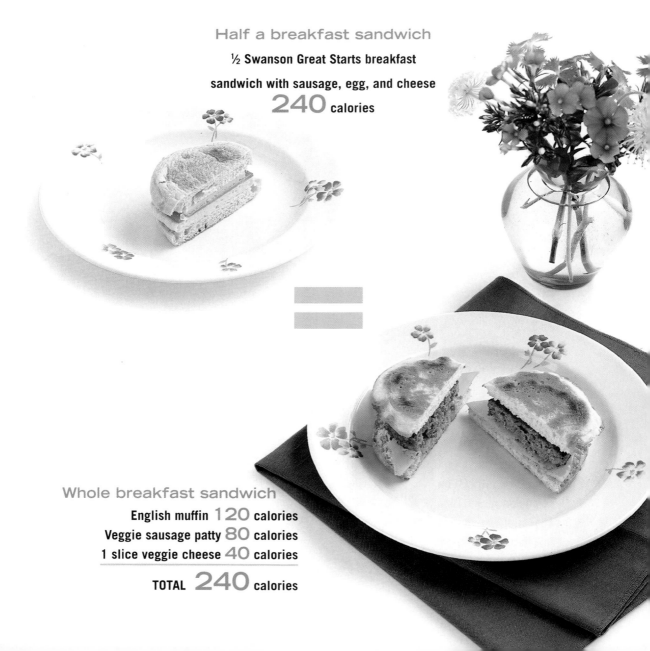

Half a breakfast sandwich
½ **Swanson Great Starts breakfast**
sandwich with sausage, egg, and cheese
240 calories

Whole breakfast sandwich
English muffin 120 calories
Veggie sausage patty 80 calories
1 slice veggie cheese 40 calories
TOTAL 240 calories

What's for Breakfast?

Soy-based products are entering the breakfast nook—just in time for you to find a healthy, low-calorie alternative to the traditional morning sausage. You'll get a calorie bargain and a health bonanza when you choose veggie breakfast links.

2½ oz breakfast sausage links
260 calories

1 package veggie breakfast links (8 oz)
260 calories

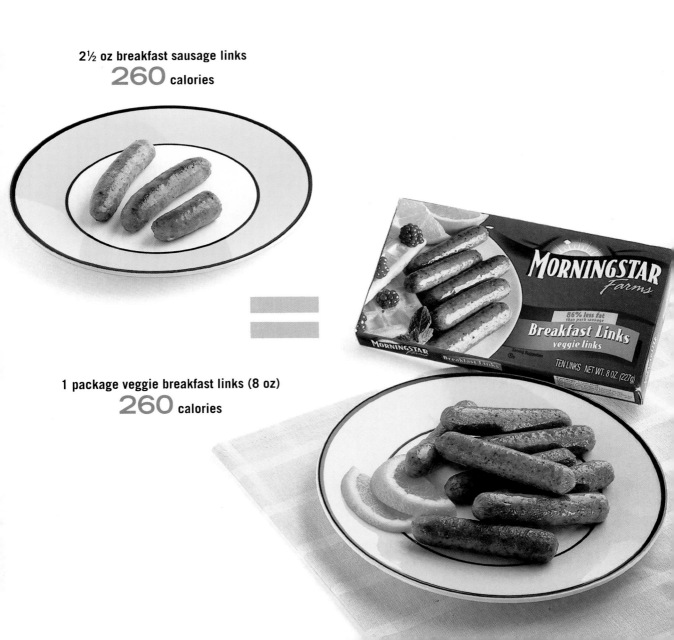

Health Bread?

Low-fat zucchini bread *sounds* like a weight-conscious choice. But if ever a picture was worth a thousand words, this is it . . .

1 slice low-fat zucchini bread (6 oz) **580** calories

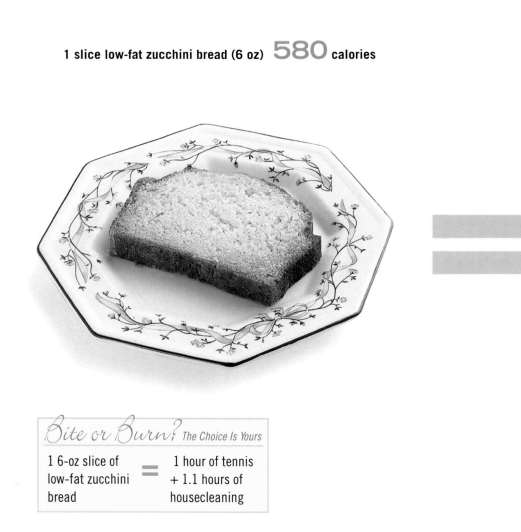

Bite or Burn? *The Choice Is Yours*

| 1 6-oz slice of low-fat zucchini bread | = | 1 hour of tennis + 1.1 hours of housecleaning |

1 box strawberries	80	calories
1 lb honeydew melon	80	calories
1 nectarine	30	calories
3 apricots	60	calories
¾ lb grapes	150	calories
1 box blackberries	80	calories
1 small seeded roll	100	calories
TOTAL	**580**	calories

Chapter 7

WEEK 2: A NEW VIEW
OF LUNCH AND SNACKS

30-Day Plan

						1
2	3	4	5	6	7	8
9	10	11	12	13	14	15
16	17	18	19	20	21	22
23	24	25	26	27	28	29
30						

By the end of Week 2, you will have:

- Figured out your emotional connection with food
- Begun to make physical activity an integral part of your lifestyle
- Tried some new lunch ideas—including soy
- Discovered a new way to snack
- Lost more weight

*B*oca burger was a curse word when I first heard it," recalls New York City firefighter Thomas Kontizas. His disdain for the soy-based "hamburger" didn't last. Now, 40 pounds lighter after making soy burgers a regular part of his eating, Kontizas says he always keeps Boca burgers in the freezer. "For lunch, I throw one on the skillet, spray it with Pam, toss in some onions, grill it all together, then top it with some lettuce and tomato and spread a dab of ketchup on it. You think I know the difference between this and a hamburger? To me, I'm having a burger for lunch!"

A lot of firefighters agree. Guys who once disdained meatless burgers, who once derided the people fluttering around the salad bar while they headed right for the hot foods se-

lection of fried chicken and ribs and meat loaf, guys who once "easily downed a couple of sandwiches for lunch," as firefighter Dean Pappas tells it, then munched "a doughnut for dessert, and had another one or two for a snack later in the afternoon"—guys like this are now eating Boca burgers, or digging into the red beans and yellow peppers from the salad bar, or ordering the portobello mushroom at the steakhouse restaurant.

For the Chicago 7's Joanne Rusch, lunch today is likely to be a plate of cut-up raw vegetables in a light dressing, or maybe soup and a potato. Heidi McInerney has discovered bialys—and how to get a low-calorie salad with light dressing at McDonald's. Like New York's Bravest, the Chisholms—Jim and Tia—

have discovered veggie burgers. Still, Tia Chisholm says she finds lunch the hardest meal of the day when it comes to making low-calorie choices.

The reasons are obvious. The American lunch tends to be either a throwaway meal—something you grab as you can—or an event, usually at a restaurant, for business or celebration. At either extreme, you're stuck with what's available—whether it's the sandwich you slap together quickly out of whatever's in the refrigerator so you can get right back to what you were doing, or the salad from the office cafeteria, or the specialty of the day recommended by the headwaiter. What's more, your dining companions, if any, may not be people before whom you want to draw attention to yourself by asking for a soy burger.

In answer to the "difficulties" of lunch, however, I offer a counter-reality. It's this: There are really an awful lot of choices for lunch—foods or food combinations you may not have thought of before, foods you may not have even known of before. I'll tell you about some of the possibilities in this chapter, and you'll see a number of additional ideas in the food demonstrations. But here's my overall message concerning lunch: With thought and imagination, you can discover—or create—an almost limitless range of nutritious, low-calorie lunches. Whether you're at work, at home, or at a five-star restaurant . . . whether you're grabbing something on the run or sitting down to a deal-making conference . . . whether you're cooking for yourself or walking the cafeteria line, lunch can be—should be—a tasty, satisfying, healthful meal that is also low in calories. In fact, lunch is a great time to put the principles of Picture-Perfect Weight Loss to work.

Through Lunchtime to Snack Time: Seven Steps to Keep the Momentum Going

The issue may be more than just wondering "what's for lunch." After all, you're in Week 2 of a 4-week program to change your life, change your relationship with food, and change the way you look and feel.

If this were a diet, and you had survived a week of it, you would probably be feeling pretty deprived. *But Picture-Perfect Weight Loss isn't about taking foods away from you; it's about adding to your food choices.* Nobody ever said you could not or should not eat any particular food for breakfast, nor will I say such a thing about lunch or snacks—not last week, not this week, not ever. Rather, I told you that if you would commit to change, I would offer you plenty of possibilities for change. The results—a thinner, healthier you—would be all yours.

Let me say it once again: You're not on a diet. You're on a journey, and you're about to move into stage two of the journey. Each stage—each of the 4 weeks of the Picture-Perfect Weight Loss 30-Day Plan—teaches you something new. At each stage, you discover more about your own behavior, and you add to your knowledge of food and nutrition. So with each week of the plan, you "evolve" to a higher level of awareness. And awareness, says the Chicago 7's Debbie Davis, more than 50 pounds lighter than when she began Picture-Perfect Weight Loss, "is everything."

Last week, I offered five steps to getting

started on your commitment to change—and to a whole new view of breakfast. This week offers a seven-step plan. It leads you to new ideas about lunch and snacking—and to ways to keep the momentum of change going.

Step 1: What Are You Really Feeling?

Make a change—any change—and the result will be a short-term improvement in people's performance. Psychologists call this the Hawthorne effect. In offices and factories, bosses know that if they change a work routine or launch a new program or put in new lighting, workers will become more productive—at least temporarily.

You experience the same thing when you rearrange your furniture or buy a new dress or put a new poster up on your office wall. Suddenly, everything seems fresh and new, and you're raring to go—full of energy, more inventive than usual, more efficient.

Maybe that's what Week 1 felt like. It was the start of a fundamental change in your life—a novelty—and you were revved up. You stepped eagerly into fresh, uncharted territory. You were curious and enthusiastic. You lost weight—you were a success.

But this is Week 2. The high of the first week is not as exalted. You're in a kind of "sophomore slump"—the bright light has dimmed just a bit. Why? And more important: What should you do next? You will need a new goal to get the energy going again—the kind of energy generated by positive change.

Part of the reason for the slump is the downside of the Hawthorne effect. Workers get used to the changed lighting pattern, and their productivity slacks off. Or your new furniture arrangement eventually stops being new, and you stop feeling a thrill every time you look at it. When it comes to Picture-Perfect Weight Loss, the novelty of your new commitment to a changed relationship with food may have worn off. You're left with the reality, with the commitment itself—long-term, lifetime, every day.

And part of the reason can be found in the Week 1 food diary you kept. Take a look at it now, paying particular attention to the descriptive measures: degree of hunger, people you were with, place, mood, activity. Can you find an emotional pattern in these measures?

Answer the question broadly. Dr. Adele Fink, the psychologist we met in chapter 6, recommends thinking about your emotional pattern in terms of four big categories of feeling: *sad*, *mad*, *bad*, and *glad*. Does your pattern show that you tended to eat higher-calorie foods when you felt sad—lonely, lost, bored, unhappy with yourself, or just plain depressed? Did you eat when you were angry, when sheer rage made you uncomfortable? Did you eat out of anxiety or fear or when feeling the bad effects of stress? Did you eat to celebrate something—or because you just felt glad? In other words, what were the feelings that "governed" your eating—that influenced your need to eat, the choices you made, the foods that satisfied you?

Taking your emotional temperature in this way is no easy exercise. But it's an important one. Here's why: There's no doubt that food very often is not just food. Dr. Fink calls food "a disconnect." That is, she explains, "we eat to not feel our feelings. We use food to stuff

The Dangers of Ma Huang

Metabolife, Stacker, and Diet-Phen for people trying to lose weight.

Ripped Fuel for the bodybuilder types.

Mormon Tea or Squaw Tea for students of herbal "remedies."

A variety of names for "natural" over-the-counter cold and allergy medications.

Whatever you call it, it's all based on the herb known as ephedra—known as ma huang in China, where it has been used for more than 5,000 years to treat symptoms of asthma and upper respiratory infections.

The U.S. Food and Drug Administration, which studied use of ephedra-based medications for nearly a decade, has said that products containing ma huang "may be hazardous to your health." The FDA found hundreds of cases of adverse reactions to ephedra—not to mention scores of deaths.

With a molecular structure similar to that of amphetamines, ephedra/ma huang can cause heart attack, stroke, seizures, fever, hypertension, paranoia, depression, numerous other catastrophic complications, and death.

Like amphetamines, ma huang products stimulate the nervous system. This can open the bronchial passages and stimulate the heart so that cold sufferers feel better. It can also promote fat-burning, which is why bodybuilders and people on diets use it. But the risk is far too high.

Ma huang is a perfect case of a benign-sounding "natural" ingredient—a Chinese herb, after all—that is unregulated, misused by manufacturers, misleadingly advertised, and downright harmful to your health. Stay away from products containing ma huang!

down the feelings we really feel instead of really feeling them." She cites a Turkish saying about people who "eat their anger"; they almost literally swallow the feeling instead of expressing it in a productive way.

We see the extreme of this phenomenon in food bingers—people with serious eating disorders—who admit that they cannot remember the taste of the food they just binged on. They know only that it dulled their feelings; in a very real sense, they anesthetized themselves with food.

You don't have to have an eating disorder to use food in this way—albeit most of us do it with less neurotic desperation. It's fairly normal—certainly not atypical—to avoid dealing with a feeling by stuffing it down with food. Sad, mad, bad, glad: See what your Week 1 diary tells you about your own use of food as an emotional crutch.

Of course, it's entirely likely that different feelings were at issue at different times during the week, so you may well find that all four categories of feeling had an impact on your eating. It's important, though, to try to find a pattern in your emotional connection to food—to explore the feelings that occur again and again, and to figure out what your real feelings are when you eat—especially when you find yourself making the higher-calorie choices.

Once you understand how you use food to disconnect from your real feelings, you can begin in Week 2 to get in touch with those feelings. Through your own awareness, you'll be able to stop using food as a disconnect. Instead of stuffing down those feelings, you'll learn to feel them—and return food to its real purpose in your life: nutrition and enjoyment.

Step 2: Break the Cycle

You have also previously met Susan Amato, the psychotherapist who works with me in my New York office and who also played a major role with the Chicago 7, in addition to maintaining a private practice. As Susan says: "Change is the essence of the entire Picture-Perfect Weight-Loss program, and to keep the ball rolling, you have to keep changing." In Week 2, Susan suggests you break the cycle of the behavior that has been giving you the most difficulty. She cites the case of one patient who found she nibbled high-calorie snacks constantly while preparing the family dinner in the evening. Susan's suggestion? Do the dinner prep work in the morning. That change alone focused the patient's mind and made her conscious every minute of what she put in her mouth.

Another patient determined that her difficulty was snacking through the evening hours. On closer examination, it turned out that she typically turned on the television the moment dinner was cleared away, and she spent the evening in front of the tube, hauling out yet another snack food at just about every commercial. The suggestion this time was to take a walk after dinner before turning on the TV. The change broke the routine, and breaking the routine gave her a new awareness about what had previously been just mindless habit.

In fact, the mere act of change—the breaking of the cycle—can produce a ripple effect of benefits. It takes your focus off whatever it is that you're finding difficult and puts the focus on your goal. And every time you change something in your routine—every time you change anything—you reinforce the concept of change. Since Picture-Perfect Weight Loss is all about change—changing your relationship with food and changing your eating habits—that's all to the good.

So breaking the cycle is an important step in keeping the momentum going.

Step 3: Find Your Voice

In Week 1, we talked about "honoring thyself"—taking time *for* yourself and taking care *of* yourself. In Week 2, it's time to take it a step further, find your voice, and assert yourself. This means that you have to stop "putting up with" things and people you know are toxic—that is, things and people that will blur your focus and drive you offtrack.

We deal with toxic people and situations nearly every day. For example, there's the coworker who talks endlessly about her problems and drains you of all energy—making you so angry you walk right over to the vending machine for a high-calorie candy bar . . . or the rude clerk at the dry cleaner's who gets you so irritated you head right for the junk food counter in the deli next door . . . or that woman from the local community organization who calls weekly, invariably as you're cooking dinner, to ask you to volunteer your time—sending you right to the cupboard for another cocktail and a generous helping of hors d'oeuvres. You know what? You can say no to the volunteer work, you can find another dry cleaning establishment or send another family member to pick up your clothes, and you can tell your pathetic coworker that you're very sorry, but you just have too much work to do right now to listen to her woes. You can do all of this nicely, civilly, with perfect courtesy. Indeed, courtesy is called for. After all, it's not your coworker's fault that you became angry and ate the candy bar; it's yours.

And that's the point. Since you know these toxic people or situations add to your frustration level, it's time to assert yourself—either by avoiding the situation or by speaking up, rather than putting up.

Here are three rules for finding your voice.

Any interest shown by your family and friends in the changes you're making for Picture-Perfect Weight Loss can be only in the form of support. That means no criticism. It also means none of that kind of "encouragement" that leads to irritation, as in: "Are you sure you want to eat that piece of pumpkin pie?" As you well know, such queries, innocent though they may be, are not helpful. Speak up, and make it clear that this is *your* life, *your* weight, and *your* program, and that you'll accept unconditional support—or silence. And the same goes for you vis-à-vis your children: It's *their* life, *their* weight, and *their* program—so give them your unconditional support, not negativism.

Set clear boundaries. Stop being a doormat. If you're like the woman in the previous chapter who leapt off the exercise bike every time a family member had a request or question, change your ways. In a family or a workplace or any situation in which humans interact with one another, it's essential to separate the areas of your life that belong to you alone from those areas into which you will accept or invite others. Only by setting these boundaries can you keep safe the effort you're making now to lose weight once and for all.

Remember that what the bathroom scale tells you is not the barometer of success. The scale measures only your weight loss. The real measure of success is your willingness to undertake the journey in the first place.

Step 4: The Week 2 Food Diary

Your Week 1 food diary was meant to serve as the boost that helped jump-start you toward Picture-Perfect Weight Loss. It asked you for details, both so you could see your eating habits etched in sharp relief and as an incentive for change. The purpose of the Week 2 food diary is to keep your awareness level high as you continue to transform your eating habits and inculcate Picture-Perfect Weight Loss into your life. Turn the page for a look.

As you can see, this diary is quicker and easier to fill out than the diary for Week 1, but it still requires you to stop and take stock and be aware of what you're eating. The first three columns are self-explanatory: Jot down the date, the time of day, and the food you are eating. The "comments" column is all yours. Write down anything you want to say: "Feeling good" or "In a rush" or "Tried this food for the first time and liked it" or "Nothing to say." It's up to you. After all, you're the one keeping track.

Week 2 Food Diary

Date	Time	Food (Preparation, Serving Size)	Comments

And that, of course, is the real purpose of this food diary. It's to keep you keeping track. You've embarked on new patterns of eating; keeping up a level of mindfulness is still important.

Most important of all is what you'll learn when you review the Week 2 food diary at the end of the week. Why at the end of the week? Because you can always justify a high-calorie or inappropriate food choice at the time you make the choice. But the end-of-the-week review gives you a real grasp of the frequency of your inappropriate choices and the rationales you create for them—and can show you how to change the behavior that led to those par-

ticular choices. It's a way to keep yourself accountable. And it's also your opportunity to review the changes you *have* made—in your eating habits, in the range of foods you're trying, and in your understanding and awareness of the principles of Picture-Perfect Weight Loss.

Step 5: Lifestyle Exercise

Just as the 30-Day Plan is aimed at instilling new habits of eating, so also is it your opportunity to lay down new lifetime habits of exercise. This is essential if you are to maintain Picture-Perfect Weight Loss and stay trim and healthy for life. I want you to be as mindful of the activity choices you make as you are of the food choices you make. The active choice should become so ingrained that you automatically choose the stairs over the elevator, park farther away from the shop rather than closer so you can walk more, and regard stopping for a red light not as a source of irritation but as an opportunity to do some sit-down stretches that flex muscles, burn calories, and ease tension.

I call this lifestyle exercise. It's the exercise you do around the house or as part of daily activities such as going to the market, completing errands, or doing your job. For Week 2 of the Picture-Perfect Weight Loss 30-Day Plan, I want you to start thinking about these physical activities, to become aware of them, and to do them with care and deliberation.

Your boss tells you to "run this memo up to Human Resources"? Take him almost literally: Eschew the elevator and walk a few flights; jog some steps if you can. It's time to rake the autumn leaves? Do it yourself, and be aware that the arm and leg motions required in raking are good aerobic exercise, while the bending down and squatting you invariably do as you scoop the leaves into lawn bags are serious stretching activities.

Lifestyle exercise embraces the three components of physical activity that are so essential to lifetime fitness: aerobic exercise, strength training, and flexibility. Why are all three essential? Aerobic exercise—walking, cycling, dancing, climbing stairs—works your heart, lungs, and circulatory system while also building your endurance. Strength training—lifting weights or carrying the laundry basket—builds muscle tissue, and built-up muscles are best at burning calories. What's more, this kind of weight-bearing exercise, as it is also called, counteracts the loss of muscle mass and the potential development of osteoporosis that are both signs of aging. So do flexibility activities—anything from a weekly yoga session to pulling weeds or hanging pictures or making the bed. Such stretching is the key to preventing injury, improving balance and coordination, and keeping you limber as you grow older.

The Gym in Your Garden

Weeding, digging, pruning, raking, mowing. Spend time working in your garden, and you can give yourself a vigorous all-around exercise workout. Scientists confirm that the tasks of gardening can strengthen your heart and lungs, enhance flexibility, and serve as resistance exercises that build muscle strength.

Two tips to think about as you garden: First, bend from your knees, not your back. Second, alternate movements. Don't spend all day squatting down to weed. Instead, do a little weeding, then stand up and switch to pruning, then switch to shoveling, then switch again to deadheading, and so on. Otherwise, you run the risk of repetitive motion injuries.

Fight Cancer with Exercise

You know that exercise promotes heart health and burns calories. Now an exercise research facility in Texas has demonstrated that regular aerobic exercise—like a brisk walk, vigorous housework, and even gardening—may also fight cancer. One study followed 20,000 men for more than 10 years and found that lower heart and lung fitness correlated with double the risk of cancer death. Another study looked at lung cancer in 25,000 men and found that the unfit had almost four times the risk faced by fitter men. The reason? Researchers suggest that since carcinogens accumulate in fat cells, exercise that lowers body fat stores can protect against cancer.

In addition, all these exercises burn calories. That's half the weight-loss battle right there, for weight loss happens when you spend more calories than you take in. Your new eating habits are aimed at reducing your calorie intake; your new exercise habits are equally aimed at paying out calories. It's a can't-miss formula for losing pounds and keeping them off.

There's even more to it than that, though. Studies repeatedly demonstrate that exercise can actually decrease appetite. In fact, several of my patients have told me that they sometimes substitute exercise for a snack when they feel hungry between meals. The exercise does just as well as the snack at taking the edge off the hunger—while offering the added benefits of fitness and stress reduction as well.

In fact, that's another important weight-loss benefit of exercise: It can lower the stress that so often influences appetite and affects eating habits.

For all these reasons, making lifestyle exercise as automatic as choosing low-calorie foods is essential to Picture-Perfect Weight Loss. And as with any physical activity, the more lifestyle exercise you do, the more you *can* do. For Week 2 of the 30-Day Plan, therefore, I'm handing down two exercise assignments.

Keep moving. Last week, you started walking. This week, make sure you do a brisk walk of at least 10 minutes every day.

Make physical activity part of your lifestyle. Start being aware of those typically "throwaway" activities you used to pay no attention to: the trip down to the laundry room in the basement—and the walk back up with your arms full of clean laundry . . . pushing that supermarket cart—and reaching up or bending down to get what you need off the shelves . . . turning your lunchtime stroll into a brisk walk . . . housework and yard work and repair work and make-work. In short, whenever and wherever there's an opportunity to burn calories, seize it: Be aware that you're doing a physical activity, and make it count.

Step 6: What's for Lunch?

It's the middle of the day, and you're hungry. You've been at work, or you've cleaned up the house, or you've been on the move, and you're really ready to eat something—especially if you didn't bother with breakfast this morning.

Makeup artist Debbie Davis of the Chicago 7 is almost invariably in transit when her lunchtime hunger pangs strike—in a taxi, on a train, in an airport—and she used to just grab a bag of potato chips or head for the nearest fast-food emporium. David Taylor, another of the Chicago 7, would make his way to the meat counter at the cafeteria and order a burger or a meat sandwich—sometimes both! Same with firefighter Tom Kontizas, our Boca burger chef from the opening of this chapter. Tom used to brush past the people lined up around the salad bar and aim right for the steam table, where he would load up his plate with "fried chicken and sliced pork with noodles."

Now, like the other fire-fighting veterans of the Picture-Perfect Weight-Loss program and like the rest of the Chicago 7, Tom, David, and Debbie have learned a whole new way to lunch. It's as satisfying as the junk food, over-stuffed sandwiches, and meat-and-starch com-binations they had grown used to, far more nutritious, and much lower in calories.

That's your basic assignment for this week: Where lunch is concerned, branch out. At least 4 days out of the 7, have something for lunch you've never had before—either because you didn't know about it, or because you simply wouldn't have considered it. And since it has to be done sometime, make one of your four "new" lunches a soy-product lunch—maybe a veggie burger or soy deli and cheese sandwich, for example.

Apart from that one requirement, however, your new lunches are up to you. Of course, your own imagination is the real determining factor for answering the "What's for lunch?" question, but here are some guidelines that all the Picture-Perfect Weight-Loss "graduates" have found useful.

Think soup and a salad. Ask any of the firefighters or police officers who have been through the Picture-Perfect Weight-Loss program, any of the Chicago 7 or Stamford 250, or any of the thousands of patients who have

Brisk Walk or Easy Stroll?

While walking-as-exercise has certainly caught on, many walkers aren't hitting the pavement frequently enough or fast enough to realize the health benefits, according to a report from the Centers for Disease Control and Prevention. It takes at least 30 minutes of moderately intense physical activity just about every day of the week to achieve health gains, but the report found that only one in three people ventured out even four times a week, and only one in four walked fast enough for their outings to count as "moderately intense." A moderately intense or brisk walk typically has a pace of 3.5 miles per hour. You'll feel short of breath and may sweat lightly, but you should still be able to carry on a conversation.

passed through my office: Your best bet for lunch is soup and a salad. Whether you're fixing lunch for yourself at home, getting takeout from the nearby deli, moving down the line at the cafeteria, or lunching out—in a diner, luncheonette, truck stop, bistro, or five-star restaurant—soup and a salad is the lunch of choice for Picture-Perfect Weight Loss. The combination is a high-fiber meal that satisfies the appetite and fills the stomach, nourishes the body, and keeps the calorie count way down.

Where soups are concerned, I don't mean a thin, clear broth, either. Rather, I am talking about a hearty concoction with plenty of body. It needn't be a low-salt soup, and it shouldn't be a "dietetic" soup—whatever that is. Go for just about anything that strikes your fancy at the time—but be aware that if your choice contains beans and vegetables, you're getting an added bonus in fiber, nutrition, and satisfaction.

On a cold winter's day, what's cozier or more comforting than black bean soup, mine-strone, or maybe a warming carrot-ginger soup? By the same token, what's more re-freshing in summer than a cool fennel soup, cold carrot soup, cold butternut squash soup, or a chilled beety borscht?

There is one kind of soup that is inappro-priate for the weight-conscious, and that is cream soups. New England clam chowder, seafood bisque, vichyssoise, and the like are best reserved for the rare occasion, but all other soups are highly appropriate daily choices. As David Taylor succinctly puts it, "A good soup is a meal in itself."

But in case it's not, add a salad. And when you do, be aware that a salad can cost you 50 calories or 1,500. A staff nutritionist in my New York office explains how easy it is "to add a thousand calories to a salad: Just sprinkle on some croutons, a spoonful or two of bacon bits, some cheese. At 50 to 70 calories per ta-blespoon," she goes on, "even small amounts of these ingredients can quickly add hundreds of calories to a salad." And watch out for the cold pastas and grains available in many salad bars today. There's nothing wrong with these foods, but—as our nutritionist says—"don't make them the focus of your salad."

Instead, load your salad with vegetables—and go easy on the high-calorie garnishes. And by vegetables, I mean all vegetables: raw, pickled, marinated . . . lettuces, carrots, red and yellow peppers, beets, mushrooms . . . delica-cies like artichoke hearts and picnic staples like coleslaw.

Be aware, too, that salad bars—which have proliferated in delis and restaurants throughout the country—typically offer choices from all three groups of recommended protein: seafood, soy, and beans. You can usually find a bin of tuna salad, another of shrimp salad, and still another of crabmeat salad. Some salad bars even provide tuna made with light mayon-naise, or an "Italian" tuna salad with chopped-up black olives and onions. The soy protein usually comes in the form of stuffed tofu "packages"—often sprinkled with finely chopped parsley or spring onions or red pepper. And the third protein choice comes in what is typically an array of different kinds and colors of beans. Pile it on. Make your salad as varied in color, texture, and ingredients—minus the high-calorie garnishes, of course—as possible. It makes lunchtime a great opportunity to get a hit of many powerful nutrients at minimal calorie cost.

Finally, be sure to keep the dressing low in calories, too. A clear oil-and-vinegar dressing is not necessarily lower in calories than the creamy-looking choice at the salad bar. In fact, a *light* ranch dressing or *low-fat* creamy Italian is quite often the lower-calorie choice. If you do use oil and vinegar, go easy on the oil; at 125 calories per tablespoon, it can quickly add calories. Also beware of classic vinaigrette at 70 to 100 calories per tablespoon. The truth is, though, that a salad as varied in ingredients and tastes as we recommend won't need all that much help from a dressing—it's delicious on its own.

By the way, if you're lunching out, ask for a light dressing or for oil and vinegar on the side. Even in the most elegant and expensive restaurants, either choice—if not both—should be available. If the waiter looks put out by the request, just ask for the standard dressing to be served separately; then apply it with moderation—but do add whatever available condiments strike your fancy.

Reinvent the sandwich. If your idea of a sandwich is two hunks of the thickest, richest bread you can find—or even pita bread or a wrap—filled with as much meat and cheese as possible, and flavored with maybe a lettuce leaf and a slice of onion, it's time to rethink the sandwich.

Instead of your usual sandwich, satisfy your craving for fillings with just a taste, fill up on the vegetable portion—lettuce, onion, tomato, pepper, and so on—and try using light bread or a roll or a bialy before going for high-calorie bread. In other words, as the Chicago 7's quotable David Taylor advises, "flip the ratio." Instead of a single leaf of lettuce and three slices of cheese, make it three leaves of lettuce and a single slice of cheese—just for the taste that you love. Instead of lots of ham or lots of chicken, how about lots of peppers and onions and tomatoes and just a hint of ham or chicken—again, with all the relish, salsa, or other condiments you enjoy.

You might also try making it a seafood sandwich rather than a poultry or meat sandwich. The difference in calories can be substantial, and you will likely be just as satisfied with a sandwich that slaps onions and peppers and smoked salmon between two slices of light bread.

Remember that the whole thrust of this chapter is that there's more to lunch than you think. So think anew. Try some fresh variations on the standard sandwich—and enjoy! And here's another tip: Try having half a sandwich and accompanying it with a cup of soup, or following it with an ample plate of fruit. In a sense, this combination gives you the best of both worlds: the taste of a sandwich with the fiber-filled nutrition and appetite satisfaction that soup and fruit provide.

Know that not every burger is a beef burger. It's the great American lunch—one of our most influential contributions to the world's cuisines (even if pounded beefsteak did originate in Hamburg, Germany, and find its way to the United States thanks to 19th-cen-

Nonmeat Burgers and Franks

Both poultry-based and vegetable-based burgers and franks offer calorie advantages over the "regular" meat versions. But how do they stack up against one another? Zoom in here for the stats on meatless burgers versus burgers made from turkey.

	Gardenburger Life Burger	Turkey Burger
Portion size	3 oz (85 g)	3 oz (85 g)
Calories	100	188
Fat	0	11.4 g
Saturated fat	0	3.1 g
Fiber	6 g	0
Protein	16 g	20.1 g
Cholesterol	0	57 mg

A comparison between veggie franks and chicken franks is equally enlightening. Check out these stats:

	Light Life Smart Dogs	Chicken Frank
Portion size	42 g	45 g
Calories	45	115
Fat	0	8.8 g
Saturated fat	0	2.5 g
Protein	9 g	5.8 g
Cholesterol	0	45 mg

Beyond the numbers, however, choosing the veggie product offers an added bonus—all those plant substances, called phytochemicals, that actually decrease your risk of cancer, heart disease, osteoporosis, and other degenerative diseases.

tury immigrants). But it is a high-calorie item, and it can also be expensive in terms of your health—especially heart health and as a risk factor for a range of other diseases. So what are the alternatives to this staple of the coffee shop, diner, deli, cafeteria, chophouse, even—under a variety of guises and foreign-sounding names—the high-priced restaurant?

One option is the turkey burger. It is a little lower in fat—and that's good because both meats contain the "bad" kind of fat—and has slightly fewer calories than a beef burger. Where a beef burger weighs in at 70 to 100 calories per ounce, meaning that a typical 6-ounce hamburger costs you anywhere from 420 to 600 calories, the turkey burger has only 60 to 70 calories per ounce, so a 6-ounce turkey burger comes in at 360 to 420 calories. Of course, that's before you add in the hamburger bun and any fixings.

Another option is a tuna steak sandwich—a piece of grilled tuna on a hamburger bun with lettuce and tomato. At some 210 calories for 6 ounces of tuna steak, it has fewer calories than beef and is much healthier. You might also want to try tuna burgers or salmon burgers; the former clocks in at 210 calories for 6 ounces, the latter at 270.

Or try a portobello mushroom sandwich, which is growing increasingly popular. It looks like a hamburger but has a special richness and superb flavor; it also soaks up the flavor of any condiments you apply, such as ketchup, mustard, relish, and marinade. And of course, since it's a mushroom, it is full of disease-fighting antioxidants and is very low in calories.

Another great choice—in terms of both calories and health—is the vegetarian burger. Filled with the nutritional power of soy and costing only about 85 to 100 calories per burger, it's an obvious choice for weight loss; it even has fewer calories than the typical hamburger *bun*. As for taste, I'll just remind you of what firefighter Tom Kontizas says: "You think I know the difference between this and a hamburger? To me, I'm having a burger for lunch!"

In fact, Tom's example is particularly instructive, and I highly recommend the kind of creative cooking he practices. I've said this before, and I'm happy to repeat it: I think soy is becoming an increasingly important part of the American diet. One signal of that growing importance is that the soy product manufacturers continue to come up with more and more interesting products exhibiting more and more variety in taste. It behooves consumers to match producers' creativity with their own imaginative ideas about preparing soy products. Do what Tom does and add onions, then flavor with ketchup. Or look to any of the condiments on the Anytime List: mustards and barbecue sauces and light salad dressings. Add garlic, other herbs, spices. Do whatever appeals to your tastes as you introduce this new alternative burger into your life—and make it an integral part of your lunchtime menu.

Check out some chili. Technically, chili is the hot pepper that flavors the dish typically made with beans and ground meat—and officially known as chili con carne, chili with meat. But the truth is that the taste is just about the same without meat, and bean chili that is spiced to taste is an excellent choice for lunch. Serve it in a bowl with chopped onion, or pour some onto a roll for a sloppy joe, or make it the hot accompaniment to a cool salad. In fact, if you add soy-based "ground beef" to the chili, you get the texture and taste of meat with the added benefits of soy protein—a highly recommended substitution that is also delicious.

For Choosy Chili Lovers

Soy has been cultivated as a food crop for at least 5,000 years and is a staple of the superb cuisines of eastern Asia—Chinese, Japanese, Vietnamese, Malaysian, and more. There are more than 2,500 varieties of soy under cultivation, producing high-protein beans in a range of sizes, shapes, and colors. Further, soy comes in many forms—as roasted soy nuts, miso, edamame, soy milk, bean curd, and even as a coffee substitute. Possibly one of the best forms, though, is a tasty, healthful, low-calorie product that can substitute for ground beef in chili, as shown here, or in sloppy joes or other dishes.

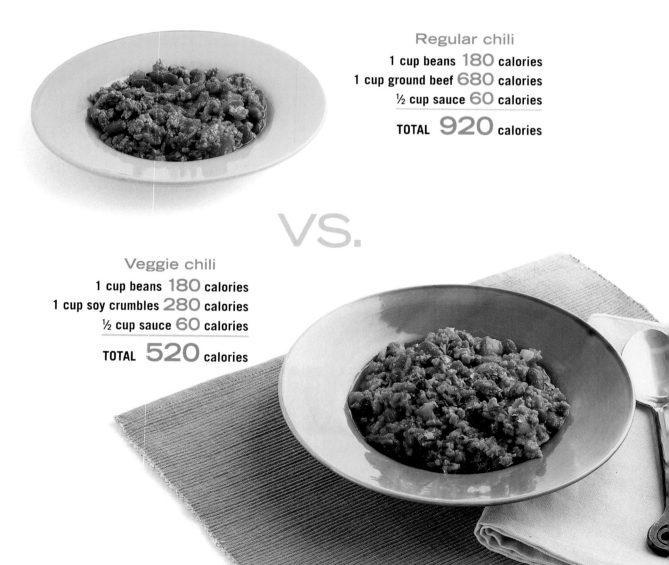

Regular chili
1 cup beans 180 calories
1 cup ground beef 680 calories
½ cup sauce 60 calories

TOTAL 920 calories

VS.

Veggie chili
1 cup beans 180 calories
1 cup soy crumbles 280 calories
½ cup sauce 60 calories

TOTAL 520 calories

Step 7: The Snack between Meals

It's 3:00 P.M. and you're hungry again—even though you had lunch a couple of hours ago. And why not? You have been pressing hard at the office, or been moving from place to place, or simply been busy. One way or the other, you've worked up an appetite for just a little something. As we've said repeatedly in this book, dismissing that urge to snack is bound to have a boomerang effect. But how can you satisfy the craving and still keep the number of calories you consume low?

Probably your best bet is fruit. Fruit contains plenty of fiber, which is good both for your health and for giving you that "full" feeling. But if fruit doesn't satisfy your sweet tooth, I recommend hard candies or low-calorie frozen desserts-on-a-stick. Hard candies like Taste Tations and Tootsie Pops are easy to keep on hand, and such frozen desserts as Fudgsicles or sorbets are easy to come by in the local convenience store. The calorie counts are right, too: A Tootsie Pop, for example, weighs in at 50 to 60 calories (two Tootsie Pops are calorically equal to one large apple), while a frozen ice pop costs only 30 to 40 calories.

If something salty is more to your liking, think about pretzel rods, at about 40 calories per pretzel. If sour is what you crave, there's nothing like a tart pickle or two. At about 6 calories per pickle (depending on the size), it's an afternoon pick-me-up you can live with, and it's good for your health, too. Or, go for a sour ball—a hard candy at its best.

Week 2 goals:

- ☐ Review your Week 1 food diary. What does it say about your feelings associated with eating?
- ☐ Break the cycle of an unhealthy habit—then keep the momentum going.
- ☐ Find your voice: Assert *your* needs.
- ☐ Start your Week 2 food diary to stay accountable.
- ☐ Walk briskly for at least 10 minutes every day, and start making physical activity an integral part of your lifestyle.
- ☐ For 4 days out of the 7, have something brand-new for lunch. Include a soup-and-salad combination and a soy product.
- ☐ Change your snack habits to fruits, hard candies, or low-calorie frozen desserts.

Size Matters

An appetizer is meant to be just a taste—a little something to take the sharp edge off hunger and whet the appetite for more. But the size of the appetizer can still matter. Check out the tiny taste of cheese and small cocktail meatball on the left. That's one appetizer choice. Another is a bowl full of nutritious soup. Same calorie count, lots more food—a healthier way to start a meal, and a more effective way to allay hunger.

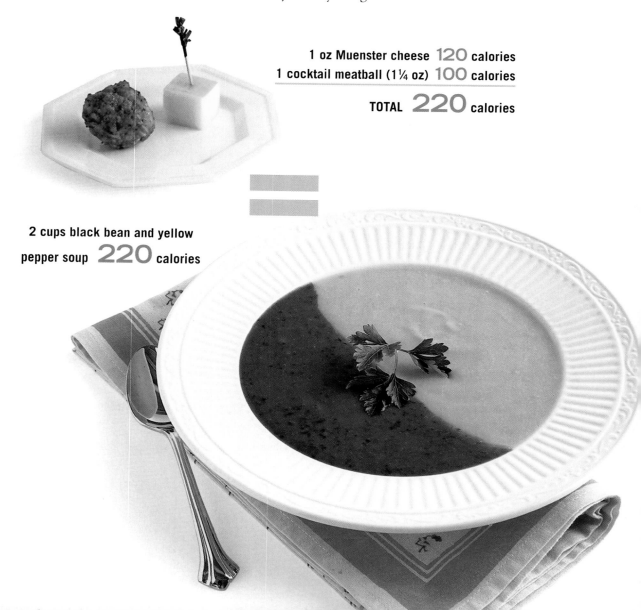

1 oz Muenster cheese 120 calories
1 cocktail meatball (1¼ oz) 100 calories

TOTAL 220 calories

2 cups black bean and yellow pepper soup 220 calories

Magic Mushroom

Next time you're hankering for a roast beef sandwich, make it something special instead and say, "Portobello, per favore!" The huge Italian mushroom is one of the trendiest foods around, favored by today's hottest chefs—not least because it is such a rich-tasting alternative to meat. On a kaiser roll, the portobello and an elegant honey mustard can cut the calorie count of a standard roast beef sandwich by nearly two-thirds while replacing a high-fat choice with a nutritious, low-fat option. Make a calorie-saving choice like this just once a day, and you're bound to experience weight loss. (You'll also be eating more nutritiously—and more interestingly.)

Roast beef sandwich

4 oz roast beef	260	calories
kaiser roll	180	calories
2 Tbsp sandwich spread	160	calories
TOTAL	**600**	calories

VS.

Portobello sandwich

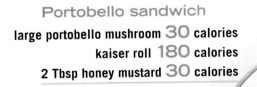

large portobello mushroom	30	calories
kaiser roll	180	calories
2 Tbsp honey mustard	30	calories
TOTAL	**240**	calories

Economics Lesson

Whether you're trying to save money or calories, the lesson is clear: For the same calorie count, you can make two bagel sandwiches, create five sandwiches on regular bread, or have enough light bread for 10 sandwiches. It's simple: More bread for less dough—and for far fewer calories.

2 bagels 800 **calories**

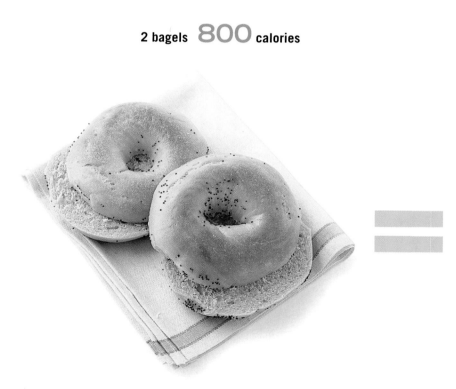

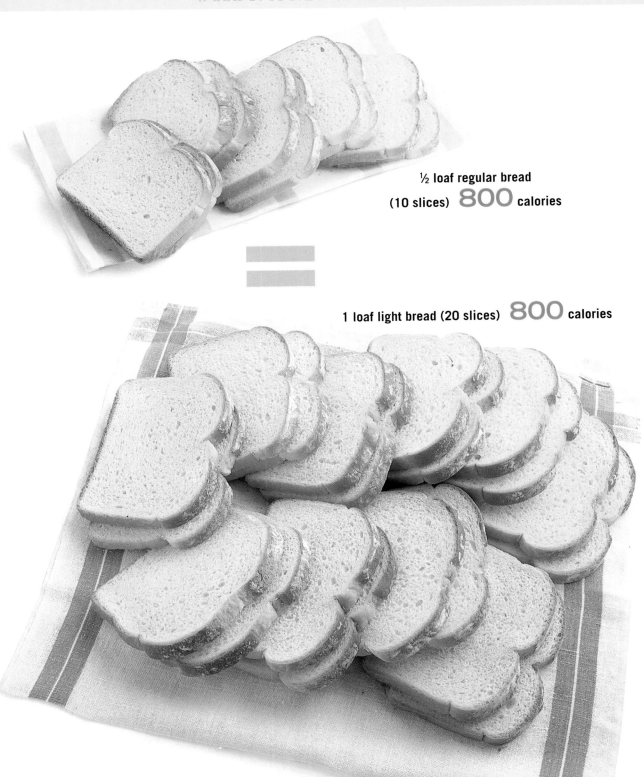

½ loaf regular bread
(10 slices) **800** calories

1 loaf light bread (20 slices) **800** calories

Viva l'Italia!

For those who can never say "basta!" to pasta or other Italian specialties, here are some alternative meal choices that can give you the same quantities, similar tastes and textures, both appetizer and dessert, healthier nutritional values, and fewer than half the calories of a more traditional bill of fare.

6 oz prosciutto and melon 590 **calories**
pasta Bolognese (4 oz pasta
and ½ cup sauce) 720 **calories**
3½ oz apple tart 480 **calories**

TOTAL 1,790 **calories**

VS.

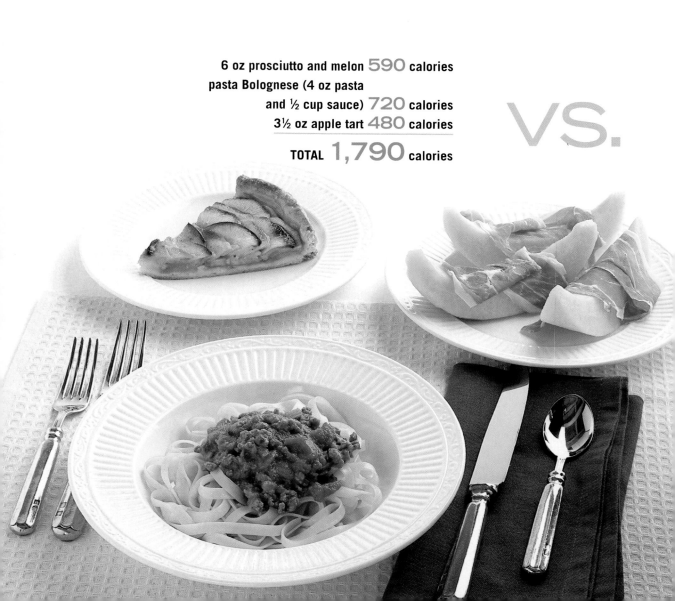

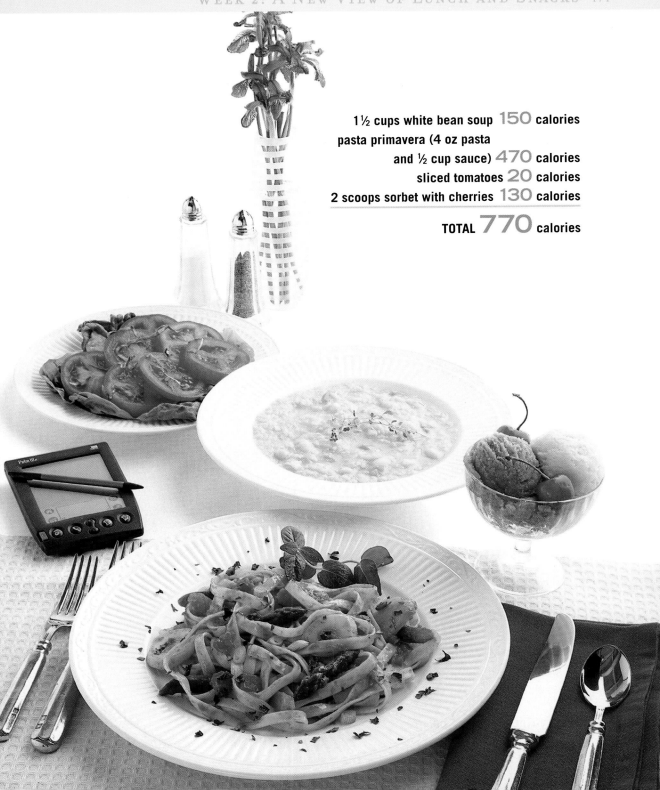

1½ cups white bean soup 150 calories

pasta primavera (4 oz pasta
and ½ cup sauce) 470 calories

sliced tomatoes 20 calories

2 scoops sorbet with cherries 130 calories

TOTAL 770 calories

It's Fried Chicken, Y'all

There are many vegetable-based chicken substitutes that are healthier and lower in calories than the real thing. But if you simply can't accept a substitute for the fried chicken you've always loved, then by all means have it. However, consider filling up on nutrient-packed vegetables and making the chicken just the crowning taste of a varied—and lower-calorie—meal.

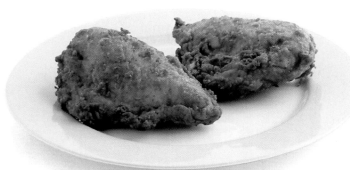

2 fried chicken breasts
800 calories

VS.

1 fried chicken breast 400 calories
1 cup coleslaw 120 calories
baked potato with salsa 180 calories

TOTAL 700 calories

For Hearty Appetites

One reason I recommend soy products for the weight-conscious is that they can eat a whole lot more food if it's soy-based—and do more for their health at the same time. Here's a case in point: half a sandwich or the full Monty when it comes to portion size—and taste!

Half a bologna sandwich with half a pickle

1 slice rye bread 85 calories

2½ oz regular bologna 240 calories

mustard and half a pickle 5 calories

TOTAL 330 calories

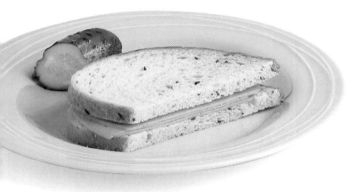

Whole veggie bologna sandwich with a whole pickle

2 slices rye bread 170 calories

5 oz veggie bologna 150 calories

mustard, lettuce, and a pickle 10 calories

TOTAL 330 calories

It's Not Fake Meat—It's Real Soy!

The beef burger on the left will barely satisfy a growing teenager, much less an adult. For the same calorie cost—but with a huge health bonus—you could actually consume four soy-based burgers, if you could manage them all. Will the Gardenburgers provide the same taste impact as the beef? Ask the New York City firefighters featured in this book. Their freezers at home are packed with soy-based products—including their new favorite lunch treat, the veggie burger!

4 oz beef burger 360 **calories**

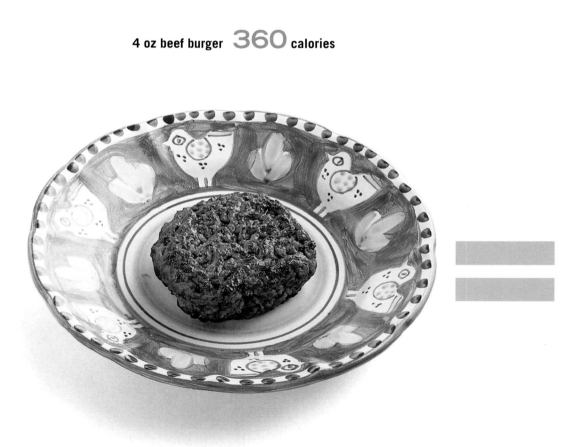

4 Gardenburgers 360 calories

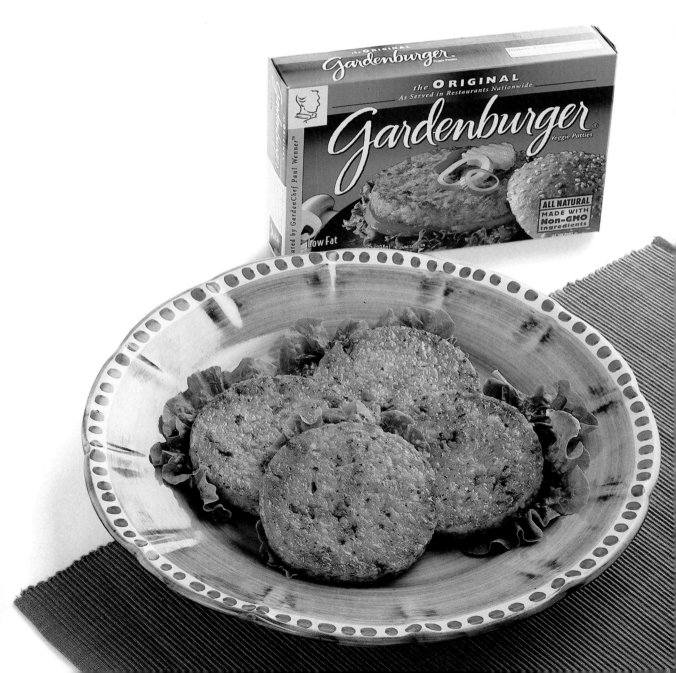

Eat Fruit, Don't Drink It

Check out the calorie count of the juice on the left. Instead, you can have your fruit and drink it, too—without wasting calories. It's proof once again that you're better off drinking a no-calorie diet beverage and taking in the rich nutrient content of fruit in the real thing.

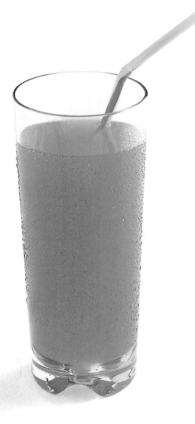

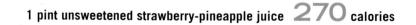

1 pint unsweetened strawberry-pineapple juice 270 **calories**

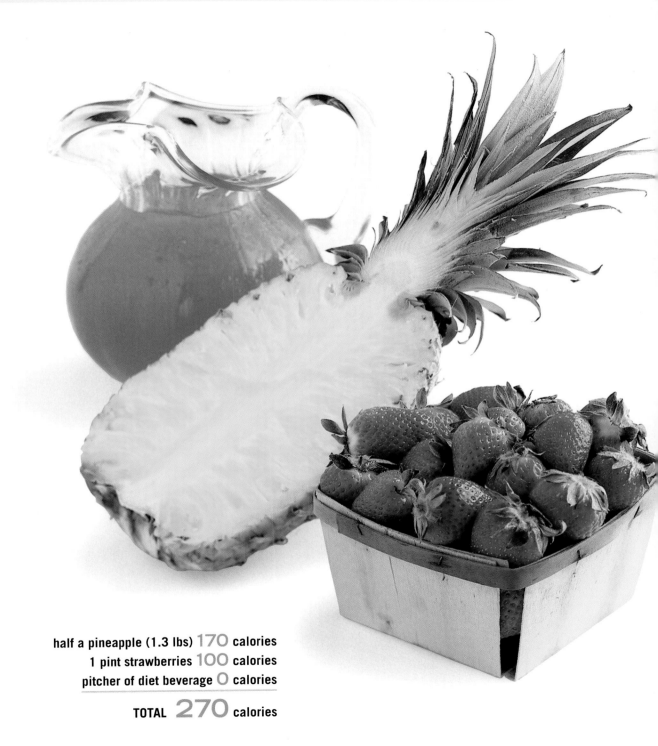

half a pineapple (1.3 lbs) 170 calories
1 pint strawberries 100 calories
pitcher of diet beverage 0 calories

TOTAL 270 calories

Snack Slices

When it comes to snacks, dried fruit is by far the lower-calorie choice over even a tiny cube of cheese. You can eat lots of fruit for a relatively small number of calories, and you'll obtain lots of fiber in the process. On the other hand, this chunk of Cheddar won't satisfy even the smallest appetite—and it's high in saturated fat, the bad kind of fat.

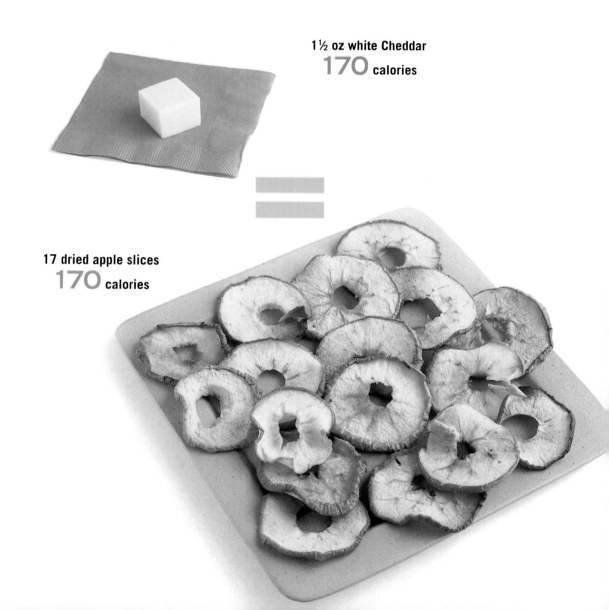

1 ½ oz white Cheddar
170 calories

17 dried apple slices
170 calories

Chomp!

When you really want to chomp on something salty, nuts are a healthful choice, but they're also high in calories. Think popcorn instead; you can take in far more food for the calories.

⅞ cup mixed nuts
800 calories

23 cups popcorn
800 calories

Virtual Illusions

What looks virtuous isn't necessarily so. We're certain the macaroni salad with its mayonnaise dressing is a high-calorie dish, but we're equally sure that the spinach fusilli salad, with its clear liquid dressing, offers a calorie saving. It's an illusion: Both salads weigh in at 350 calories.

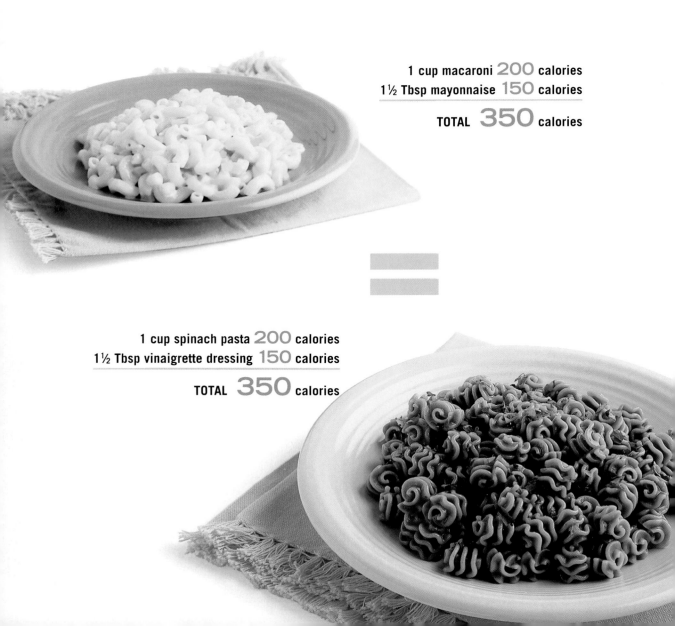

1 cup macaroni 200 calories
1 ½ Tbsp mayonnaise 150 calories

TOTAL 350 calories

1 cup spinach pasta 200 calories
1 ½ Tbsp vinaigrette dressing 150 calories

TOTAL 350 calories

Not All Dried Fruits Are Equal

Take a look. Some of the following dried fruit choices—papaya, pineapple, and cranberries—have added sugar. Banana chips, which are fried, have added fat. You pay a calorie penalty for eating them that you won't pay if you get your dried fruit enjoyment from the snacks on the right.

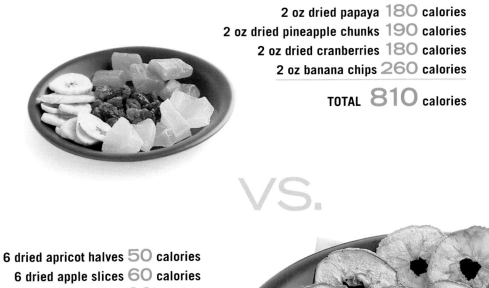

2 oz dried papaya 180 calories
2 oz dried pineapple chunks 190 calories
2 oz dried cranberries 180 calories
2 oz banana chips 260 calories

TOTAL 810 calories

VS.

6 dried apricot halves 50 calories
6 dried apple slices 60 calories
3 dried pear halves 90 calories
3 dried peach halves 50 calories
3 dried figs 80 calories
6 dried plums 140 calories
3 dried mango slices 60 calories

TOTAL 530 calories

Not So Smoothie

Advice to the weight-conscious: Eat your calories, don't drink them. Of course, this doesn't mean you shouldn't drink if you're thirsty, but if you need to drink, consider a diet beverage, and make your calories mean something.

Healthwise, too, the real fruit beats the drink every time. While the smoothie offers some fiber, you get much more from the actual papaya—and for a lower calorie count.

If it's a "hit" of sweetness you crave, go for the sorbet, which offers great taste but is low in calories.

12 oz papaya smoothie made with whole milk or yogurt, papaya, and honey or sugar 350 **calories**

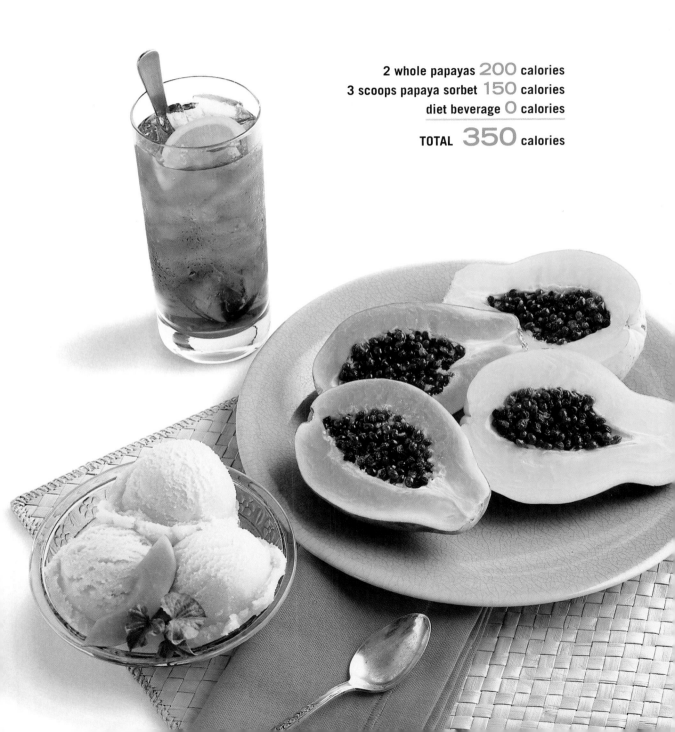

2 whole papayas 200 calories
3 scoops papaya sorbet 150 calories
diet beverage 0 calories

TOTAL 350 calories

Classic Saboteur

Here it is: the classic self-deception. This small package of reduced-fat cookies looks like just the thing when you need a quick hit of sweetness. "Quick" is right. You'll down the cookies in no time—and you'll pat yourself on the back for eating a reduced-fat snack, even though it wasn't very satisfying. Instead, for one-eleventh the calories of the SnackWell's cookies, try a butterscotch candy. It will take longer to consume and will satisfy you much more. And given its calorie cost, you can go ahead and enjoy several.

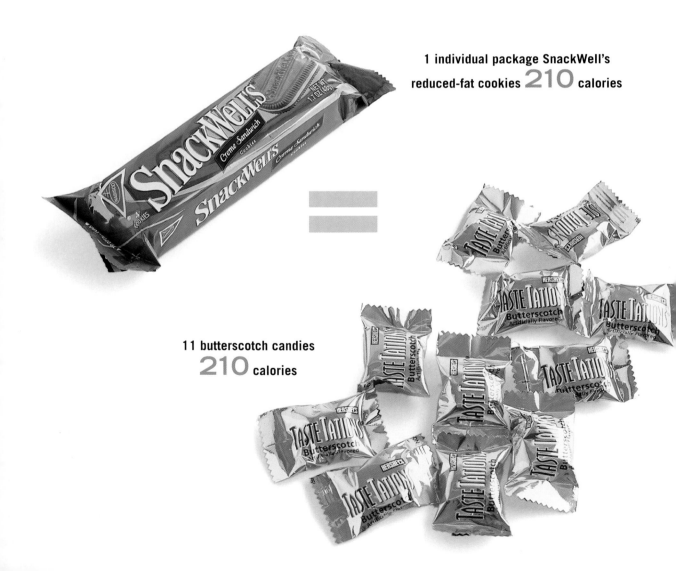

1 individual package SnackWell's reduced-fat cookies 210 calories

11 butterscotch candies 210 calories

Lasting Pleasure

You know how fast the M&M's disappear, or how quickly that handful of gummy worms goes down. Then you want more. But even a single Tootsie Pop can be enjoyed for a good long while—and leave you feeling satisfied. And three Tootsie Pops would last a very, very, very long while and leave you feeling triply satisfied.

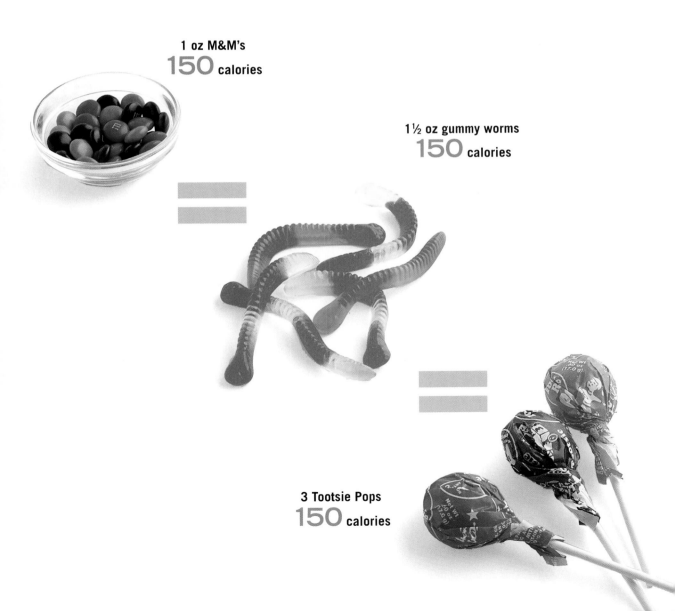

1 oz M&M's
150 calories

1½ oz gummy worms
150 calories

3 Tootsie Pops
150 calories

Combinations Compared

If you love the chocolate-and-vanilla combination, the cookie on the left is one way to get it—but look at the calorie count. Instead, how about one of each of the cones on the right— one chocolate and one vanilla. In fact, given the calorie differential, you can easily indulge yourself in two of each—or even more!

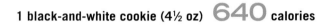

1 black-and-white cookie (4½ oz) 640 **calories**

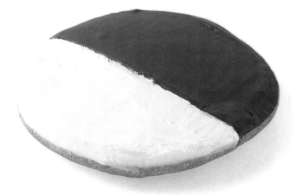 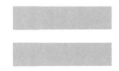

4 vanilla fat-free frozen yogurt cones 320 calories
4 chocolate fat-free frozen yogurt cones 320 calories

TOTAL 640 calories

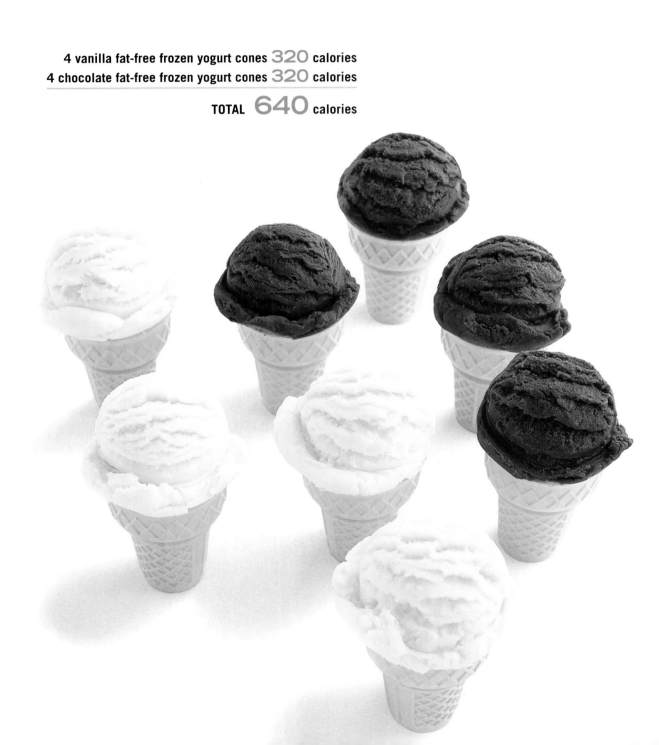

Cookie Consequences

Do you want a little or a lot of raspberry taste? For a little, you'll pay a big penalty in fat and calories with the Linzer cookie on the left. Stick to the real thing; it'll take almost 2 quarts of raspberries *plus* topping to equal the calories of the cookie.

Bite or Burn? The Choice Is Yours

1 Linzer cookie	=	65 minutes of swimming laps

1 Linzer cookie (4 oz) **520** calories

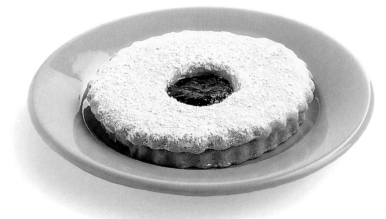

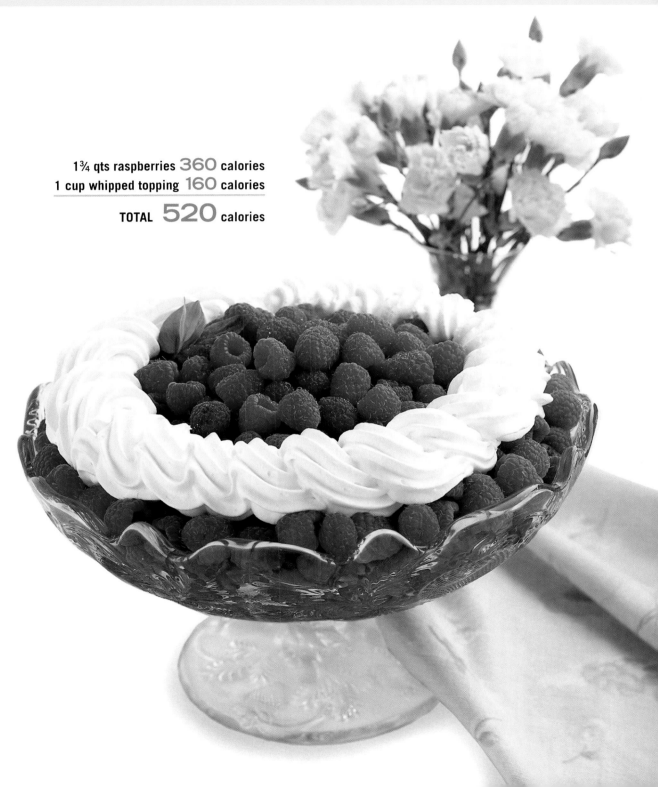

1¾ qts raspberries **360** calories
1 cup whipped topping **160** calories

TOTAL **520** calories

Licorice Licks

It's a fact: Little pieces tend to go down more quickly. If what you crave is the flavor of licorice, think about getting it in a licorice stick or two, or in hard candies—or in a combination of the two.

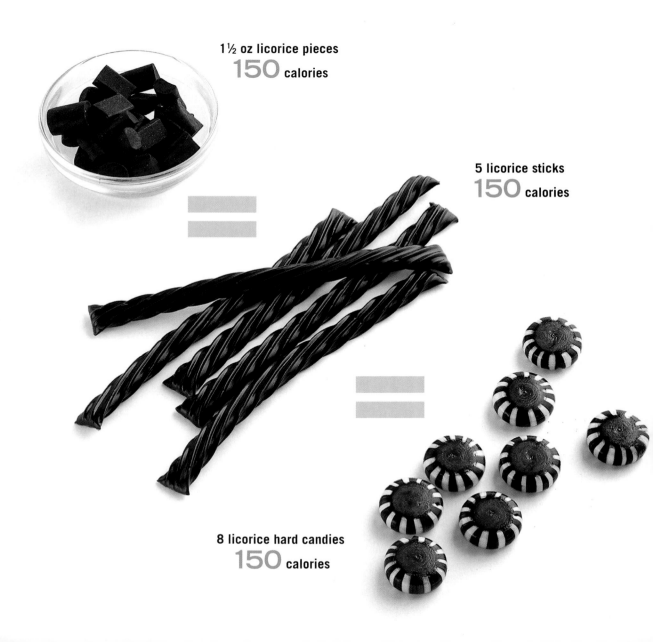

1½ oz licorice pieces
150 calories

5 licorice sticks
150 calories

8 licorice hard candies
150 calories

Chapter 8

WEEK 3: WHAT'S FOR DINNER?

30-Day Plan

						1
2	3	4	5	6	7	8
9	10	11	12	13	14	15
16	17	18	19	20	21	22
23	24	25	26	27	28	29
30						

By the end of Week 3, you will have:

- Reassessed, reconfirmed, and recommitted yourself to Picture-Perfect Weight Loss
- Learned to explore the unfulfilled needs that may influence your eating habits
- Chosen a recreational activity or sport
- Turned dinner into an opportunity for realizing the full potential of Picture-Perfect Weight-Loss choices

It's dinnertime, and all across America, tablecloths are being unfurled across the smooth surfaces of dining room tables . . . plates and flatware are being pulled from cupboards and drawers . . . children are being called in from play or admonished to log off or close the book, wash up, and come to dinner. A sense of peace settles over the household and everyone in it—all are filled with the sense that this family meal is a reward, the prize that caps the day, a time for good food, good talk, a good feeling of togetherness.

And if you believe what I've just written, there's a bridge I'd like to sell you.

Not that the family dinner *doesn't* happen this way; it does—in some families, some places, sometimes. But it is happening less and

less. Increasingly, the typical family—say a family of four—operates on four separate schedules, especially if the children are teenagers, and that can mean four separate dinner menus at four separate times. And more and more, when the family does sit down together, it's only briefly and rarely in a relaxed manner. Phone calls typically interrupt the conversation, and in some cases, the television might even stay on, making conversation utterly impossible. Or, dinner may be only the first stop in a long evening of events and obligations. There's little time to taste the food, much less savor it. It's no wonder women across America have lost interest in preparing and cooking dinner for their families under such circumstances.

That's one reason why I'd like to make a plea to the readers of this book to reinstate the family dinner. In our culture, after all, dinner tends to be the main meal of the day. Let it also be a time when the family can sit and talk—and since it comes at the end of the day, everyone should have plenty to say! And for those undertaking the Picture-Perfect Weight-Loss program, let dinner be an occasion to articulate your commitment to the program's principles loud and clear. Make it the meal where you demonstrate the full potential of healthful, low-calorie foods—for yourself, and for your family as a whole. Turn it into an opportunity to show your kids the right way to eat. And let it even be the place where you let your imagination run free and demonstrate the creativity you know you possess when it comes to cooking. Who knows? Maybe the whole family sitting down together to a Picture-Perfect Weight-Loss dinner will have the added benefit of bringing the family closer—and starting a new *family* tradition of Picture-Perfect nutrition.

Still, I'm a realist, so I understand that the relaxed family dinner—thought out beforehand, deliberately shopped for, carefully prepared—may not always be possible. Instead, your situation may be like Heidi McInerney's of the Chicago 7. A part-time optician with three small children, her work schedule and her husband's mean that they often simply can't have dinner as a family. And because Heidi is—actually, *was*—"the only heavy person in a thin family," as she puts it, when they do all eat together, her meal tends to be different.

Or maybe your life is like David Taylor's.

After a long, tiring day at the office—and, as a single man, with no family to come home to—David used to decide what he was having for dinner on the way home from work, picking up whatever struck his fancy at the time—or whatever seemed easiest.

Then there are the firefighters, for whom dinner is a group event—and one that is frequently interrupted by an urgent alarm. Says Thomas Kontizas: "Firemen are fast eaters because we hate to come back to a cold meal. So we race through meals. Nobody talks; we just shovel in as much food as we can while we can. Then, with the edge off the hunger, we take a second portion, and that's the one we enjoy!"

However you eat dinner—whether you sit down to a prepared family meal or grab takeout on the way home or eat as if an alarm might go off any second—you can still manage to make healthful, low-calorie choices the Picture-Perfect Weight-Loss way.

At the Halfway Mark

This chapter is about more than coming up with new answers to the classic question, "What's for dinner?" For as Week 3 gets underway, you're at the halfway mark of the 30-Day Plan, and that's usually a time when people take a breath and reexamine what they're doing. Fine. Let's reexamine it together. In fact, let's make the reexamination step 1 of a five-step assignment for this week.

Step 1: Reassess, Reconfirm, Recommit

If you've been conscientious about your "assignments" for Weeks 1 and 2, if you've been making new food choices, exercising regularly, filling out your food diary, and paying attention to your emotional patterns of eating, then you have surely begun to lose weight. Typically, it is in Weeks 3 and 4 that my patients tell me—invariably in a tone of surprise, if not astonishment—"I don't even feel like I'm dieting!"

Of course, that's because they aren't dieting. If this were a diet, and you were depriving yourself of satisfying food, or weighing and measuring your portions, or steeling yourself never again to eat chocolate or ice cream or cheese, then by the halfway mark, you would probably be thinking to yourself, "I don't think I'm going to be able to do this."

Well, you're not on a diet, not depriving yourself, not restricting portion size, not giving up anything forever. But you are undertaking a fundamental change in your relationship with food, and while you are certainly losing weight, you may be losing it slowly.

What's more, you may have made inappropriate choices a couple of times. Maybe you just couldn't resist a lavish dessert after dinner the other night. Or maybe you just got tired of the same salad bar lunch and went for a cheeseburger one day. You know what? So what! A cheeseburger for lunch doesn't mean you've lost the whole day; pick up the Picture-Perfect Weight-Loss program again at dinner. A single "mistake" is all part of the learning process. If it's okay to make mistakes when you learn to play the violin, to take just one example, it's okay to make an inappropriate food choice in learning Picture-Perfect Weight Loss, too.

Further, that single inappropriate choice is not a harbinger of failure to come; what you

did last Thursday does not mean that you will make the same inappropriate choice next Thursday or Thursday 2 months from now. Inappropriate choices are not signs of a weak character, of someone who is hopelessly incapable of changing her relationship with food. Change isn't always a walk in the park, and Picture-Perfect Weight Loss isn't even asking you to change everything—or anything—all at once. In fact, it assumes that the odd cheeseburger and occasional lavish dessert are part of life. They're not grounds for guilt or self-doubt or self-criticism.

Maybe you've been on a dozen diets in your life—maybe more. It's because they haven't worked for the long term that you're reading this book. But failed diets of the past have nothing to do with the changed relationship with food you're learning now. This is a new time, and you're undertaking a new initiative—a lifetime initiative. You're ready for change, and you've made a good beginning—even with "mistakes" and inappropriate choices. This is a process, a journey. And like any journey, it doesn't move smoothly on a straight line. There are bumps and potholes along the way.

You know the old proverb that says "Well begun is half done"? It works just as well in reverse: "Half done is well begun." You are halfway to making Picture-Perfect Weight Loss the guide to your eating habits for life. Keep at it.

And the kids?

If your child has undertaken Picture-Perfect Weight Loss, the halfway mark can be a particularly vulnerable time. After all, to kids, 2 weeks can seem like a lifetime. They can easily slide back into their old habits, which may look to them like a reward for the time and effort they've already expended. What's more, kids tend to lose weight more slowly than adults, so if you're doing the program with your kids, there may be a noticeable disparity between your weight loss—substantial and quick—and theirs. To a lot of children, this can look like failure on their part. It means that what *you* do at this time is even more important.

And what should you do? First of all, as I said in the previous chapter, make sure that anything you say to your child about his or her participation in the program is positive. That doesn't mean you have to be shy about talking with your kids. In fact, the halfway point is a good time to engage your child in conversation about the program, and it's a perfect opportunity for you to validate your child's own experience—the slower progress and whatever there may be of program fatigue.

In a very real sense, a child's experience with a program like Picture-Perfect Weight Loss *is* harder than an adult's. Even more than grown-ups, kids tend to measure things "by the numbers." It's a lot harder for them to see that success is in the endeavor, not in what the scale shows. It's also harder for kids to exercise control over their food choices. Nine times out of ten, they're lunching in the school cafeteria, where the definition of "vegetables" may still be former President Reagan's idea—ketchup. After school, they can easily be dragged along with the crowd to the corner deli or local diner for a high-calorie snack. Do you remember what peer pressure felt like when you were a kid? It's tough to resist.

Validate these difficulties when you engage your child in conversation about his or her Pic-ture-Perfect Weight-Loss progress. You might start with your own concerns by saying, "Lunchtime is a real problem for me. How about you?" Let your child talk through the problem, then remind her of the changes she has made, that she's succeeding in what she set out to do, that her goal is possible. Don't compare your child to any other—especially not to a sibling—nor to yourself. Be positive, proud of your child, encouraging. And be sure to ask if there's anything you can do for her, anything she needs you to get for her. Let her know that you're there to help, but be sure she understands you're not "in her face." Remember that, like you, kids have to undertake Picture-Perfect Weight Loss *for* themselves, *by* themselves.

Step 2: What's Underneath the Feelings You've Been "Stuffing Down"?

Last week, you worked at getting in touch with what you were really feeling—you learned to *feel* your feelings. In Week 3, it's time to understand the unfulfilled needs beneath those feelings.

When you were stuffing down your feelings, you were trying to fill your needs with food. It didn't work; all that happened was that you put on unwanted weight. The reason it didn't work is that the need was not physiological; it wasn't really food you hungered for—it was something else. In Week 3, work on figuring out what it is you're *really* hungry for.

Start with the emotional needs we all share—the need for love and companionship; the need to succeed and be admired; the need to be productive, competent, useful. If you are wildly successful on the job and spend 14 hours a day at it, only to come home to an empty house and a pantry full of high-calorie foods, chances are you are lonely—and trying to fill the loneliness with work and food. If you are perceived as sweet but "a doormat," you probably eat to make up for your lack of assertiveness. Also, it's not uncommon to find that underneath a feeling of inadequacy is a fear of intimacy—both physical and emotional; being overweight offers what Dr. Fink calls "a protective barrier" against such intimacy. For adolescents, the problem is often their need for peer group approval; if they don't get it easily, many teenagers eat instead—even though this may lead to even more disapproval from their peers.

In any event, it's only when you know the need that you can find the right way to fill it.

If it's companionship you need, for example, join something. Take a course. Volunteer for a community group or political organization. Attend your local house of worship. Wherever your interest lies, join the relevant organization; there you'll meet like-minded people. And you can fill that gaping need inside you—not with food but with acquaintances who may become friends, lovers, or lifetime companions.

Step 3: The Week 3 Food Diary

The food diary worksheet for Week 3 helps you gain an understanding of the need you are satisfying by eating. Here's what the Week 3 food diary looks like:

Week 3 Food Diary

Date	Time	Food (Preparation, Serving Size)	Why am I allowing myself to eat this now?

Columns one through three are straightforward and familiar. Note the day of the week, the time, and what you're eating. Column four is the key, however. If you're eating a healthful, low-calorie, Picture-Perfect Weight-Loss choice, leave column four blank. But if you have just eaten inappropriately, your comments should prompt further exploration: Are you eating mindlessly? Are you eating the way you used to? If so, why are you reverting to the old habits that made you gain weight when what you are trying to do is lose weight? Why are you undermining your own goal? What need are you trying to satisfy with food? In short, what's really going on? Write it down.

As always in filling out the food diary, both timing and scrupulous honesty are essential. At the end of the week, when you review your diary, pay particular attention to the inappropriate choices you made. Let them guide you to an understanding of your own particular psychology of eating.

Step 4: Exercise through Recreation

You've now spent 2 weeks exercising regularly. You started by simply moving, and last week you broadened your awareness of lifestyle exercise—and your participation in it. In Week 3, I'm going to ask you to explore a range of recreational activities so that you can find one—or more—that you can enjoy for a lifetime.

Did you play a sport in high school or college? Now's a good time to take it up again. Have you always wanted to learn to play tennis—or maybe golf? This is the moment to start taking lessons. You live alone and you like team sports? Join the local Y or gym or com-

munity center. I guarantee you there's a nearby volleyball league, or a pickup game of basketball, or a group of soccer moms—that is, the kind of moms who *play* soccer.

Take a yoga class. Try tai chi. Learn karate or kickboxing or Tae Kwon Do. Go bowling. Try roller-blading; everybody else does. Dig your baseball glove out of the trunk, oil it, and warm up with a game of catch in the backyard—before going on to find a diamond and some like-minded friends. It's winter? Dig deeper in the trunk and pull out your ice skates. Try paddleball or handball, skiing or snowshoeing.

In other words, find something—some recreational activity that you enjoy, that you know how to do or would like to know how to do, that can exercise your body and clear the cobwebs out of your mind and that you can do for the rest of your life. Then start doing it—slowly, easily, only as far and as much as you can. Next week, I'll ask you to get more serious about your choice; this week is for playing around, so don't worry about your skill level or your creaking muscles. With time, you'll limber up and improve your skills. And you will have given yourself a tool against aging and *for* mind-clearing and trimness and energy and weight loss—for life.

Step 5: What's for Dinner? Eat the Pyramid

When I say, "Eat the pyramid," I don't mean it literally, of course. What I do mean is that dinner is the perfect opportunity to put to work Dr. Shapiro's Picture-Perfect Weight-Loss Food Pyramid—and enjoy healthful, low-calorie eating at its best. Unlike breakfast,

If You're a Greens Greenhorn . . .

Ready to try some of the unfamiliar greens said to be so good for you? If you've shied away because you worried about the supposedly bitter taste of some, or the mushy texture of others, be aware that the right cooking procedures remove both those possibilities. And the rewards of going for the green can be outstanding: They're loaded with nutrients—including folate, fiber, iron, and other minerals—and they contain disease-fighting phytochemicals that can be particularly helpful in warding off eye troubles.

Here are some cooking tips:

Beet greens, spinach, and Swiss chard work wonderfully in salads; if you'd rather cook them, it takes only a very few minutes. After washing them, place the still-wet leaves in a pot and stir over medium-high heat for 3 to 5 minutes until they wilt. Drain.

Beet greens do well with garlic sautéed in a little olive oil. Add a hint of anchovy paste, too. Sautéed or stir-fried garlic also gives spinach a kick. So do stir-fried ginger and such seasonings as soy sauce, rice vinegar, and sesame seeds. Swiss chard cooperates wonderfully with sautéed onion, peppers, and, of course, garlic.

Collards, kale, mustard greens, and turnip greens—the so-called bitter or "assertive" greens—need blanching. Trim the tough stems, then place the greens in boiling water and cook, uncovered, about 8 to 12 minutes—less for the mustard and turnip greens. Drain, press out the moisture, chill under cold water, and then drain again.

Sautéing garlic and onion is also a great way to perk up the flavor of the assertive greens. Apple cider vinegar and hot pepper sauce are particularly good on mustard and turnip greens. All these greens go well with beans and peas. Sprinkle with lemon juice, too.

which calls for a particular first-thing-in-the-morning taste and texture, or lunch, which is often dependent on what's available on the coffee shop or deli menu, dinner is the one meal you can control "from soup to nuts" and your one chance to be as creative a cook as you want to be. Take advantage of it.

Most diets typically tell you to make dinner the smallest meal of the day—despite the fact that in our culture, it is traditionally the main meal. Such portion control is a mistake—in more ways than one. First, studies show that

when you take in the bulk of your calories is relatively unimportant to weight gain or loss. It's the total overall amount of calories that counts, not the hour of the day you consume them. On the other hand, "saving" calories during the day so you can "reward" yourself at dinner is equally a mistake. If you deny your appetite through breakfast and lunch, it will be much too powerful at dinner: You'll tend to make inappropriate choices, eat too much, and eat too quickly. The result can be the exact opposite of what you want.

So eat breakfast if you're hungry, have a substantial and satisfying lunch, and snack in the afternoon if you need to. As much as possible, try to fill up on protein and high-fiber foods. They take the edge off your appetite and lessen the craving for high-calorie foods.

Then, sit down to dinner, relax, and eat the pyramid—that is, eat as the pyramid suggests. You can turn to page 130 to refresh your memory about the specifics, but here are the basic guidelines.

- Fill up on vegetables—alone, in salad, in soup—and fruits as much as possible. These form the base of the pyramid.
- Get your protein in the form of soy, beans and other legumes, and seafood. (Be aware, however, that the government has suggested limiting intake of swordfish, shark, king mackerel, and tile because of high mercury levels and suggested that pregnant women totally avoid swordfish.)
- Make grains and starches take third place on your dinner plate—and make them whole grains whenever possible.
- Take in essential fats through olives, seeds, nuts, and some oils—in moderation.

Keep in mind that frozen dinners can be a fine choice—although in my view, most offer too little in the way of vegetables. My solution? Supplement your frozen dinner with an extra plate of vegetables or a salad or soup—or all three!

Go frozen on desserts—if fruit won't do. Try the fudge bars, fruit bars, and sorbets recommended on the Anytime List (see page 113). Or, satisfy your sweet tooth with a hard candy.

Week 3 goals:

☐ Remind yourself why you're undertaking Picture-Perfect Weight Loss.

☐ Start trying to uncover the feelings you've been "stuffing down."

☐ Fill out your Week 3 food diary.

☐ Try out a lifetime recreational activity.

☐ Change your relationship with dinner by "eating the pyramid."

Soup for Starters

There's nothing like soup to take the edge off the appetite *and* supply you with vitamins and minerals. The chunky tomato basil soup offers many of the same taste sensations you enjoy in the mozzarella appetizer—minus the cheese itself, with its high fat content and high calorie count.

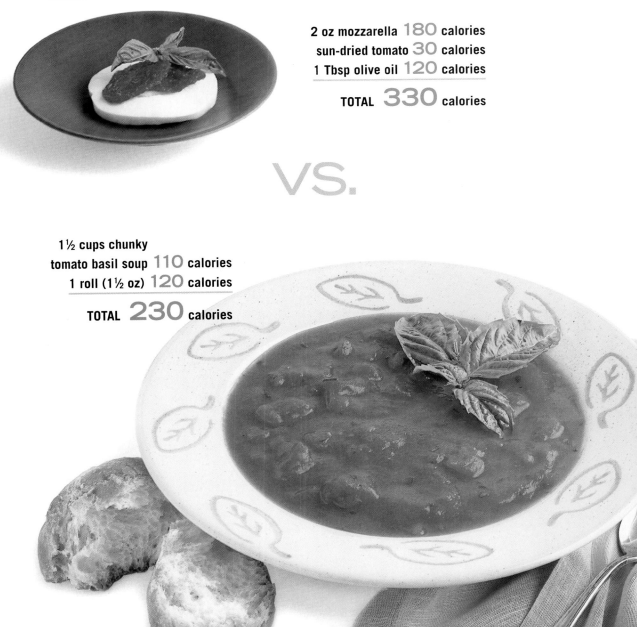

2 oz mozzarella 180 calories
sun-dried tomato 30 calories
1 Tbsp olive oil 120 calories

TOTAL 330 calories

VS.

1½ cups chunky
tomato basil soup 110 calories
1 roll (1½ oz) 120 calories

TOTAL 230 calories

Salsa the Border

Yes, there are a lot of calories in a lot of Mexican food—just check out the numbers for the taco salad and chicken quesadilla—but by no means in all Mexican food. After all, this is a cuisine known for beans, seafood, and vegetables. Put them all together, as on the plate at the bottom of this demo, and you have a feast of exotic tastes and textures for a very low calorie cost.

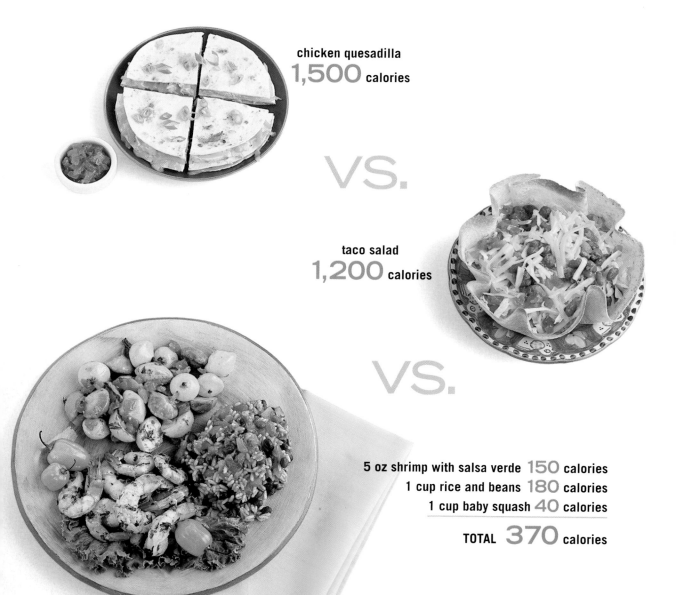

chicken quesadilla
1,500 calories

VS.

taco salad
1,200 calories

VS.

5 oz shrimp with salsa verde 150 calories
1 cup rice and beans 180 calories
1 cup baby squash 40 calories

TOTAL 370 calories

Pyramid Power

Remember Dr. Shapiro's Picture-Perfect Weight Loss Food Pyramid? (See page 130 for a refresher.) Here's an example of just how it works. The bulk of the meal pictured at the bottom of the page comes from the base of the pyramid—the several different vegetables that also give the meal such a variety of tastes and textures, and protein from fish. Note also that the potatoes are prepared using light creamy dressing, which is a creative way to add taste and texture at a low calorie count.

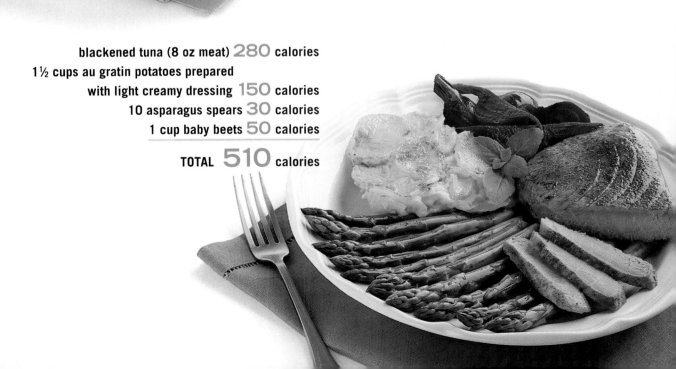

2 lamb chops (8 oz meat) 560 calories
1½ cups au gratin potatoes 570 calories
3 asparagus spears 10 calories

TOTAL 1,140 calories

VS.

blackened tuna (8 oz meat) 280 calories
1½ cups au gratin potatoes prepared
with light creamy dressing 150 calories
10 asparagus spears 30 calories
1 cup baby beets 50 calories

TOTAL 510 calories

Paltry Poultry

Most people assume that chicken is a healthy, low-calorie answer to meat. But other low-calorie choices let you eat lots more food. For example, consider the platter pictured on the right. With tofu and vegetables, it is healthy, filling, low-calorie, and an ample portion for the heartiest appetite. I call it a picture-perfect contrast to the paltry chicken thigh on the left.

3 oz chicken thigh 220 calories

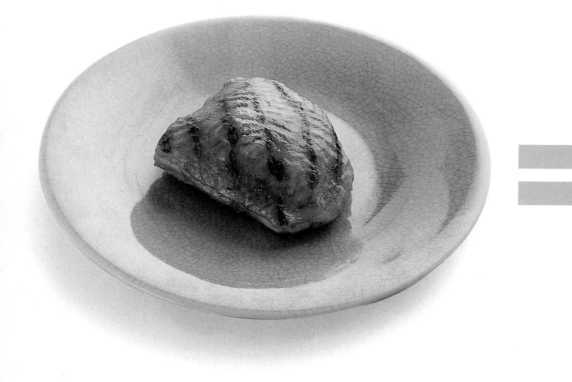

1 stuffed red pepper, with corn and tofu 130 calories
3 slices grilled red onion 30 calories
3 slices grilled acorn squash 40 calories
3 slices grilled zucchini 20 calories

TOTAL 220 calories

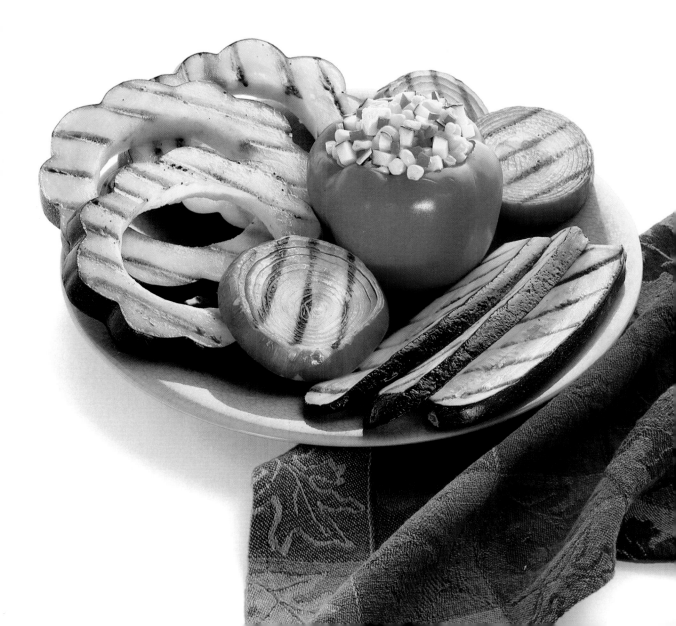

Protein Profile

We Americans love our steaks and burgers, chicken and prime rib. But the weight-conscious should be aware that there are calorie differences among these foods depending on the cut of meat and/or the manner of preparation. Barbecued poultry has less fat and fewer calories than the fried version. Similarly, when it's beef you want, you'll save a few calories on filet mignon over prime rib. (Of course, there are calorie differences between side dishes and bread accompaniments, too.)

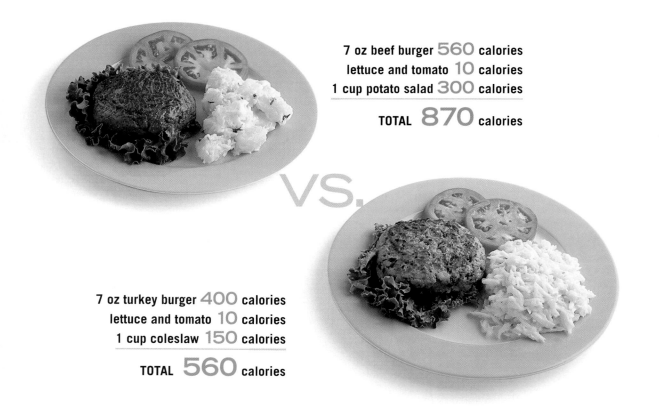

7 oz beef burger 560 calories
lettuce and tomato 10 calories
1 cup potato salad 300 calories

TOTAL 870 calories

VS.

7 oz turkey burger 400 calories
lettuce and tomato 10 calories
1 cup coleslaw 150 calories

TOTAL 560 calories

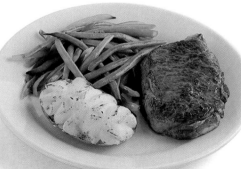

7 oz prime rib 630 calories
stuffed potato with cheese 350 calories
1 cup French cut green beans 40 calories

TOTAL 1,020 calories

VS.

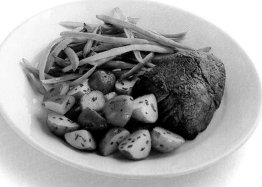

7 oz filet mignon 480 calories
1 cup new potatoes with chives 120 calories
1 cup French cut green beans 40 calories

TOTAL 640 calories

7 oz fried chicken leg and thigh 640 calories
2 oz corn bread 180 calories
1 cup macaroni salad 450 calories

TOTAL 1,270 calories

VS.

7 oz barbecued chicken leg and thigh 510 calories
¼ cup barbecue sauce 60 calories
2 oz dinner roll 160 calories
corn on the cob 90 calories

TOTAL 820 calories

Summer Evening

The spartan meal on the left looks like something someone "on a diet" would have on a summer's evening. Everything on the plate is low-fat, unadorned, bland. Even the dessert is fat-free—with berries for a garnish. But in fact, nothing about this meal is conducive to weight loss. It is not a low-calorie meal. Further, it's high in refined carbohydrates—not the greatest thing for weight loss or general health—and it's low in fruits and vegetables that are rich in the fiber that helps weight loss.

By contrast, the colorful meal on the right, with its diverse tastes and bigger portions, is a healthy and low-calorie choice. The scallops on the skewer are a better protein choice than the chicken, while the vegetables and fruit supply plenty of nutrients *and* take the edge off the appetite.

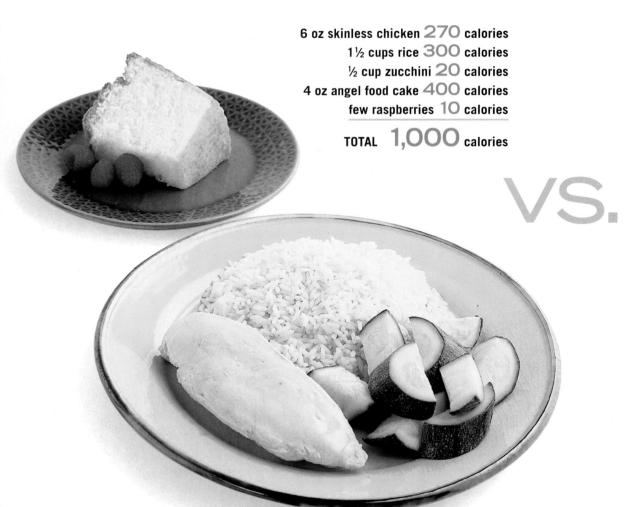

6 oz skinless chicken 270 calories
1½ cups rice 300 calories
½ cup zucchini 20 calories
4 oz angel food cake 400 calories
few raspberries 10 calories

TOTAL 1,000 calories

VS.

6 oz scallops with teriyaki sauce 180 calories
2 cups zucchini and eggplant with marinara sauce 90 calories
1 cup green, yellow, and red peppers 40 calories
1 cup button mushrooms 40 calories
1 scoop vanilla fat-free frozen yogurt 60 calories
1½ cups raspberries 60 calories
half a melon 60 calories
1 biscotto 100 calories

TOTAL 630 calories

Protein and Veg

How are you going to get your protein and vegetables? Eight ounces of beef and French fries are one way; 8 ounces of chicken and fries are another, slightly less caloric way. But hold the beef and poultry and just look at what happens: When you take in your protein as 8 ounces of fish, you get more food, more variety in taste, more healthful nutrition, and far fewer calories. In fact, the meal pictured on the lower right is a perfect Picture-Perfect Weight-Loss meal: fish for protein, lots of vegetables, more food overall, and still a goodly portion of the French fries you simply won't be deprived of.

4 medium barbecue spareribs
(8 oz meat plus ½ cup sauce) 800 **calories**
20 large French fries 400 **calories**

TOTAL 1,200 **calories**

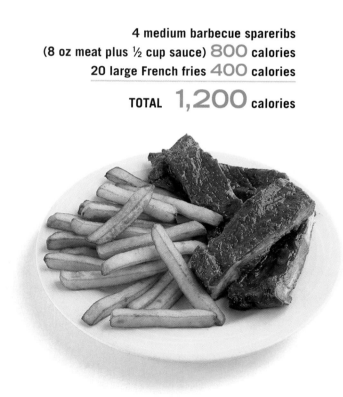

VS.

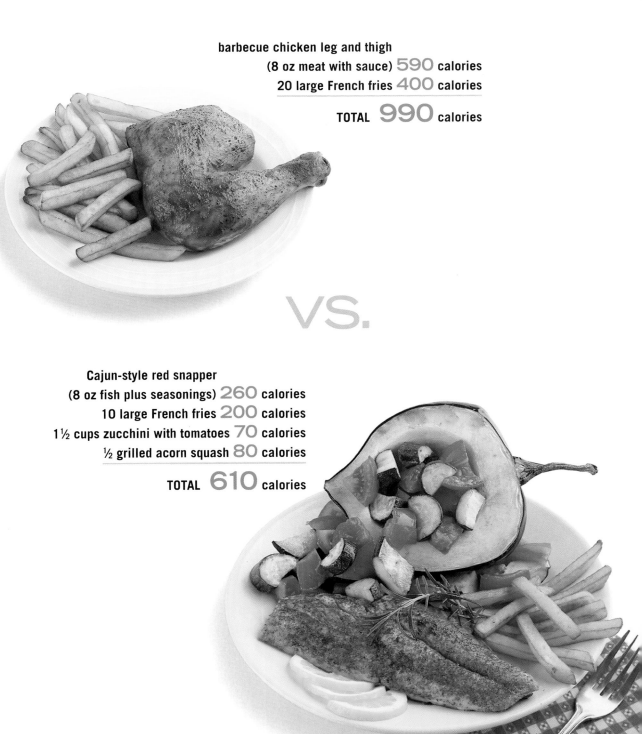

barbecue chicken leg and thigh
(8 oz meat with sauce) 590 calories
20 large French fries 400 calories

TOTAL 990 calories

VS.

Cajun-style red snapper
(8 oz fish plus seasonings) 260 calories
10 large French fries 200 calories
1½ cups zucchini with tomatoes 70 calories
½ grilled acorn squash 80 calories

TOTAL 610 calories

Protein Picks

It seems that with protein foods, the lower the calorie count, the higher the health benefit. So what'll it be for protein tonight? Three and a half ounces of rib steak or 7 ounces of grilled tuna? What will you choose for dinner tomorrow? A modest portion of grilled chicken or a hearty Salisbury steak, veggie style? It's your choice—for weight loss and for health.

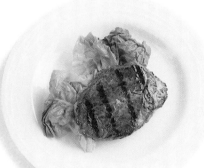

3½ oz rib steak
250 calories

OR

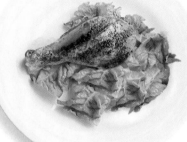

4 oz dark

meat chicken
250 calories

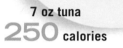

7 oz tuna
250 calories

OR

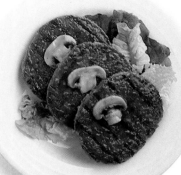

7 oz veggie Salisbury steak
250 calories

Pasta Proving Ground

Pasta is a treat the weight-conscious eat only rarely, so it's important to know that not all pasta dishes are created equal. Calorically, pasta is pasta, but the *penne alla vodka* on the left is defined by its rich, cream-based sauce, and it's the cream—not the vodka —that adds calories and saturated fat, the bad kind. Go for linguine with red clam sauce, which is far less caloric, more nutritious, and of course, very tasty!

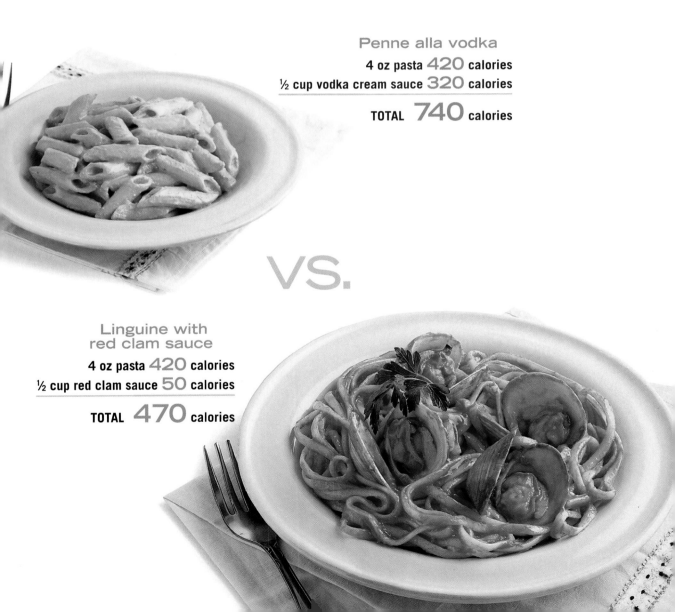

Penne alla vodka

4 oz pasta 420 calories
½ cup vodka cream sauce 320 calories

TOTAL 740 calories

VS.

Linguine with
red clam sauce

4 oz pasta 420 calories
½ cup red clam sauce 50 calories

TOTAL 470 calories

Flavors of Japan

Japanese cuisine has become immensely popular in America, largely because it offers so many healthy, low-calorie options as well as exotic taste sensations. But don't be fooled: There are high-calorie foods in Japanese restaurants, like this chicken tempura, which is deep-fried and calorically over-the-top. Stick to soy and seafood alternatives and treat yourself to a full meal—like this rich-tasting feast of miso (soy-based), sushi and sashimi, and a seaweed salad with vinegar dressing.

3 oz chicken tempura　430 calories

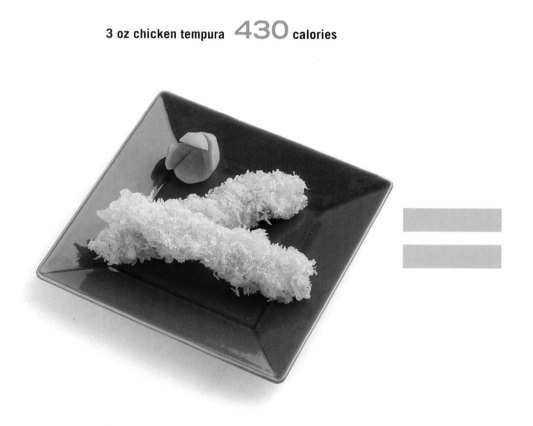

1 cup miso soup **40** calories
12 oz sushi and sashimi **360** calories
1 cup salad **30** calories

TOTAL **430** calories

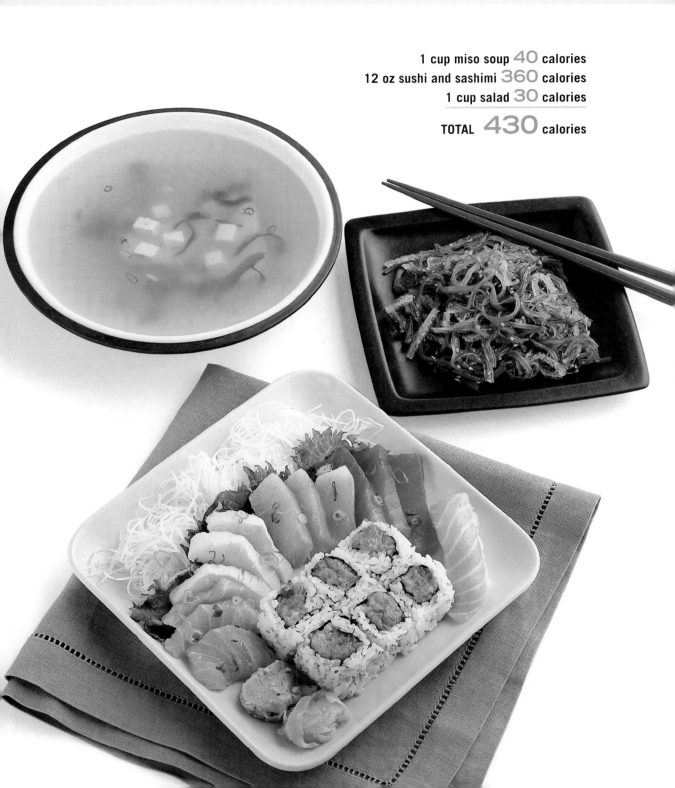

Better Than Burritos

Go to a Mexican restaurant, and it's all too easy to fill up on high-calorie appetizers like nachos or chips with guacamole before you even start on your combination plate of burritos slathered with cheese and sour cream. But there's a lot more to Mexican cuisine than these items. It's as varied, colorful, and interesting as the nation it comes from. Check out the meal on the right: From soup to entrée to side dish to salad, it's delicious, nutritious, varied, filling, and a definite calorie bargain.

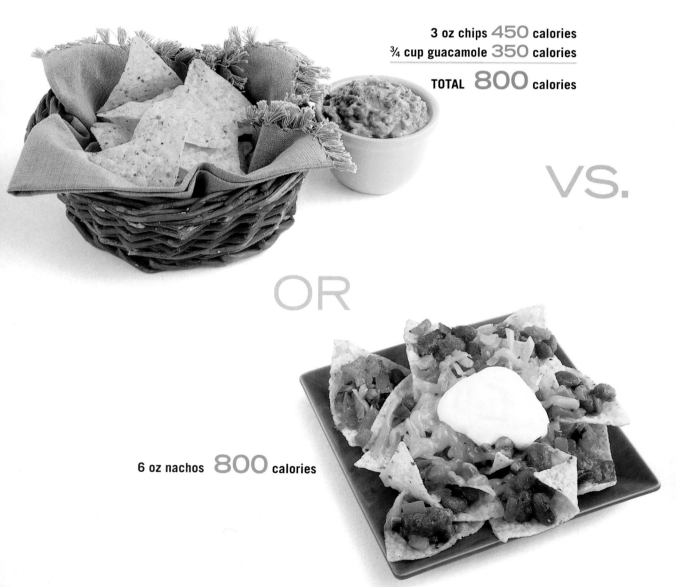

3 oz chips 450 calories
¾ cup guacamole 350 calories

TOTAL 800 calories

VS.

OR

6 oz nachos 800 calories

1½ cups pumpkin soup 100 calories
5 oz shrimp with salsa verde 150 calories
1 cup rice and beans 180 calories
1 cup baby squash 40 calories
jicama salad 30 calories

TOTAL 500 calories

Chinese Choices

One of the world's great cuisines, Chinese food offers choices for a range of appetites. Some choices, however, can be high in calories—just look at these standard appetizers. But so much more is available that the weight-conscious should have no trouble finding alternatives. The full meal shown on the right, for example, has the calorie count of *each one* of the appetizers. The lesson? Enjoy the rich, filling variety of the full meal—and save the calories.

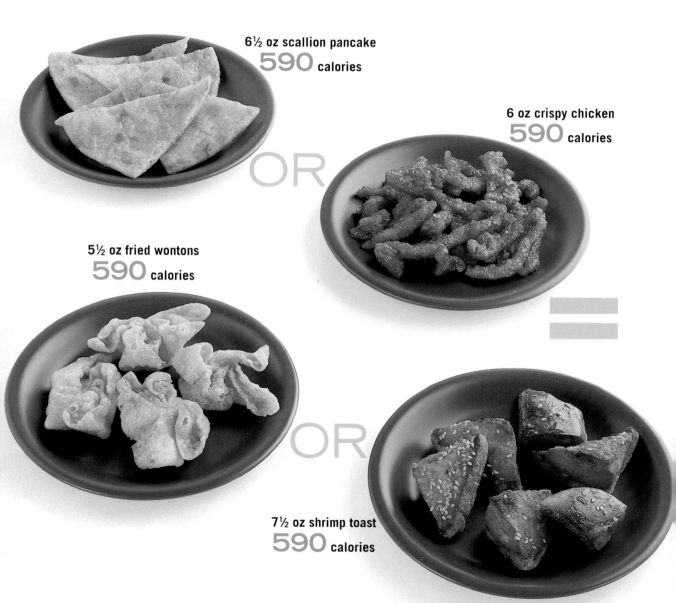

6½ oz scallion pancake
590 calories

6 oz crispy chicken
590 calories

5½ oz fried wontons
590 calories

7½ oz shrimp toast
590 calories

1 ½ cups vegetable wonton soup 100 calories
Szechuan seafood and vegetables
(2 cups Szechuan vegetables,
4 oz seafood, 1 Tbsp oil) 320 calories
½ cup rice 100 calories
4 litchis 40 calories
1 fortune cookie 30 calories

TOTAL 590 calories

Principled Actions

The meal below shows the basic principles of Picture-Perfect Weight Loss in action. The result is more food, healthier food, a feast for the eyes and the palate, and substantially fewer calories than the meal on the left.

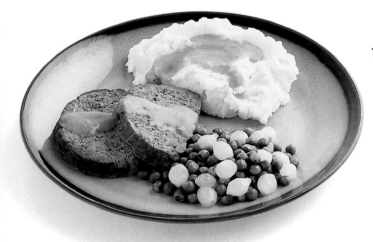

2 slices meat loaf (8 oz)	640 calories
1 cup garlic mashed potatoes	300 calories
½ cup gravy	120 calories
½ cup peas and pearl onions	60 calories
TOTAL	1,120 calories

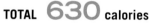

VS.

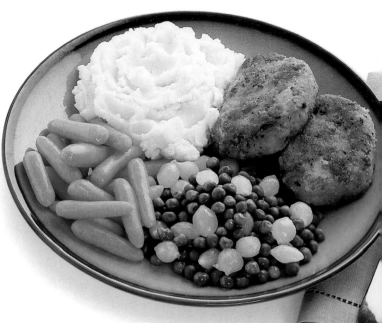

2 baked salmon croquettes (8 oz)	360 calories
1 cup garlic mashed potatoes prepared with garlic, broth, and light dressing	100 calories
1 cup peas and pearl onions	120 calories
1 cup baby carrots	50 calories
TOTAL	630 calories

A Difference Aired

Compared to most desserts, a chocolate soufflé seems light as air, hardly *there* at all. Yet it packs a lot of calories and fat. For an equally festive treat, try strawberries dipped in chocolate. They're very nutritious and tasty, and so rich and substantial you're satisfied with just a few.

1 cup chocolate soufflé 240 calories

8 chocolate-dipped strawberries 240 calories

Starch Binge

The bowl of rice looks bare, healthy, and a touch impoverished. In comparison, the plate of starchy food on the right seems like a real binge. Yet all the foods on the plate together are the caloric equivalent of the single portion of rice. Even more to the point, the potatoes and corn are nutritionally superior to the rice, which offers you nothing but refined-carbohydrate calories. Bottom line? The starch binge provides more food, more nutrition, more fiber, and more diversity of taste—for the same amount of calories.

1 pint (4 oz dry weight) white rice **440** calories

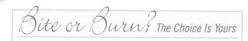

Bite or Burn? The Choice Is Yours

| 1 pint white rice | = | 1 hour of white-water rafting + 15 minutes of waterskiing |

8 boiled new potatoes 160 calories
1 baked sweet potato 180 calories
1 ear of corn 100 calories

TOTAL 440 calories

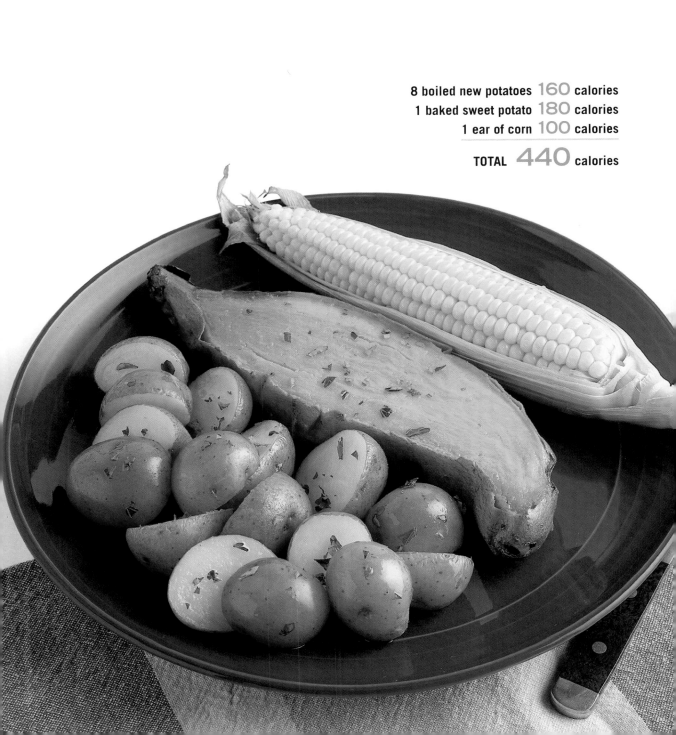

Green with Envy

Ponder this: 135 of the 240 calories in the premium pistachio ice cream come from fat. In fact, it's the fat that makes that little scoop so high in calories. You can avoid both the high calorie count and the fat by choosing the frozen dessert on the right—and still get the pistachio taste you crave.

½ cup premium pistachio ice cream
240 calories, 15 g fat

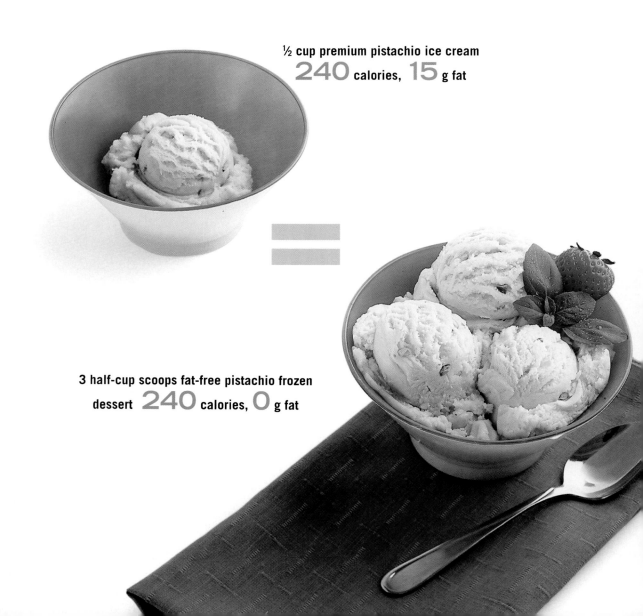

3 half-cup scoops fat-free pistachio frozen dessert 240 calories, 0 g fat

Sweet or Sour?

Lemon or chocolate? Just about every weight-conscious person would avoid the chocolate and choose the lemon—and just about every weight-conscious person would be wrong. Sure, chocolate is the supreme indulgence. And this tiny slice of lemon tart, especially when compared to that hulking wedge of chocolate layer cake, looks like the virtuous choice. But numbers don't lie: There's no calorie advantage to the lemon tart. So have it, by all means, if you love lemon pastries, but if you're choosing it because you think you're saving calories, think again—and plunge into the chocolate cake.

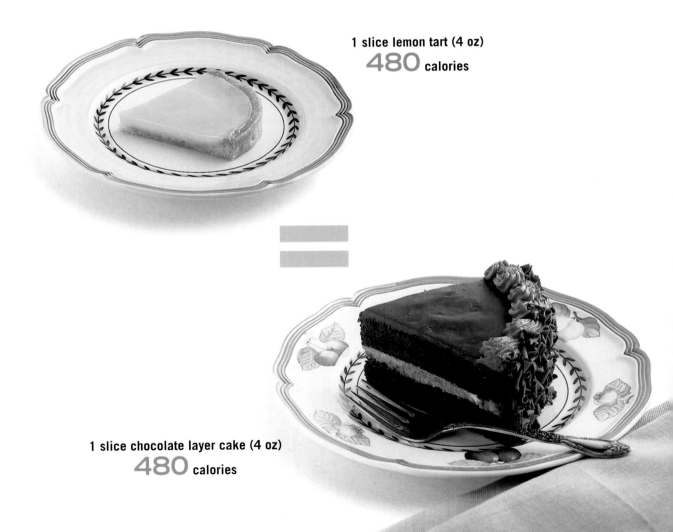

1 slice lemon tart (4 oz)
480 calories

1 slice chocolate layer cake (4 oz)
480 calories

Dolce Vita

Dolce is Italian for "sweet" and Italian for "dessert," and it's possible to get both at a low price in calories. For example, here is a low-calorie alternative to sinfully sweet cannoli: Simply fill ready-made waffle cups with Italian ices. Even one will satisfy your taste for la dolce vita.

1 cannoli (3 oz) 340 **calories**

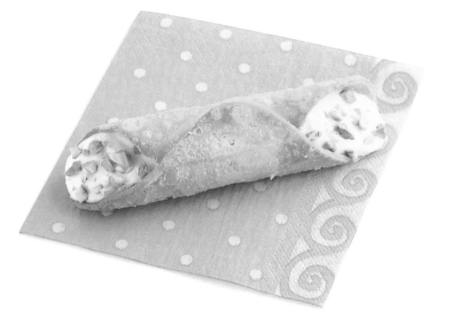

3 waffle cups 150 calories
12 oz Italian ice 190 calories

TOTAL 340 calories

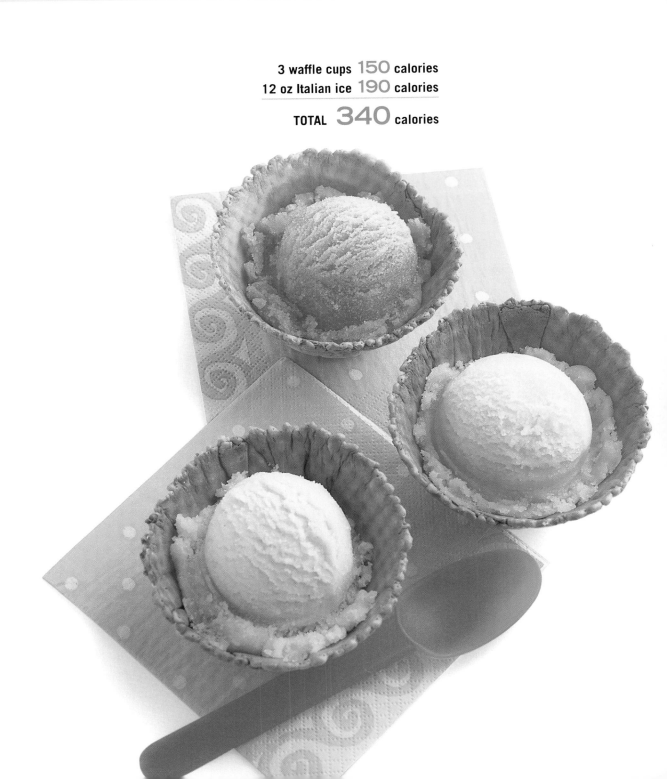

Lucky 13

Just because you're weight-conscious is no reason to give up the lush taste of a blueberry dessert. But unless you're a karate champ or rugby player, think about getting that lushness from one of the 13 stem glasses pictured on the right. Calorically, it trumps a piece of pie 12 times over.

1 wedge blueberry pie 450 calories
4 oz rich vanilla ice cream 200 calories

TOTAL 650 calories

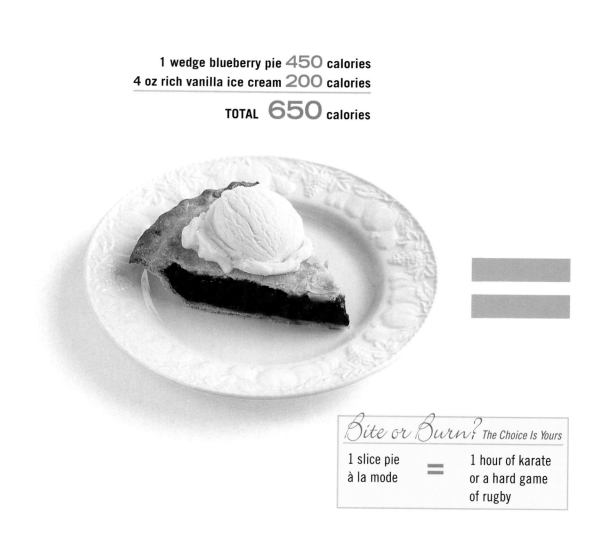

Bite or Burn? The Choice Is Yours

| 1 slice pie à la mode | = | 1 hour of karate or a hard game of rugby |

13 cups berries 520 calories
13 Tbsp topping 130 calories

TOTAL 650 calories

Chapter 9

WEEK 4: LET'S EAT OUT!

30-Day Plan

						1
2	3	4	5	6	7	8
9	10	11	12	13	14	15
16	17	18	19	20	21	22
23	24	25	26	27	28	29
30						

By the end of Week 4, you will have:

- Learned how to read any menu in any restaurant—and find the appropriate Picture-Perfect Weight-Loss choice
- Practiced using your voice to get your needs met
- Structured an exercise program you can follow for a lifetime
- Completed your "course" in Food Awareness Training

nlike diets, which require you to accommodate your lifestyle to your eating, one of the core principles of Picture-Perfect Weight Loss is that your eating must accommodate itself to your lifestyle. And certainly an integral part of today's lifestyle is eating out. Where Picture-Perfect Weight Loss is concerned, the "party line" on eating out is pretty simple. It's this:

Wherever you go, from the most sophisticated five-star bastion of haute cuisine to the fastest fast-food place—and at all the stops in between—you can find a reasonable low-calorie choice on the menu, a choice that lets you adhere to the principles of Picture-Perfect Weight Loss *and* satisfy both your appetite and your tastebuds.

When I say you can find the choice "on the menu," I mean precisely that. You don't have to insist that the fish be "dry-broiled." You don't need to order the vegetables "steamed—no butter." You may if you wish, but the point is that Picture-Perfect Weight Loss asks you to enjoy the rich variety of possibilities that eating out makes available—without restrictions or guilt, without drawing attention to yourself as having "special needs," but with an eye to good health, good nutrition, and of course, weight loss.

Make It Fun

Part of the fun of eating out the Picture-Perfect Weight-Loss way is the challenge of finding the choice or choices that are most appropriate for your weight-loss goal. Often, this means trying something you've never tried before in a restaurant. Good! Reaching out for fresh options is essential to achieving and maintaining Picture-Perfect Weight Loss.

Later in this chapter, I'll present a range of menus and show you the Picture-Perfect Weight-Loss choices on each. In addition, the food comparison demonstrations throughout this book will educate you about restaurant choices as well as about your own at-home food preparation choices. But of course, menu items are always changing. They change with the seasons. They change as old trends yield to new. In addition, a chef's creativity or changing consumer tastes can alter the bill of fare at the fanciest restaurant or the simplest. So as always, what counts in making the Picture-Perfect Weight-Loss choice when eating out is mindfulness and attention to all that you're learning in this book about the eating habits appropriate to weight loss.

It reminds me a little of that craze a few years ago over the children's book *Where's Waldo*. Remember it? Think of finding the menu choice that's right for you as something like the search for Waldo. Scan the menu carefully. At first, it may not look like there's anything on it that you could reasonably want to eat. Look again. Think. Maybe you'd like to put together two appetizers instead of one entrée. What about side dishes? Perhaps there are vegetables on the menu you've never heard of—maybe odd-sounding mushrooms or something with a foreign name. Try them. Maybe there's a fish listed that you've never tasted. This could be the moment. Use your imagination and all your awareness; the search

for your meal can turn into an intriguing exercise—your opportunity to "work out" your very own meal. And the result just might be a new addition to your range of Picture-Perfect Weight-Loss possibilities.

Glitches?

Suppose the dish you really want is the fresh Atlantic salmon. The problem is it's served with a rich, creamy sauce that you know will add a heap of calories and won't really add that much to your enjoyment. You have two choices. Your first choice is to order the salmon with the sauce. Period. After all, no food is forbidden. If the sauce with all its calories is worth it to you, go ahead and have it. So long as you're eating mindfully, there are no rules or prohibitions. If the sauce with all its calories is not worth it to you, though, move on to choice two.

Choice two, of course, is to order the salmon with no sauce—or with sauce served on the side. People are often reluctant to do this. Perhaps they're afraid of offending the chef who has expended his creative genius concocting this sauce. Perhaps they don't want to "bother" the waiter. Perhaps they simply don't want to draw attention to their own needs and wants—or to the fact that they are eating differently.

But in fact, this is just the time to speak up.

Your Needs, Your Voice

I've said that Picture-Perfect Weight Loss is a journey, and that the trip is often as much about emotions as about a number on a scale. In Week 2 of the journey, we talked about the importance of finding your voice and putting

Vegetarianism on Rise, Even among Felons

The number of vegetarians in the United States is increasing, and even the Bureau of Prisons has taken note of the fact. To be sure, the term "vegetarian" covers at least two categories of eater: vegans, who eat no meat, poultry, fish, eggs, or dairy products; and ovo-lacto vegetarians, who do eat eggs and dairy. In addition, there are semi-vegetarians, who occasionally have either meat, poultry, or fish—or all of them.

The Vegetarian Resource Group tracks the growth in vegetarianism and reports the following:

◆ Some five million Americans—2.5 percent of the population—eat neither meat, poultry, nor fish
◆ 4.5 percent of the population eat no red meat
◆ 6.7 percent eat no eggs

For vegetarians serving time in federal prisons, a "no-flesh/heart healthy alternative" diet has been available since October 2000, according to the Bureau of Prisons, in order to "meet the changing dietary habits of the Bureau's inmate population."

---

an end to tolerating people and things you know are toxic. In Week 3, we talked about the importance of identifying the unfulfilled needs you might be trying to fill with food. Now it's time to put it all together. It's time to speak up for yourself to get those unfulfilled needs met. Exercising your voice on your own behalf with a waiter is pretty basic, but it's a good start.

Often, the reluctance to make your wishes known—even to the perfectly nice person whose job it is to wait on you in a restaurant—really springs from deep emotional roots. Psychologists have observed that many overweight people tend to want to live up to others' expectations. Of course, we're all brought up to please people—our parents, our teachers, our friends, and later in life, our spouses and bosses. But with some people, the desire to please becomes something like a negation of the self, as these people put their own needs and wants "on hold" in favor of doing what they think others want—on the theory that doing so will make these people like them.

A lot of people who are overweight fall into this trap. They don't want to bother anyone, prefer to avoid confrontation, and try to be invisible. But as my staff psychotherapist Susan Amato reminds me, "*Everyone* has to ask for what they need." That's a basic rule of life—whether you're thin or fat, tall or short, old or young. In a restaurant setting, asking for what you need can be as basic as inquiring about the ingredients of a sauce, requesting that the sauce be served on the side, or sending the dish back if it's served wrong. It can—and should—all be done politely and courteously, of course: "Excuse me, maybe I wasn't clear, but I need the sauce served on the side."

It comes down to a pretty simple formula, and I leave it to psychologist Adele Fink, Ph.D., to articulate it. She puts it like this: "Get your needs met—and exercise your voice to do it." You need to feel good about yourself. One way you're doing that is by losing weight. One way you're working to lose weight is to fill up on vegetables rather than bread. If all those needs translate into the need for the bread basket to be removed from the table, for example, speak up and ask the waiter to remove it.

Of course, the words are simple—"Please take the bread away"—but often, exercising your voice is not. Dr. Fink's suggestion? Practice. Rehearse in front of friends or your pet or the mirror. Talk to the television set or direct your words out the window. The point is to say the words out loud. In a sense, you're warming up your assertiveness muscles, long unused and out of practice. Getting those muscles limber and strong is something that's important not just for weight loss, but for everything in life. Remember: It's all really about what you can gain for your whole self, not just about the pounds you'll lose.

Fast Foods— Everybody's Favorite

As I wrote in chapter 1, fast food is one of the culprits in the rising tide of obesity around the world. "Fast" tends to mean high in calories and high in fat—and the bad kind of fat at that—two consequences that are probably inevitable when food is mass-prepared and mass-produced for speedy delivery and low cost. And fast food is spreading everywhere; it's one of the great American exports—although whether for good or ill is a matter of debate.

Kids love fast food, of course, and fast-food places cater to children and to families with children. In fact, for many families—especially those with young children—a trip to "Mickey D's" or Pizza Hut or Boston Market or the like is about the only eating-out experience possible, both in terms of affordability and convenience. Ever try to drag a couple of little kids to an elegant, "grown-up" restaurant? That's the sort of experience almost no one enjoys—not the kids, not the parents trying to keep the kids in order, not the restaurant staff, and often not the other diners, either. As a result, fast-food restaurants will probably continue to dot the global landscape for many years to come.

The good news from the fast-food front is that the message of health and nutrition has penetrated even there. New chains are starting up aimed specifically at health-conscious eaters who yearn for tasty, affordable "fast food." These new chains are dedicating the bulk of their menus to healthy foods—mass-marketing such choices as soy-based sloppy joes and air-baked fries. Says Rosemary Deahl, owner of Chicago's wildly popular HeartWise Express, "The key is to make sure the food doesn't taste like anyone has compromised to eat here." At HeartWise, at Florida's fledgling Healthy Bites Grill and Evos restaurants, and at southern California's new Topz chain, that's exactly what's luring increasing numbers of customers.

Meanwhile, back at the mainstream fast-food chains, finding the low-calorie foods means choosing from a growing number of options in soups, vegetables, salads with light dressings, and grilled instead of fried seafood. But even with these choices, eating low-calorie is a case of *caveat emptor* —let the buyer beware! For example, Pizza Hut now features salad bars with a beautiful array of fresh fixings—but no low-fat dressings. The result is not low-calorie at all. Some possible solutions? Carry your own bottle of light dressing. Or, have a small amount of the available dressing. Or, if oil and vinegar are provided, use the least amount of oil necessary.

A second example: McDonald's offers such items as a vegetable sandwich on pita bread; salad shakers, which are often available with light dressing; and veggie burgers. These efforts at healthful eating are all to the good. On the other hand, the Chicken McGrill, also billed as an effort at healthful eating that eschews frying, actually consists of a very small piece of grilled chicken on a hamburger bun with a slice of tomato, a leaf of lettuce, and mayonnaise! It contains 470 calories and 18 grams of fat—not the best choice for folks concerned about their weight and their health. Maybe McDonald's feels "burned" by the failure of an earlier offering, the McLean burger. But the McLean was perceived as a "health-food" or "diet" offering, and was marketed as such, scaring people off before they ever got a taste. (How well I know this syndrome: All the firefighters to whom we served veggie sausages absolutely loved them—until they learned they were soy products! Eventually, they swallowed their resistance to the name—and have been swallowing the food with enjoyment ever since.)

Here's another example that really points up the kind of awareness you'll need when you're eating out at a fast-food restaurant: Taco Bell offers a taco salad with salsa that on its own—

minus taco shell and dressing—contains 217 calories. Add the shell, and it's 648 calories; add the dressing, and you pour on another 240 calories for a total of nearly 900 calories. While this is another case where you might bring your own dressing and have a tasty salad at a low calorie count—and at a nice low price as well—the point is that you need to be aware of what's really going on.

Still, the fact remains that many fast-food establishments are going out of their way to make fast food healthy and low in calories for those, like you, to whom these attributes are important. Boston Market, for example, offers a skinless chicken entrée and a white meat turkey entrée. Actually, the real treasure at Boston Market is found in the side dishes—a truly outstanding selection of vegetables: barbecue baked beans, black beans, green beans, squash, broccoli, potatoes, steamed vegetables, coleslaw, cucumber salad, fruit salad. Here's a place where making a meal out of side dishes can prove highly rewarding.

Subway is another good bet. You've probably seen the television commercials celebrating the weight-loss benefits of eating at this popular chain. Well, I agree. Subway offers such items as tuna salad or seafood and crab salad—and light mayonnaise to go with them. Their vegetable salads come with fat-free dressings. And the turkey breast sandwich is decidedly lower-calorie. Perhaps most impressive of all is that Subway's veggie delight sandwich is actually made with soy cheese. This means that soy products are now part of mainstream fast-food menus— not just of the menus of ethnic chains. I think Subway's use of soy and its very sub-

The Picture-Perfect Weight-Loss Guide to Fast Food: A Survival Kit

Need a guide to Picture-Perfect Weight-Loss choices at some of the nation's most popular budget eateries? Here's how you can enjoy a convenient, low-cost, low-calorie meal—from a pancake breakfast; to a range of sandwiches, soups, and salads; to side dishes; to dinner entrées of everything from seafood platters to plateloads of pasta.

Fast-Food Eatery	Picture-Pefect Weight-Loss Best Bets
Au Bon Pain	Soups, vegetarian chili, garden and Caesar salads with low-calorie dressings, fresh fruit
Bennigan's	Baked potatoes, fire-roasted salsa shrimp, grilled shrimp, O'Cajun grilled seafood platter, grilled salmon Caesar salad with low-fat or fat-free dressing, vegetable stir-fry
	Side orders: Bailey's broccoli, corn and black beans, coleslaw
Olive Garden	Minestrone, linguine alla marinara, penne romana, capellini pomodoro, pasta primavera, ravioli stuffed with portobello mushroom, seafood portofino, shrimp primavera
Perkins Restaurants	Buttermilk 5, fruit pancakes, short stack, potato pancakes, Belgian waffle—all with low-calorie syrup!
Ruby Tuesday's	Serious salad bar, soups, baked potatoes, Creole catch, veggie burger, grilled portobello mushroom sandwich
Wendy's	Baked potatoes, salad bar with light dressings, classic Greek and vegetable-stuffed pita sandwiches
	Side orders: applesauce, sliced cantaloupe, cottage cheese, sunflower seeds and raisins, vegetables

stantial efforts to offer healthy, tasty, low-calorie choices should be applauded by consumers—and emulated by other fast-food franchises.

Bottom line? We may be witnessing a revolution in fast food made specifically for the health-conscious and weight-conscious. Until the revolution is fully realized, however, you can find healthful, low-calorie choices when you eat at mainstream fast-food restaurants if you look carefully and choose wisely.

The Portion-Size Issue

One of the more pernicious trends in recent fast-food history is the "supersizing" phenomenon. It means that you don't just get a lot of high-calorie, high-fat fried foods; you get a gargantuan amount of high-calorie, high-fat fried foods.

The trend has spread, too. Steakhouses and family restaurants have joined in, with competing claims of "man-size" chops and steaks or "family-size" portions on side orders.

Interestingly, many of today's "designer" restaurants have done just the opposite. While their prices may have grown bigger, you're not paying for portion size but for the artistic "presentation" of a dish. Beautiful and appetizing as the presentation may be, a portion may consist of just a small amount of whatever is at the center of the dish—and an almost pathetic portion of vegetables. In fact, the vegetable may be little more than a garnish.

The truth about portion size, though, is that it doesn't matter. Restaurant portions, big or small, may have little to do with standard serving sizes. And they have nothing at all to do with what's right for you. The "correct" food portion for you is however much it takes to satisfy your appetite.

The Eating-Out Guide

As much as you can, satisfy your appetite with generous helpings of soup, salad, vegetables, and fruit. That's the key to eating out as well as the key to eating at home. Do you love the fresh baguette that's served at your favorite French bistro? Don't avoid it, but eat a smaller piece of it along with your pea soup, salad, and a side dish of vegetables as you wait for your main course. Instead of the biggest T-bone the steakhouse has to offer, try a smaller cut of beef—and stuff yourself with shrimp cocktail, soup, and a salad.

In other words, as I've advised before, flip the ratio. Load up on the appropriate choices and lighten up on the inappropriate choices. You'll still enjoy the tastes you love, and you'll still eat till you're satisfied.

A Three-Step Assignment

It's your last full week of the Picture-Perfect Weight Loss 30-Day Plan. By now, the principles of Picture-Perfect Weight Loss should be almost second nature to you. Your changed relationship with food—your new way of eating—should be getting very close to being automatic. Prove it to yourself this week with a three-step assignment.

Step 1: Go Out to Eat

Go out to eat, drop your old preconceptions about foods on the menu, and "find Waldo" on the menu. Maybe you'll choose your favorite restaurant—one you possibly haven't been to since you began the 30-Day Plan. This time, when the waiter asks if you're going to have "the usual," surprise him by saying no and ordering something entirely new and original and different.

Or go someplace you've never been before. It's a fresh menu, and you're bringing to it a fresh eye—a new way of looking at menu choices thanks to your new awareness of food and your changed relationship with it.

Step 2: Exercise—Make It a Habit

Your changed relationship with food is accompanied by new habits of exercise. You've now been active for 3 weeks—and I'm pretty sure you feel better and look better as a result. Just think: If 3 weeks of basic movement can do this, imagine what a lifetime of physical activity might accomplish.

This week, make exercise a habit for life.

Meditate to Exercise Longer

Remember the old Latin proverb about "a healthy mind in a healthy body." Well, now it turns out that a *relaxed* mind can help the body exercise more. How? Studies show that meditation can actually keep a body exercising longer before exhaustion sets in.

Researchers instructed 11 of 31 male runners in meditation, which they were to practice several times a week. After 6 months, the meditative runners showed a dramatic decrease in blood levels of lactic acid following exercise. It's lactic acid buildup that makes you feel your muscles "burn" during intense exercise; the lactic acid interferes with muscle contraction and pretty much forces you to stop the exercise. Delaying the production of lactic acid, as the meditation did, makes it possible to exercise longer.

How? By structuring a regular exercise program for yourself. If you've thought about joining a gym, this is the week to do it. Take a class or sign on with a personal trainer; for whatever kind of exercise regimen you undertake at the gym or health club, it's important that you learn to do it the right way. This is particularly the case with weights or machines, where doing things the wrong way can actually prove harmful.

You don't have to go to a gym, however. Maybe you've decided instead to formalize the walking you've been doing the last 3 weeks—to pick up the pace and lengthen the distance over time. Fine. Set a schedule. Maybe you're thinking of taking it up a notch to jogging, or even, eventually, to running. Structure a plan. Think it through. Write it down.

Or perhaps you've decided to do yoga or tai chi. Or maybe you've decided to follow a workout show that airs each morning on your local TV station, or as was suggested in the previous chapter, you've chosen to make golf the center of your exercise program, or cycling, or the basketball you were pretty good at in high school. Excellent. Remember to ease into it. Don't push yourself beyond your own comfort zone. Keep in mind that progress moves in increments, that you'll add more reps or stretch your muscles farther or be able to jog past the corner next week, and you'll do still more and go even farther the week after that—and so on. Remember that you're in this for life; don't rush it.

Please don't think I'm suggesting that you pick an activity this week and stick to that particular activity for life. Not at all. You may find that 6 months or a year of regular cycling on country roads, delightful as it seems at first, eventually becomes boring. The solution? Find an alternative activity. In fact, as you become stronger and more skilled, you will eagerly seek out fresh exercise options.

It isn't a particular activity or sport or exercise regimen you must commit to; it's the fact of exercise. Just as you've established a new relationship with food, you must also establish a new relationship with physical activity. Just as you're committing yourself to a new way of eating for life, so also must you commit yourself to regular exercise for life. The specifics may change with time—*will* change, in fact, and probably *should* change—but the habit of physical activity must be an integral part of your life *for* life. Maintaining weight loss and staying healthy depend on it.

The point this week is to formalize your exercise: Structure it into a program, set a schedule, and start using the vocabulary of someone who exercises regularly. That vocabulary might include such phrases as "I can't meet you until later because I have to do my workout" or "I'll call you back after I've done another 20 reps" or "Meet you at the corner for a power walk." In a way, you're saying out loud that exercise is an essential part of your life—and that helps validate your commitment to it.

Whatever exercise program you undertake, it should adhere to the following two guidelines.

Exercise regularly—and focus on it. Research indicates that even brief periods of low-intensity to moderate-intensity physical activity have weight-loss and health benefits. Still, try to work up to at least 40 minutes of exercise at a time at least every other day. Your workout should be broken up as follows:

10 minutes of warmup

20 minutes of activity

10 minutes of cooldown

It's also important to pay attention to the exercise you do while you're doing it. Even if 10 minutes is absolutely all you can manage today, give the activity your full focus for every one of the 10 minutes. This is your time. Make it count.

Include aerobics, strength training, and flexibility training in your exercise routine. Here's a classic example: some brisk walking or cycling for warmup aerobics, 20 minutes of weight-bearing exercise, and then 10 minutes of stretches to cool down. Of course, it's up to you to mix and match—there's nothing wrong with one day being all aerobics, the next a yoga class for flexibility, and the next all weight-lifting.

Step 3: Your Personal Food Awareness Worksheet

By the end of this week, you will have graduated from the Food Awareness Training course that is at the heart of Picture-Perfect Weight Loss. That makes Week 4 of the 30-Day Plan a good time to create your own personal Food Awareness worksheet. It will show you how far you've come in changing your relationship with food, and it will serve as a signpost that continues to point you in the direction you want to go.

Fill out the Food Awareness worksheet anytime during this last week of the program. Think about it carefully. It looks simple, and it is, but it's a very important exercise, so don't rush it.

In the left-hand column, write down the 10 lowest-calorie foods you've incorporated into your life over the past 3 weeks. By "incorporated," I don't mean just "tasted"; I mean foods that you have made a part of your regular diet. Some may be entirely new to you. Others may be new only in the sense that they have gone from being foods you nibbled at occasionally to foods that are truly incorporated into your eating habits—maybe you're eating more vegetables now, or more fish, or making sure you have some fruit every day, or discovering hard candies and low-calorie Popsicles.

In the right-hand column, write in at least six high-calorie foods you believe you ought to eat less often, or find other choices for, or in some way ease out of your eating habits.

I'm not going to set down any guidelines about what should or should not be included in either column. If you think in specifics—hot fudge sundaes, the two vodka martinis before dinner, southern fried chicken—that's fine. If you think in broader categories—desserts, alcohol, fried foods—that's fine, too. It's your worksheet; it should reflect your perceptions.

If you come up with more than 10 low-calorie foods and more than 6 high-calorie foods, that's also fine, but please find no fewer than those minimum numbers. Remember that you have all week to decide what should go on the Food Awareness worksheet, so take your time and think it through.

At the end of the week, when the worksheet is complete, have a good look at it. Look at the column on the left. See how far you've come over the 4 weeks of the Picture-Perfect Weight Loss 30-Day Plan. Clearly, it is entirely possible to come up with new food choices and new ways of eating. You really *have* changed your relationship with food.

Look at the right-hand column from the perspective of that accomplishment. If the six or more foods listed here show you the dimensions of the task still ahead of you, the left-hand list is assurance that the task is eminently

My Personal Food Awareness Worksheet

New Low-Calorie Foods (at least 10)

1. _____
2. _____
3. _____
4. _____
5. _____
6. _____
7. _____
8. _____
9. _____
10. _____

High-Calorie Holdovers (at least 6)

1. _____
2. _____
3. _____
4. _____
5. _____
6. _____
_____
_____
_____
_____

doable. After all, you've already accomplished an even more substantial task.

Take another look at the right-hand column. Sometimes, just writing down the names of these high-calorie foods makes them stand out in your mind. It may enhance your awareness so that the task of minimizing their place in your life or reaching out for new alternatives becomes much easier to accomplish. The list is a good thing to keep in mind whether you're at home, on the job, or eating out.

So with that in mind, let's look at some menus from a range of restaurants.

Picture-Perfect Weight-Loss Haute Cuisine: A Primer on Dining Out

Let's start with really fine dining at some top-notch gourmet restaurants in New York City. These are the types of places most of us go to only for special occasions or as a particular treat. Why start with these restaurants? You know what the song says about New York: "If you can make it here, you can make it any-where"—and it's true of eating as well. With this primer showing you how to enjoy low-calorie, weight-conscious meals at the *hautest* of *haute cuisine* restaurants in New York, you can achieve Picture-Perfect Weight Loss wherever you dine.

For people "on a diet," an evening at such a restaurant can be a difficult—even a painful—experience. If they stick to the diet, they end up ordering the dullest item on the menu, then dutifully downing their bland meals—and drawing attention to their dieting—while surreptitiously drooling over the tasty, inventive creations everyone else at the table is enjoying. If they don't stick to their diets, they're plunged into guilt and gloom as they contemplate the penance of deprivation they will have to start paying the next morning. Either way, dieters can be forgiven for deciding to stay home, save the money, and forgo one of life's great pleasures—dining out on fabulous food.

But take a look at the following menus I've assembled from some of my favorite New York restaurants, representing a range of cuisines. Note the highlighted choices. They're the dishes that are consistent with the principles of Picture-Perfect Weight Loss, with "eating the pyramid," and they yield an almost mind-boggling number and range of choices. Deprivation? Hardly. A "limited menu"? Not on your life. All sorts of tastes are offered, answering all sorts of appetites. The bottom line? The most weight-conscious diners can enjoy their dining-out experience to the fullest. That means eating superb food—from appetizer through main course and side dishes to dessert—food that is characteristic of the particular cuisine or that fully explores a particular chef's inventiveness. It means that nothing is eliminated—not fat (the good kind) or sauces or rich taste. It means acting just like everybody else around the table—figuring out what you feel like eating, choosing something delicious, and savoring and celebrating your selection. All the while you'll know that you've made a healthful, low-calorie Picture-Perfect Weight-Loss choice—one among several, most likely, on the menu.

Note: Due to space limitations, the menus shown on the following pages have not been reproduced in full.

Jean-Georges

Internationally renowned chef Jean-Georges Vongerichten is perhaps New York's leading chef—and one of the world's great cuisine innovators. Born in Alsace, trained in France and the Orient, Jean-Georges creates inventive dishes that are known for their intense flavors and satisfying textures. With restaurants around the world and four in New York, the signature Jean-Georges is the four-star flagship of the fleet.

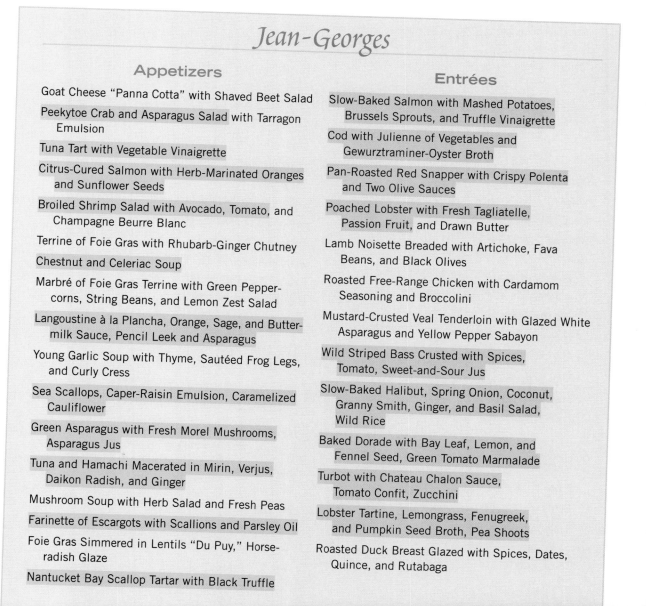

Jean-Georges

Appetizers

Goat Cheese "Panna Cotta" with Shaved Beet Salad

Peekytoe Crab and Asparagus Salad with Tarragon Emulsion

Tuna Tart with Vegetable Vinaigrette

Citrus-Cured Salmon with Herb-Marinated Oranges and Sunflower Seeds

Broiled Shrimp Salad with Avocado, Tomato, and Champagne Beurre Blanc

Terrine of Foie Gras with Rhubarb-Ginger Chutney

Chestnut and Celeriac Soup

Marbré of Foie Gras Terrine with Green Peppercorns, String Beans, and Lemon Zest Salad

Langoustine à la Plancha, Orange, Sage, and Buttermilk Sauce, Pencil Leek and Asparagus

Young Garlic Soup with Thyme, Sautéed Frog Legs, and Curly Cress

Sea Scallops, Caper-Raisin Emulsion, Caramelized Cauliflower

Green Asparagus with Fresh Morel Mushrooms, Asparagus Jus

Tuna and Hamachi Macerated in Mirin, Verjus, Daikon Radish, and Ginger

Mushroom Soup with Herb Salad and Fresh Peas

Farinette of Escargots with Scallions and Parsley Oil

Foie Gras Simmered in Lentils "Du Puy," Horseradish Glaze

Nantucket Bay Scallop Tartar with Black Truffle

Entrées

Slow-Baked Salmon with Mashed Potatoes, Brussels Sprouts, and Truffle Vinaigrette

Cod with Julienne of Vegetables and Gewurztraminer-Oyster Broth

Pan-Roasted Red Snapper with Crispy Polenta and Two Olive Sauces

Poached Lobster with Fresh Tagliatelle, Passion Fruit, and Drawn Butter

Lamb Noisette Breaded with Artichoke, Fava Beans, and Black Olives

Roasted Free-Range Chicken with Cardamom Seasoning and Broccolini

Mustard-Crusted Veal Tenderloin with Glazed White Asparagus and Yellow Pepper Sabayon

Wild Striped Bass Crusted with Spices, Tomato, Sweet-and-Sour Jus

Slow-Baked Halibut, Spring Onion, Coconut, Granny Smith, Ginger, and Basil Salad, Wild Rice

Baked Dorade with Bay Leaf, Lemon, and Fennel Seed, Green Tomato Marmalade

Turbot with Chateau Chalon Sauce, Tomato Confit, Zucchini

Lobster Tartine, Lemongrass, Fenugreek, and Pumpkin Seed Broth, Pea Shoots

Roasted Duck Breast Glazed with Spices, Dates, Quince, and Rutabaga

All' Italiana

Want to eat Italian? You can't do better than these three New York landmarks: Cipriani, founded by a scion of the family that launched the legendary Harry's Bar in Venice; Felidia, the elegantly appointed northern Italian restaurant founded by Lidia Matticchio Bastianich, well-known for her book and TV series, *Lidia's Italian Table*; and Bellini, whose under-30 owner, a former lawyer, travels yearly to Italy to keep up with the latest in regional specialties. Because Italian food features fresh ingredients in season and makes wide-ranging use of legumes and fish for protein sources, the number and variety of Picture-Perfect Weight-Loss choices it offers are astounding, whether for *antipasti*, main *piatti*, delicious *contorni*, or of course, *dolci*.

Cipriani

Appetizers and First Courses

Polenta with veal ragù or caciocavallo cheese

Vegetable peperonata

Fagioli in Saor

Sliced goat cheese, Acacia honey, and pears

Asparagus alla vinaigrette

Cold turkey with tuna sauce

Cold marinated salmon with asparagus

Small insalata del doge

Prosciutto cotto di Parma

Prosciutto di Parma with rucola or melon

Fried calamari with tartar sauce

Clams alla Veneziana

Fresh tuna tartare with mache salad

Tonno scottato with fennel vinaigrette

Soups

Minestrone soup

Pasta e fagioli

Cold carrot soup

Traditional fish soup

Pasta

Baked green or white tagliolini with ham

Potato gnocchi with tomato and basil

Tagliatelle with chanterelle mushrooms

Lasagnette pasticciate al forno

Tagliardi with veal ragù

Homemade Spaghetti Chitarra mussels and clams

Spinach and cheese ravioli with butter and sage

Veal cannelloni alla Piemontese

Risotto with homemade sausage

Risotto alla Milanese

Main Courses

Fried calamari with tartar sauce and green salad

Monkfish with broccoli di rapa

Large tuna tartare with mache salad

Large tonno scottato with fennel vinaigrette

Medallion of salmon alla Veneziana

Branzino Mediterraneo al forno with vegetables

Halibut in a light leek sauce with rice pilaf

Veal kidneys with risotto alla Milanese

Free-range chicken spezzatino alla Pizzaiola

Veal Piccatine al limone with rice pilaf

Veal Milanese with vegetables

Veal chop with fresh rosemary and vegetables

Roast veal shank alla Cipriani with vegetables

Felidia

Zuppe e Minestre

Minestra di Fagioli e Cozze con Cicoria e Ditalini di Ceci al Torchio
Minestra of fresh cranberry beans and chicory with Mediterranean mussels, chickpea ditalini pasta "al Torchio"

Zuppa Branzino con Couscous
Light San Marzano tomato and Mediterranean bass broth with couscous

Zuppa di Finocchi Selvatici e Verdure con Fidelini e Granchio
Wild fennel and spring herbs soup with broken Fidelini and crab

Pesci

Branzino Al Forno con Spinaci "Al Pane"
Mediterranean bass served with spinach "al pangrattato"

Rombo "Tutto Sedano" con Riduzione di Funghi e Sherry
Pan-roasted turbot "all celery" puree and braised, dry porcini and sherry wine reduction

Astice con Porri e Fave in Brodetto
Roasted Maine lobster with baby leeks and fava bean Brodetto

Primi Piatti

Bigoli Integrali con Melanzane, Pomodoro, Ricotta Salata e Basilico
Whole wheat Bigoli with eggplant, orange tomatoes, basil, and salt-cured ricotta

Risotto con Frutti di Mare
Superfino Carnaroli rice with rock shrimp, scallops, clams, crab, and light tomato broth

Pasutice in Brodetto d Astice
Diamond-shaped pasta in light tomato-lobster sauce with peperoncino

Antipasti Caldi e Freddi

Insalata di Polipo alla Griglia con Pomodorini, Cipollotti e Germogli di Capperi
Grilled octopus salad with New Jersey grape tomatoes, scallions, and caperberries

Baccala Dorato con Pure di Ceci, Salsa di Olive e Panelle
Golden panfried salt cod, chickpea puree, gaeta olives, orange zest horseradish sauce, and "Panelle"

Insalata di Barbabietole e Mele con Caprino Vinaigrette di Balsamico
Roasted baby beets and Granny Smith apple salad with Coach farm goat cheese and balsamic vinaigrette

Soppressata di Lingua Vitello con Fegato Grasso, Salsa Verde e Rossa al Rabarbaro
Duck foie gras and calf tongue "soppressata," rhubarb red and green sauce

Ortiche All'Aglio con Ricottina Calda All'Olio del Garda
Wilted nettles with garlic and warm ricotta with fattoria il Pardiso

Bellini

Antipasti and Zuppe

Carpaccio di tonno con finocchio
Thinly sliced raw tuna topped with shaved fennel and brushed with truffle oil

Sapore di Capri
Mozzarella, sliced tomato, and roasted pepper with virgin olive oil

Carpaccio di manzo con carciofi
Thinly sliced raw beef with raw artichoke and Parmesan shavings

Calamari ai ferri con verdure
Grilled Atlantic squid with diced sautéed squash, eggplant, and tomato

Polenta e funghi
Cornmeal diamonds and sautéed shiitake mushrooms topped with Gorgonzola fondue

Ricotta di Bufala Indorata Fritta
Lightly panfried imported buffalo ricotta with baby arugula salad and tomato

Grigliata di verdure
Grilled assorted vegetables infused with extra-virgin olive oil and balsamic vinegar

Purea di funghi selvatici con porri e patate
Creamless mushroom soup with leeks and potato

Pasta

Ravioli con ragù di granchio
Seafood-filled ravioli with crabmeat ragout

Scialatielli con gamberi e zucchini
Milk- and cheese-based pasta with rock shrimp and zucchini in a lobster sauce

Cavatelli con salsiccie e cime di rapa
Semolina flour twists with roasted sausage and bitter broccoli sautéed with garlic and olive oil

Ravioli di Melanzane e pecorino
Ravioli filled with eggplant, pecorino, and mozzarella with tomato and basil sauce

Malfatti con carciofi
Unevenly shaped pasta with sautéed artichokes, capers, and gaeta olives

Ziti Aumme Aumme
With plum tomatoes, basil, fried eggplant, and melting mozzarella

Fusilli all'ortolana
With sautéed mushrooms, zucchini, and vine-ripened cherry tomatoes

Farfalle alla vodka
With sweet peas and chicken in a vodka sauce enriched with cream

Penne alla principessa
With asparagus, sausage, and roasted pine nuts in a light cream sauce

Tortellini della Nonn
With tomato, peas, and julienne of prosciutto in a cream sauce

Linguini in white clam sauce

Bucatini all'Amatriciana

Linguine con frutti di mare

*Pasta available in appetizer portion

Pesce (Fish)

Gamberoni Bellini
Jumbo shrimp sautéed with white wine and tomato and topped with mozzarella

Salmone alla Griglia
Grilled salmon served with shiitake mushrooms and Dijon mustard sauce

Dentice all'acqua pazza
Snapper simmered in water, flavored with garlic, olive oil, and cherry tomatoes

Tonno al pepe nero
Seared tuna encrusted in crushed black pepper

Morton's

A Chicago original that now has more than 50 locations all over the world, and a favorite of New York sports figures, show biz celebrities, and politicians, Morton's is the quintessential upscale chophouse, offering generous portions of the very best steaks. But make it salmon steak, concentrate on the equally outsized platters of vegetables—including steamed vegetables—and go for a range of rich appetizers, and Morton's becomes a weight-conscious diner's delight. Have a look.

Morton's of Chicago

Appetizers

Jumbo Lump Crab Cake, *Mustard Mayonnaise Sauce*

Jumbo Shrimp Cocktail

Bluepoint Oysters on the Half Shell

Smoked Pacific Salmon

Jumbo Lump Crabmeat Cocktail, *Mustard Mayonnaise Sauce*

Broiled Sea Scallops Wrapped in Bacon, *Apricot Chutney*

Shrimp Alexander, *Sauce Beurre Blanc*

Sautéed Wild Mushrooms

Lobster Bisque

Salads

Morton's Salad

Spinach Salad

Caesar Salad

Sliced Beefsteak Tomato, *Purple Onion or Blue Cheese*

Entrées

Double Filet Mignon, *Sauce Béarnaise*

Porterhouse Steak

New York Strip Steak

Rib Eye Steak

Cajun Rib Eye Steak

Sicilian Veal Chop

Broiled Center Cut Swordfish Steak, *Sauce Béarnaise*

Jumbo Lump Crab Cakes, *Mustard Mayonnaise Sauce*

Domestic Rib Lamb Chops

Shrimp Alexander, *Sauce Beurre Blanc*

Chicken Christopher, *Garlic Beurre Blanc Sauce*

Farm-Raised Salmon

Whole Baked Maine Lobster

Vegetables

Creamed Spinach

Steamed Fresh Asparagus, *Sauce Hollandaise*

Sautéed Fresh Spinach and Mushrooms

Steamed Fresh Broccoli, *Sauce Hollandaise*

Sautéed Wild Mushrooms

Sautéed Mushrooms

Sautéed Onions

Potatoes

Baked Idaho Potato

Hash Brown Potatoes

Mashed Potatoes

Lyonnaise Potatoes

Potato Skins

Dawat

The name means "invitation to a feast," and Dawat lives up to its name. This restaurant offers a tantalizing tour of the many cuisines of India—in a menu created with the help of famed actress and chef Madhur Jaffrey. The variety of tastes is staggering, and since India's religious tradition places a premium on vegetarian cooking, Indian menus, like Dawat's, offer a great many choices to the weight-conscious.

Dawat

Specialties from the Tandoor (Clay) Oven

Tandoori Shrimp
King-size shrimp marinated in mild spices

Tandoori Fish Tikka
Chunks of seasonal fish, marinated in an aromatic herb mixture

Tandoori Chicken
Chicken marinated in yogurt and mild spices

Seekh Kebab
Minced lamb with aromatic herbs, wrapped around a skewer

Whole Tandoori Fish
Whole fish and fiery, quick-cooking ovens are meant for each other. The fish is marinated in yogurt and flavored with dill-like ajwain seeds before it is roasted.

Seafood

Scallops Caldin
Crusty scallops with a green coriander chili sauce, a Goan specialty.

Fish in a Mustard Sauce
Chunks of tilefish in a spicy sauce of crushed mustard seeds and mustard oil

Kerala-Style Konju Pappaas
Shrimp in a coconut sauce, flavored with aromatic curry leaves and smoked tamarind

Parsi-Style Patra-ni-Machhi
Salmon smothered in a fresh coriander chutney wrapped in a banana leaf and steamed. Served with basmati rice.

Special Menu

Hyderabadi Patthar Kabab
Thin slices of marinated lamb.

Tandoori Grilled Vegetables
A delightful plate of marinated seasonal vegetables and fresh cheese grilled in our tandoor and served with chickpeas.

Lamb Chops "Gurnar"
Our tandoori chef's exquisite lamb chops marinated in garlic, ginger, yogurt, and saffron and then baked quickly in a clay oven

Moola—Shilpa
Mussels and clams cooked in a curry leaf sauce in the style of Maharashtrian fishermen

Chicken Badami
Chicken pieces in a rich almond-flavored sauce

Black-Eyed Peas and Corn
A delicious mixture of black-eyed peas and corn, flavored with tomatoes, dill, and curry leaves

Sarson Ka Saag
Fresh mustard greens and spinach cooked in a Punjabi village style

Breads

Nan
A light, flat bread made from a dough of superfine flour and baked in a clay oven

Keema Nan
A nan stuffed with ground lamb and baked in a clay oven

Garlic Nan
A special, multilayered nan bread from the tandoor, flavored with garlic

Nan-E-Dawat
A rich, flat bread stuffed with nuts and dried fruit and baked in a clay oven

Tandoori Roti
Whole wheat bread baked in a clay oven

Tandoori Paratha
Rich, multilayered whole wheat bread, baked in a clay oven

Poori
Whole wheat puffed bread, deep-fried

Accompaniments

Papadum
Light, airy wafers

Kheera Raita
Yogurt and grated cucumber

Timatar Raita
Yogurt with tomato and mint

Boondi Raita
Yogurt with tiny chickpea-flour dumplings

Vegetarian Specialties

Paneer Makhani
Fresh homemade cheese, tomato sauce

Sautéed Shiitake Mushrooms
With curry leaves and green coriander

Mattar Paneer
Fresh homemade cheese cubes cooked with green peas

Saag Paneer
Fresh homemade cheese cubes in a spicy spinach sauce

Bhindi Masala
Okra-flavored with browned onions and dried mango

Baked Eggplant
Thin slices of eggplant coated with a mild sweet-and-sour tamarind sauce and baked

Maharashtrian-Style Farasvi Bhaji
Green beans cooked with freshly grated coconut

Labdharay Aloo
Potatoes with ginger and tomatoes in a thick sauce

Tadka Dal
Slow-simmered matpe beans and red kidney beans, sautéed with tomatoes, ginger, cumin, and onion

Vegetable Jal Frazie
Mixed vegetables with cottage cheese, mildly spiced

Dal Saag
Split pea lentils sautéed with spinach, onions, ginger, and spices

Zeera Aloo
Spicy potatoes flavored with whole and ground cumin seeds

Desserts

Gajrela
Caramelized grated carrots, studded with pistachios and served with whipped cream

Rasmalai
Sweet, spongy cottage cheese dumplings, flavored with cardamom and rose water

Special Kheer
Cooling rice pudding, flavored with cardamom and garnished with pistachios

Gulab Jamun
A light pastry made from dry milk and honey

Mango or Coconut Ice Cream

Kulfi
Traditional Indian ice cream

Asia de Cuba

It doesn't get any hipper than Asia de Cuba, which caters to the young Hollywood crowd, high-fashion models, television glitterati, and anyone who loves the fusion of Asian and Latin cuisines. Located in Morgans Hotel—created by the ever-stylish Ian Schrager, who cofounded the legendary Studio 54—Asia de Cuba looks impressively elegant, and the same can be said for the menu. Everyone tries the famous tunapica, citrus-infused raw tuna with olives, currants, almonds, and coconut with soy lime vinaigrette. And that's just an appetizer!

Asia de Cuba

Appetizers

Tunapica
Tuna tartare picadillo sauce with Spanish olives, black currants, almonds, and coconut with soy lime vinaigrette over wonton crisps

Thai Beef Salad
Seared carpaccio of spicy beef with avocado, shredded coconut, orange segments, and Asian salad with hot and sour dressing

Cangrejo and Asian Mushroom Cakes
Crab cakes with scallops and shiitake mushrooms with chipotle remoulade

Peking Duck Salad
Grilled sweet corn arepa, Asian greens, and cabrales blue cheese vinaigrette

Cuban Black Bean "Soup" Dumplings
Roasted tomato-ginger sauce and citrus palmetto salad

Asian Pesto Grilled Shrimp
Wok-charred tropical fruit and crisp lotus root chips

Lobster Potstickers
Vanilla bean spiced rum and lobster coral sauces, roasted sprout salad

Entrées

Szechuan Peppercorn Crusted Sirloin
Stir-fried Chinese broccoli, yucca crisps, and guava demi-glace

Palomillo of Marinated Lamb
Pan-seared with sofrito of stir-fried peppers, onions, and Japanese eggplant watercress salad with orange oil

Rum Grilled "Chuletta" of Pork
Marinated centercut pork chop served with Shanghai bok choy

Hunan Whole Wok Crispy Fish
Stuffed with crab escabeche, red pepper sauce

Miso Glazed Salmon
Wild "chofan" of vegetables and Chinese long beans

Pan-Seared Ahi Tuna
Served rare with crunchy wasabi mashed potatoes and chimichurri sauce

Seasame Crusted Seared Diver Scallops
Thai coconut rice, mango salad, and passion fruit vinaigrette

Anise Scented Corn Tamal
With wild mushroom chow mein

Side Orders

Stir-Fried Coconut Rice

Wok-Sautéed or Bamboo-Steamed Asian and Caribbean Vegetables

Cuban Black Beans

Lobster Boniato Mash

Black Bean Croquettes

Indochine

The tropical look of this upscale French-Vietnamese restaurant makes you think Catherine Deneuve might walk by at any moment, and so she might, for Indochine attracts a mature, very classy crowd—including audience members and actors from the famed Public Theater across the street. Offering a menu at once authentic and uniquely the creation of chef Huy Chi Le, Indochine is a treat for all the senses.

Indochine

Mixed Green Salad
With lemongrass vinaigrette and fried ginger

Fried Spring Rolls
With shrimp, bay scallops, and fresh crabmeat and mango-tamarind dipping sauce

Pan-Fried Vegetable Ravioli
Filled with asparagus, water chestnuts, and black mushrooms, with soy-lime sauce

Spicy Beef Salad
Thinly sliced filet of beef with basil, mint, lemongrass, crisp shallots, and a spicy oil-free dressing

Salad of Grilled Marinated Shrimp
With green papaya, jicama, daikon, cucumber, carrots, peanuts, and a Vietnamese ginger vinaigrette

Baby Squid Salad
With an oil-free spicy tamarind dressing, hijiki, shallots, and mint

Summer Roll of Vegetables and King Crab
With black bean sauce

Grilled Eggplant
With lime juice, ginger, and sesame seeds

Grilled Brook Trout
Stuffed with Asian basil and black bean sauce

Seared Arctic Char
With a pesto of preserved lemon and coriander seed, on a bed of cumin-spiced cabbage

Amok Cambodgien
Filet of sole with coconut milk, cabbage, and lime leaves, steamed in a banana leaf

Steamed Filet of Sea Bass
With ginger, scallions, and asparagus

Grilled Whole Prawns
Marinated in ginger and scallions on a bed of rice angel hair noodles

Spicy Shrimp
Sautéed with long beans, diced fresh tomato, and basil

Vietnamese Bouillabaisse
Sea scallops, prawn shrimp, baby squid, mussels, and cabbage, in a lime leaf and galangal sauce

Boned Roast Duck
With ginger and steamed Asian greens

Chicken Breast Stuffed with Shiitake Mushrooms
Kaffir lime leaves, coconut milk, with water spinach and lotus root chips

Assorted Grilled Vegetables with Fresh Herbs

The Russian Tea Room

Few places say "New York" as glamorously as the Russian Tea Room. Standing "slightly to the left of Carnegie Hall," as the famous ad used to say, the RTR has long been a glittering home for the city's cultural and literary communities. In 1995, it was purchased by theatrical producer/restaurateur Warner LeRoy, who revitalized this icon and reopened it—bigger, better, and more glamorous than ever—in 1999. Now run by Warner's youngest daughter, Jenny LeRoy, the classic establishment draws eager crowds of hip, young trendsetters. Blintzes, blini, and caviar—and still plenty of choices for Picture-Perfect Weight Loss.

Russian Tea Room

First Course

Baked Potato with Caviar

Hot Borscht
Braised meats, beets, horseradish dumplings, caramelized bacon onion potato pirozhki

Pelmeni
Siberian veal and beef dumplings in chicken broth, mustard, dill, and sour cream

Summer Pea Soup
Apple peekytoe crab salad, crispy potatoes, sevruga caviar

Tsar's Salad
Russian Caesar salad

Mixed Green Salad

Mussels a la Russe
Black bread crouton, Russian mustard

Smoked Salmon
Blini, crème fraîche

Oysters of the Day

Potato Galette
Smoked salmon, sevruga caviar, baby cress salad

Main Course

Coulibiac of Salmon
In puff pastry with champagne sauce

Lobster Blinchiki
Rolled blini, lobster-mushroom fricassee, lobster bisque

Stuffed Striped Bass
Sautéed summer vegetables, citrus vinaigrette

Chicken Kiev
Panfried Russian fingerling potatoes with bacon and asparagus

Duck Tabaka
Pommes fondantes, baby beet greens, port sauce

Beef Stroganoff
Beef tenderloin, mustard cream sauce, and dill ribbon noodles

Braised Lamb Shank
Vegetable caviar, dried fruits

Roasted Veal Chop
Sautéed summer vegetables, sour cherry sauce

Pan-Seared Cornmeal Cake
Fricassee of wild mushrooms and asparagus, natural jus

Blini Royale
Napoleon of blini, smoked salmon, scrambled eggs, sevruga caviar

Blintzes
Blueberry, cherry, cheese

Tea Room Chopped Salad
Red onion, cucumber, Feta cheese, smoked chicken, peas, asparagus, tomatoes, eggs, haricots verts, romaine and arugula, meyer lemon herb vinaigrette

Seafood Chopped Salad
Red onion, cucumber, Feta cheese, calamari, crabmeat, baby shrimp, lobster, peas, asparagus, tomatoes, eggs, haricots verts, romaine and arugula, meyer lemon herb vinaigrette

Georgian-Spiced Seared Halibut
Potato puree, baby leeks, red wine sauce

Pan-Seared Scallops
Asparagus, peas, mushrooms, upland cress, barley risotto

Tuna Tartare
Avocado, breakfast radish, pickled melon, citrus vinaigrette

Crab Salad
Crispy soft shell, peekytoe crab salad, asparagus, tomato, lemon caper vinaigrette

Grill

Tuna Steak
Haricots verts salad, tomatoes, yogurt, and mint

Swordfish
Haricots verts salad, tomatoes, yogurt, and mint

Russian Mustard Glazed Chicken
Georgian vegetable rice pilaf

Shrimp Shashlik
Apple celery remoulade, baby spinach

Desserts

Strawberry Napoleon
Vanilla crème brûlée, muscat ice cream, sweet basil sauce

Frozen Pistachio Nougat
Mixed berries, orange pepper tuile, passion fruit coulis

Blueberry Baklava
Vanilla ice cream, lemongrass dipping sauce

Valhrona Chocolate Wheel
Mint ice cream, strawberry surprise

Melon Soup
Frozen yogurt

Sorbets
Mango, strawberry-guava, or chocolate

Soufflé Duo
Lemon soufflé, vanilla whipped cream
Chocolate soufflé, crème anglaise

Ocean Grill

Cool, dark, and absolutely swinging, this seafood restaurant in a beautiful building on Manhattan's trendy Columbus Avenue—near the American Museum of Natural History—is one of a trio of fish houses owned by aquatic impresario Steve Hanson. Like Hanson's other entries, Blue Water Grill on the East Side and the downtown Atlantic Grill, the Ocean boasts a raw bar and consistently fresh seafood. The word "grill" in the name is an important giveaway: That's mostly how the fish dishes are prepared.

Ocean Grill

Appetizers

Lobster Bisque

Crispy Point Judith Calamari

Bamboo-Steamed Dumplings with Spicy Asian Dipping Sauce

Sesame-Crusted Lobster Roll with Sweet Pepper Glaze

Maryland Crab Cake with Roasted Red Chile Basil Sauce

Maine Lobster Crêpe with Lobster Sauternes Emulsion

Chilled Jumbo Shrimp Cocktail with Three Sauces

House Entrées

Lobsters: Steamed, Broiled, or Grilled

Three Peppercorn Seared Yellowfin Tuna with Soba Noodle Stir-Fry and a Miso-Ginger Vinaigrette

Chervil-Rubbed Atlantic Salmon with Pencil Asparagus, French Fingerling Potatoes, and Sautéed Wild Morel and Cremini Mushrooms

Blackened Swordfish with Sweet Potato-Crabmeat Hash

Maryland Crab Cakes with Roasted Corn Salsa and Roasted Red Chile Basil Sauce

Classic Seafood Cioppino with Shrimp, Scallops, Clams, Mussels, Calamari, and Sea Bass with Garlic Croutons

Poached Mahi Mahi with Golden Leek Mashed Potatoes and a Savory Lobster, Corn, and Asparagus Ragout

Pine Nut–Crusted Chilean Sea Bass with Grilled Eggplant, Zucchini and Spaghetti Squash, Marinated Red Pepper, and a Sweet Roasted Garlic Sauce

Alaskan "Singing Bay" Scallops, Littleneck Clams, Prince Edward Island Mussels, and Trumpet Pasta in a Garlic–White Wine Sauce

From Our Wood-Burning Grill

Atlantic Salmon

Yellowfin Tuna

Florida Grouper

Pacific Mahi Mahi

East Coast Swordfish

Gulf Shrimp and Sea Scallops

Heartbeat

In Heartbeat, famed restaurateur Drew Nieporent and chef Michel Nischan have created a place where heart-healthy food is the mission—and where just about every menu item is a Picture-Perfect Weight-Loss choice. Organic ingredients claim the spotlight without the addition of butter or cream. It's high-quality, low-calorie food—beautifully prepared and presented.

Heart Beat

Summer Squash Soup

Green Salad with Young Seasonal Lettuce

Asparagus with Lemon and Mustard

Asian Pear Salad with Tamari Pecans and Maytag Blue Cheese

Chilled Oysters on the Half Shell with Osetra Caviar

Seared Tuna with Citrus and Fennel

Sashimi of Fluke and Sweet Shrimp

Maryland Lump Crab Cake with Lemon and Basil

Pistachio Roasted Baby Chicken with Asparagus and Morels

Greenmarket Vegetables with Fire-Roasted Pepper Sauce

Pan-Roasted Monkfish with Fava Beans and Porcini Mushrooms in Spring Garlic Broth

Wild Pacific Salmon with Sweet Pea Sauce

Steamed Black Bass with Lime and Bok Choy

Grilled Rack of Lamb with Cherry Horseradish and Fresh Mint Salad

Filet of Naturally Fed Beef Tenderloin with Wild Mushrooms and Baked Yukon Potato

Dry-Aged New York Strip Steak with Fingerling Potatoes

All of our entrées can be prepared simply plain, with organic seasonal greens, lemon, and lime.

Sides

Grilled Asparagus with Corn Béarnaise

Virgin Whipped Potatoes

Sautéed Porcini with Garlic

Brown Rice

Picture-Perfect Weight Loss Nationwide: Eating Well across the United States

As the previous menus illustrate, New York City offers some of the world's finest cuisine. But that's not to say that there aren't equally wonderful restaurants in all parts of the country. In fact, some of the world's most innovative and imaginative chefs are at work all across the United States, and their creations prove that you can find Picture-Perfect Weight-Loss choices anywhere and everywhere. Read on for some examples.

Los Angeles: Campanile

Housed in a building designed by Charlie Chaplin, Campanile is the apex of Cal-Med cuisine, where the ingredients and forward thinking of the Golden State meet the rich culinary traditions of the Mediterranean. It's the perfect setting for an appetizer of summer ice oysters with champagne mignonette, or of grilled sardines on spaghetti with pine nuts, currants, and *cavolo nero*. For a main course, think about grilled rare tuna with ragout of sprouted legumes, arugula, and romesco. Then cap the meal with a dessert bowl of Persian mulberries.

Pittsburgh: The Steelhead Grill

Another entry in the restaurant portfolio of award-winner Drew Nieporent (this time with Pittsburgh chef Greg Alauzen), The Steelhead focuses on absolutely fresh seafood, "grilled, steamed, or sautéed." That makes it near-perfection for Picture-Perfect Weight Loss, from its seared rare tuna salad with warm soy wasabi dressing to its Steelhead minestrone soup to the Steelhead cioppino with shrimp, littleneck clams, and sea scallops—and more just like it.

Seattle: Flying Fish

The inventive Flying Fish menu features lots of Pacific seafood and an Asian accent in many of its dishes, but that's just for openers. How about an appetizer of lobster ravioli with morel mushrooms and leeks? Or an entrée of pine nut and sun-dried tomato risotto with halibut and portobello mushrooms? Or maybe the spicy lobster with a hoisin chili glaze?

Houston: Café Annie

An elegant setting—richly paneled mahogany walls, checkered limestone floor, leather banquettes, high ceiling—enfolds one of the nation's most innovative menus, with a range of choices for the weight-conscious. You might start with the black bean terrine, fresh tomato salsa, and minced avocado, or with a mussel soup with cilantro, serrano chiles, and ancho chile jam garnish. Then how about the yellowfin tuna—seared rare—in a sauce of fresh tomatoes and extra-virgin olive oil with avocados and a black olive tapenade? Or maybe wood-grilled shrimp with sweet garlic cloves and sprigs of cilantro, accompanied by thin-cut fries? Cleanse your palate with a fresh fruit sorbet for dessert.

Washington, D.C.: Kinkead's

In their kitchen open to full view, Kinkead's chefs focus on modern American cuisine—and, no doubt, on the power elite chowing down in the dining room. A fistful of appetizers includes jumbo lump crab cake with mustard sauce and corn pimento relish, or a platter of snap peas, grilled shiitake mushrooms, and Thai basil. An arugula fennel salad features tuna carpaccio, pine nuts, and basil. For your entrée, how about the horseradish- and walnut-crusted flounder with cauliflower flan, baby carrots, shiitake mushrooms, and sherry beet sauce? That's just one suggestion in a realm of possibilities.

San Diego: Azzura Point Restaurant, Loews Coronado Bay Resort

Elegant and exotic—decorated in taupe, gold, persimmon, and mureno green—Azzura Point offers sweeping ocean views and, naturally, a focus on fish and farm-fresh vegetables. Ahi a la Niçoise, baby romaine hearts, or poached spot prawn make a tasty prelude to a dish of potato gnocchi with English peas and black truffles or to a range of seafood main courses. Top it all off with a California peach parfait with peach lemon verbena sorbet—and white chocolate ice cream!

Philadelphia: Striped Bass

Given its raw bar featuring clams and oysters from various locations, the caviar sampler allowing tastes of a variety of caviars, and appetizers and entrées that feature beautifully prepared fish and fresh vegetables, the exceptional Chef's Table menu at this all-seafood restaurant looks almost as if it had been designed specifically with Picture-Perfect Weight Loss in mind. Try the seared dayboat sea scallops for an appetizer, served with pickled chanterelle mushroom, flageolet beans, haricots verts, and chives. Or the seared copper river salmon with marinated artichokes, fresh herbs, and balsamic vinegar. For a main dish, how about pan-roasted black bass with watercress-potato

puree, or roasted lobster with porcini mushrooms, garlic butter, and pearl onions? Executive chef Terence Feury has even created a Tasting Menu, offering a little bit of a lot of fish and vegetable dishes—a wonderful idea!

San Francisco: Delfina

In a city that is world-renowned for its numerous superb restaurants, Delfina stands out—primarily for the inventiveness and unique style of chef-proprietor Craig Stoll. Starting out as a neighborhood storefront eatery, Delfina today is a sleek, hip, well-appointed restaurant that nevertheless maintains the lack of pretense of its beginnings as well as its commitment to local, seasonal ingredients and simple preparation. Seafood-based appetizers run to such treats as grilled fresh Hawaiian plantation shrimp with warm white bean salad, fresh-cured anchovies, or salt cod *brandade*—or try the warm porcini salad with dandelion and red wine vinaigrette. For a main dish, sample gnocchi with morels and corn—or a range of fish entrées, from local king salmon to local sand dabs.

Boston: Sonsie

Rated the best place in Boston for people-watching, Sonsie, on elegant Newbury Street in the Back Bay section of town, is also a gourmet's delight, especially if the gourmet is weight-conscious. A range of seafood-based appetizers is supplemented by the likes of Vietnamese vegetable spring rolls. The steamed Chinese dumplings or the fish and shellfish "zuppa" with pasta are good choices, as are such main dishes as charred salmon, baked wild mushroom crepes with artichoke, or wok-seared tuna. Of special interest are the many beautiful side dishes, from Yukon Gold potato puree to spinach leaves with extra-virgin olive oil to thick portobello slices with garlic and parsley.

Atlanta: Pano's and Paul's

A top-of-the-line Atlanta restaurant known for luxury and its clubby atmosphere, Pano's and Paul's offers a range of generously portioned, beautifully prepared fish entrées: Atlantic salmon fillet with red wine–braised French lentils; or sautéed Chilean sea bass with baby artichokes, Fingerling potatoes, and white asparagus; or the yellowfin tuna seared in a cracked pepper coriander crust with English peas and Hanshiminji mushrooms. If you think you'd like an appetizer as well, try the platter of fava beans and morel mushrooms.

Dallas: The Mercury

The atmosphere is rustic but elegant, with polished dark woods, soft fabrics, and fine art—something for just about all the senses. For the sense of taste, the weight-conscious find a range of choices: appetizers like Gulf shrimp cocktail with salsa cruda and avocado mousse, or blue crab and asparagus salad, or smoked salmon, or a selection of soups. There's even a wild mushroom risotto. Entrées include such unusual offerings as glazed black cod with fresh mango and hot mustard sauce; truffle-crusted halibut with asparagus-and-leek papardelle, morels, and tomato broth; and a portobello mushroom "sandwich" on sourdough bread with basil aioli, onions, and warm yellow tomatoes.

Miami: Norman's

Norman Van Aken is one of the country's most impressive innovators of New World cuisine, fusing Latin, Asian, and Caribbean flavors, and this restaurant in a two-story freestanding Mediterranean building is his headquarters. Here, he has concocted such appetizer treats as yucca-stuffed crispy shrimp or "clear" gazpacho and crab cocktail with smoky truffle ice, sherry foam, and Grey Goose vodka. There are main dishes like skate wing teriyaki on a tiny shrimp ramen noodle pad thai, and a spinach and beet lasagnette with wild mushrooms and wilted arugula—not to mention pan-cooked fillet of Key West yellowtail with asparagus spears or spice-crusted wild striped bass.

Week 4 goals:

☐ Eat a meal at a restaurant: Find and order the Picture-Perfect Weight-Loss choices on the menu, and use your voice to speak up for your needs.

☐ Decide on your choice of exercise, structure a program, and commit to your workout schedule!

☐ Assess your Food Awareness progress: Recognize what you've accomplished and evaluate the task still ahead.

☐ Practice "reading" menus the Picture-Perfect Weight-Loss way.

Chapter 10

DAY 30: CELEBRATE!

30-Day Plan

						1
2	3	4	5	6	7	8
9	10	11	12	13	14	15
16	17	18	19	20	21	22
23	24	25	26	27	28	29
30						

By the end of today, you will have:

- Celebrated the end of the Plan and the start of your changed relationship with food
- Learned how to "get through" holidays the Picture-Perfect Weight-Loss way

It's Day 30 of the Picture-Perfect Weight Loss 30-Day Plan—time to celebrate.

And celebrating sets the stage for focusing on low-calorie ways to enjoy all of life's happy occasions: special events, holidays, parties of every kind. To help with this, I'll offer tips and advice from patients who have successfully negotiated the dangerous shoals of holiday temptations, avoiding or surviving potential pitfalls.

Your Final Assignment

Before we get to the discussion of eating for special occasions, there is still a little bit more work to do to finish up our 30-Day Plan. Today, you have a simple, two-step assignment.

Step 1: Weigh Yourself

Climb onto the scale, check your weight, and then find the page in your personal food diary/journal where, 30 days ago, you wrote down your starting weight. Note the difference between the two numbers.

Of course, the weight loss of these first 30 days is probably not a complete surprise to you. My bet is that your clothes fit a bit more loosely, your energy level is up, and you feel better about yourself—more understanding of your emotional life and more mindful of your eating, more confident in a newly strong body. As I said earlier in the book, this is not about numbers on a scale.

Still, seeing the weight loss measured quantitatively—hard numbers on a piece of paper—can really bring home to you how far you've traveled in these first 30 days. You're in quite a different place from where you were a mere 4 weeks ago—and not just in terms of pounds. Congratulations!

Before you close your journal, though, note also that there's plenty of room on this page to continue jotting down your weight in the weeks, months, even years to come. The point, of course, is that this first weight loss is only the beginning. You haven't come to the end of anything; you've made a successful start.

Step 2: Celebrate!

The progress you've made so far is worth marking in some congratulatory way. After all, you have set in motion profound and fundamental changes in your life. You have refashioned your eating habits, introduced a range of new food options into your daily menu, changed your relationship with food. You have begun regular physical activity, and you have committed yourself to a program of exercise as an integral part of your life and your lifestyle. You have learned how to probe what might be the underlying causes of your former weight gain, and you have begun to analyze your own needs and to understand that they are best met by nutritious, low-calorie eating that ensures weight loss and good health for life. This is a very great deal to have accomplished in a mere 30 days; it's an accomplishment that deserves to be celebrated.

But how? At the end of fad weight-loss diets, most people celebrate by treating themselves to all the foods they've been deprived of by the diet. They'll have a blow-out meal—or a blow-out couple of days—filling up on those personal favorites they weren't "allowed" to eat during the diet. That, of course, is simply the first step down what is invariably a slippery slope to regaining all the weight they've lost—and probably more.

We've talked about this repeatedly in this book—how deprivation simply doesn't work, how diets may actually have the opposite effect from what is intended. The research on this renders absolutely consistent results, and those results are compelling—namely, that the weight loss achieved by dieting is temporary for virtually all dieters, even those who are certain they can beat the statistics. I can't put it better than a National Institutes of Health study group did when it concluded that "as much as two-thirds of the weight lost [is] regained within 1 year" of a diet and "almost all by 5 years." The reality, said the study group, is that "achieving and maintaining a healthy weight is a lifelong challenge" that can only succeed if and when an individual's "pattern of eating and activity is . . . permanently altered."

You've now taken the first step toward permanently altering your pattern of eating and activity, and it would be a fool's errand to celebrate that achievement by reverting to your old pattern. Remember: "If you do what you did, you get what you got."

The fact is, though, that life is full of celebrations, and celebrations almost without exception include food and alcohol. For birthdays, graduations, weddings—from birth to death, and *including* birth and death, people the world over come together to eat and drink. You can't go through life avoiding these occasions because of the high-calorie eating they promote. Nor can you go through life afraid of such occasions. Picture-Perfect Weight Loss is about changing your relationship with food, not your lifestyle. So how does Picture-Perfect

Health Tip: Enjoy Your Food

Researchers from Sweden and Thailand have found that enjoying food is key to realizing the health benefits of the food. When a simple Thai dish was served to women of the two cultures, it was found that the Thai women absorbed significantly more iron from the dish than did the Swedish women, who found the food too spicy. This is evidence that the brain is the first step in digestion, instructing the stomach to start issuing the gastric juices and thus starting the digestive process. By contrast, not liking the way a food looks or tastes can actually reduce the spontaneous muscle-driven movement of foods through the digestive tract.

Bottom line: Enjoying food is important to healthy eating and to satisfying your hunger. No wonder the dietary guidelines of Great Britain, Australia, Korea, Thailand, Vietnam, and Norway all recommend that people enjoy what they eat. It's good for you!

Weight Loss "get you through" celebrations, holidays, special occasions, even those religious observances that call for ritual foods or big family meals?

You know the answer already. *Your changed relationship with food keeps working whatever the occasion.* It's as viable on a normal Tuesday as on the Tuesday of your 50th birthday, as operative during the dull, hard-working month of March as during the high-partying month of December. No food is forbidden, and special occasions are special occasions, but there is almost always an alternative to the high-calorie option—and now you know how to find it, and you are empowered to choose it.

The Holidays

I know: It's practically unpatriotic or a mortal sin not to overeat and overdrink on national and/or religious holidays. Think about Valentine's Day with its promise of a romantic dinner at a fabulous restaurant, the hard-drinking partying on St. Patrick's Day, Easter with its emphasis on gifts of candy and sweets, the Fourth of July barbecue, the Labor Day picnic. How is one to "get through" such holidays as these, holidays that almost depend on eating—even on specific foods—as integral to the way they're celebrated?

Above all, how are the weight-conscious to get through that autumn-winter season known as "The Holidays," the dreaded season that starts with Thanksgiving and progresses in a rising crescendo of rich food to Christmas, Hanukkah, Kwanza, and then the show-stopping gourmet overkill of New Year's? For my patients and others trying to lose weight or maintain weight loss, I know that this time period can cause a real sense of unease—even apprehension.

Of course, the holidays are typically a period of stress and anxiety as much as of joy and celebration for a great many people—those not concerned about weight loss as well as those who are. There is so much going on, so much expected of people, so much expected of the time of year itself. We're *supposed* to have fun and feel wonderful; we have an *obligation* to be joyous, and that sense of obligation is the cause of a lot of stress and anxiety.

Part of the obligation may mean getting together with family—something that is easy for some people, but not at all easy for others. What's more, the general atmosphere is one of fun, partying, and good times, so people feel required to enjoy every minute of the holiday weeks—or at least to look like they're enjoying every minute, and that, of course, is another contributor to stress.

Further, the party atmosphere is everywhere. There are the office parties, the holiday lunches with clients, the cocktail parties at the neighbors', the party you really must give this year. For those who may be having a rough time emotionally, this constant round of social gatherings can simply act as a reminder of how awful they feel—and serve as another cause of anxiety.

For the weight-conscious, there's the added burden of wondering, "How am I going to get through all the eating?" During the season between Thanksgiving and New Year's Day, there is so much special-occasion food available on a regular basis that the issue is not so much the particular food offered at one dinner or one party, but rather what I call the pile-on effect:

the number of events at which food is the centerpiece and where eating and drinking are the main activities.

The pile-on effect also means that there are more factors you can use to justify eating high-calorie foods. Maybe you feel you really owe it to your client to take him out for a very special meal at a very special restaurant. Or, your client has gone to a lot of trouble and expense to take *you* out for a very special meal at a very special restaurant. How can you say no? Once at the restaurant, can you really order a side dish and a salad? Or, it's Thanksgiving or Christmas or New Year's Day or vacation time or a party—you name it—and eating this food or that meal is a family tradition or a once-a-year event or it's your favorite food or it's good business to eat up—pick one—and so on and on and on. All are fine justifications for eating high-calorie foods, but during the holidays, there are more and more occasions warranting these justifications; they pile on in rapid succession, day after day.

Tips for Holiday Weight-Loss Maintenance

In short, during the holiday season, both the types of food served and the circumstances in which they're served offer the weight-conscious serious grounds for concern. Still, the Picture-Perfect Weight-Loss philosophy remains the same—make the low-calorie choices where possible, don't waste calories unnecessarily, make sure you keep up your exercise program, avoid deprivation, eat a variety of foods, and remember that no food is forbidden. Here are some specific tips to make it easier to implement the philosophy:

First, it's probably slightly more efficacious to do your exercise workout before the big holiday meal. On Thanksgiving Day, for example, do your jogging or play your game of touch football in the morning, and then eat a light snack. This will keep you from arriving at the meal starved. As we know, that backfires.

In fact, do what some politicians do before they head out for a round of meetings, parties, or fund-raisers: Eat before you go. Take the edge off your hunger with a piece of fruit, for example, washed down with a couple of glasses of a low-calorie beverage.

Once you're at the party, keep in mind that studies show people do eat more at buffets. Since you're not all that hungry anyway, having snacked before coming here, try to keep your distance from the food area where the guests are densely grazing among the hors d'oeuvres, imported cheeses and sausages, exotic breads, calorie-laden dips, and mayonnaises. If this is a cocktail party, remember that a meal will follow—where you can almost surely find low-calorie choices.

Finally, a word about alcohol. There is research to support the proposition that drinking alcoholic beverages may actually increase appetite. In fact, studies show that drinking prompts people to eat more, eat faster, eat for a longer time, and keep on eating even after they are full. In addition, alcoholic drinks tend to be high in calories. And you probably don't need a research study to know that drinking can certainly decrease your resistance to temptation—including the temptation of high-calorie foods. So booze offers a triple whammy to the weight-conscious: It is high in calories, makes you eat more, and probably incites you to eat high-calorie foods.

But what if the fact is that you like liquor, wine, or beer, and you believe that at a cocktail party, or dinner, or most social gatherings worth the name, drinking is part of the fun. What's the solution?

My standard advice on this subject is pretty simple—and highly effective. Make the first drink a seltzer or mineral water or even plain water—dolled up with a twist of lemon or lime if you like. Why? Because the first drink tends to go down very quickly; it's all too easy to gulp it almost without noticing, then move on to a second, third, and even a fourth drink.

What my patients find is that making that first drink a glass of cool, clear club soda offers the exact same social effect as a double bourbon on the rocks—without the potentially dangerous effect on eating habits. You'll still be standing around with an elegant glass in your hand. You'll still be sipping away just like all the other guests. In fact, you'll be sipping more slowly, making it last even longer. Finally, when you've drunk it down, order your glass of wine or your cocktail or your bottle of beer—or even better, make the second drink a club soda, too. And if the party is a dinner, be sure to ask for water as well as alcohol; then alternate between the two as the meal progresses. It's a way to pace your drinking as well as to lessen its impact on your eating.

Grilling Lesson

As one of my patients once said: The steak and turkey burger on the left look like the amount of food you would eat while deciding what to eat. If so, you'd be nibbling on high-calorie foods that are not particularly healthy. Contrast that now with the vast amount of food on the right, the caloric equivalent of those meager meats on the left. The lesson is simple: For the same number of calories as those meager meats, you could eat an astonishing amount of food—more varied, far healthier, and much more filling food. *If* you could eat it all. It's worth thinking about when you haul out the backyard grill this summer—or at any time of the year.

6 oz steak 490 calories
4 oz turkey burger 240 calories

TOTAL 730 calories

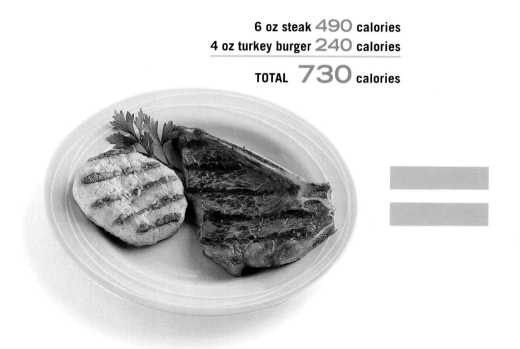

4 oz grilled tuna 140 calories
veggie burger on bun 190 calories
veggie frank on light bun 120 calories
3 small ears corn 90 calories
2 grilled tomato halves 20 calories
2 grilled red onion slices 20 calories
2 grilled eggplant slices 20 calories
2 grilled portobello mushrooms 30 calories
2 grilled summer squash slices 20 calories
assorted marinades and condiments 30 calories
¾ lb assorted melon 50 calories

TOTAL 730 calories

Served "Al Fresco"

It's a hot summer day, and you're in the mood for deli—and lots of it. If you also want to eat a healthy and low-calorie meal, think about the choices on the right. You get not only a deli-taste sandwich, but a second sandwich as well; the two together cost fewer calories than the single sandwich on the left—and are much healthier.

In addition, you fill up on loads of interesting and savory vegetables—as opposed to the virtuous-looking but seriously high-calorie small salad on the left. (Note that 1 cup of the pasta salad is almost four times as calorie-laden as the 2 cups of vegetable salads on the right.) The meal on the right also gives you a cooling, tasty, and very nutritious bowl of soup.

Watch out on the beverages, too. Exercise caution when you see the words "naturally flavored" or "naturally sweetened"; such beverages can contain hidden sugar calories.

3 oz prosciutto	270 calories
4 oz Gruyère cheese	460 calories
baguette (5 oz)	400 calories
a few leaves of greens and a drizzle of olive oil	120 calories
1 cup pasta and vegetable salad	350 calories
1 bottle sparkling water beverage with all-natural fruit flavor (20 oz)	200 calories
TOTAL	**1,800** calories

VS.

1 pint chilled red pepper soup 100 calories
1 marinated portobello mushroom 20 calories
1 poppy seed roll (2 oz) 160 calories
red onions, greens, and salsa 20 calories
8 slices veggie deli
and veggie cheese 160 calories
Italian bread (3 oz) 240 calories
creamy mustard, greens,
and sliced tomato 20 calories
1 cup pickled beet salad 50 calories
1 cup marinated artichoke hearts 40 calories
diet beverage 0 calories

TOTAL 810 calories

Take Me Out to the Ball Game

Sushi at a ball game? It's happening more and more. The point is that even at the ballpark, it's possible to find healthy, lower-calorie choices. Of course, if part of your idea of going to a ball game is to have a hot dog and beer, go for it—but do so mindfully. And if you're eating the hot dog just because it's part of the ritual—rather than something you're really hungry for—maybe it's time to look around for other options.

hot dog with bun and mustard 330 calories

French fries 400 calories

beer 150 calories

TOTAL 880 calories

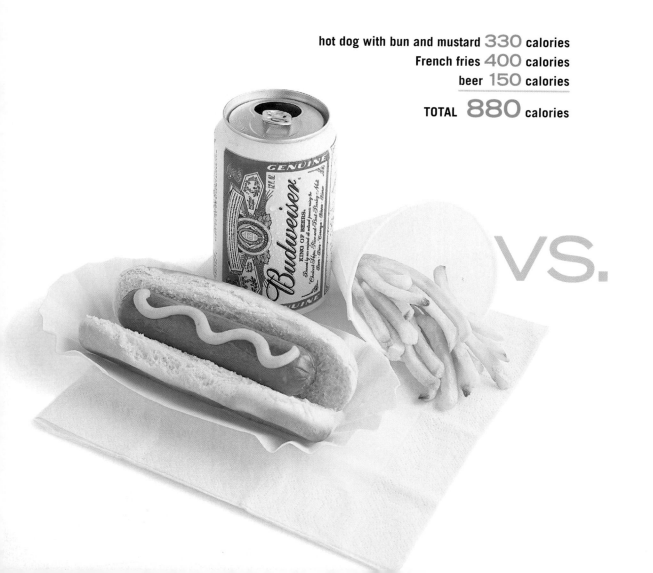

7 pieces sushi 240 calories
1 potato knish 200 calories
2 cups fruit 100 calories
diet soda 0 calories

TOTAL 540 calories

Stadium Munchies

What could be more virtuous than a small chicken Caesar salad? The very sound of it, not to mention its appearance—healthy green lettuce, pale chicken—speaks volumes about health and nutrition and, of course, weight loss.

So it probably comes as a surprise to hear that the fun food shown here—peanuts and a beer—carries the same calorie count. Nutrition-wise, in fact, the 50 peanuts are a far healthier protein source than the chicken. With their high content of essential fatty acids, fiber, vitamins, and minerals, peanuts are a boon to heart health. And, washed down with beer, they're a lot more fun than a Caesar salad, too.

small chicken Caesar salad
450 calories

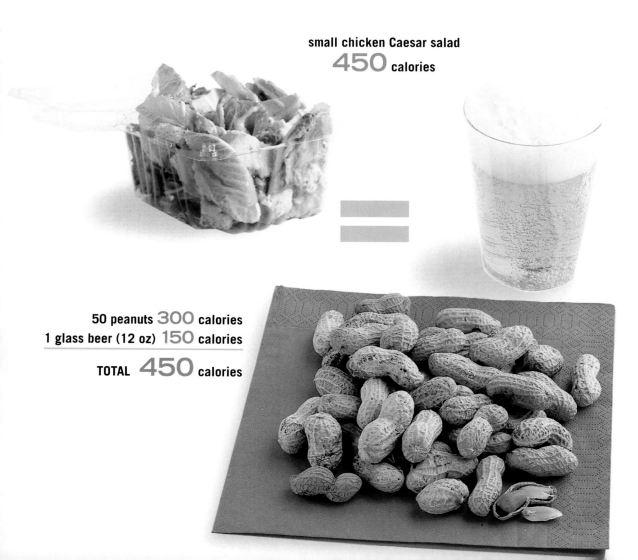

50 peanuts 300 calories
1 glass beer (12 oz) 150 calories
TOTAL 450 calories

Slice of Pizza?

It's no secret that pizza is in no way a low-calorie snack. But if you are going to allow your-self this treat, consider the calorie difference between pizza with meat and cheese and a slice with cheese only. The 200-calorie gap is enough to hold a cup of beer—even a little more!

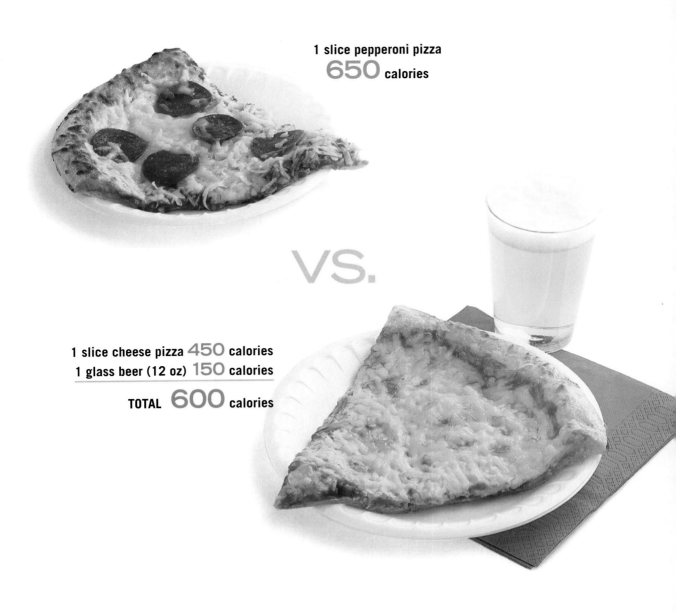

1 slice pepperoni pizza
650 calories

VS.

1 slice cheese pizza 450 calories
1 glass beer (12 oz) 150 calories

TOTAL 600 calories

Upscale Appetizers

Like appetizers? The smoked salmon choice gives you a far bigger portion, plus diverse tastes and a real health hit. Salmon is an excellent source of omega-3 fatty acids, which are essential for heart health, your immune system, even disease-fighting. The salmon's "good" fat contrasts favorably with the pâté and cheese's high concentrations of "bad" saturated fat. It means the pâté and cheese square offer a little bit of food at a high cost of the least healthy kind of calories.

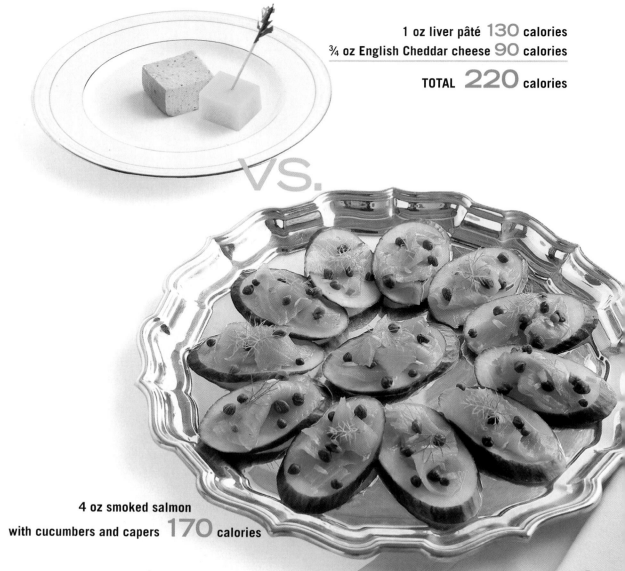

1 oz liver pâté 130 calories
¾ oz English Cheddar cheese 90 calories

TOTAL 220 calories

VS.

4 oz smoked salmon
with cucumbers and capers 170 calories

Hors D'Oeuvres

Smoked sturgeon offers as luxurious and indulgent a taste as a wedge of Brie, yet its calorie count and nutrition power make it a perfect choice for hors d'oeuvres—in fact, a Picture-Perfect choice. Add the tomatoes stuffed with crabmeat, also low-calorie and nutritious, and you have a generous helping of a delicious appetizer. By contrast, the cheese is not the healthiest choice—for reasons that go beyond its high content of saturated fat. And when you consider that you'll surely eat a full meal afterward, it's certainly no calorie bargain, either.

3 oz Brie 300 calories

3 oz smoked sturgeon 100 calories
6 tomato cups stuffed
with crabmeat 200 calories

TOTAL 300 calories

Cute Quiches

These mini-quiches *are* adorable. And they're tempting, like so many of the hors d'oeuvres passed around on platters at parties. But because they're so easy to pop into your mouth mindlessly as you chat with someone, they're dangerous stuff and can add significant calories. Fortunately, there *are* alternatives, and in today's world, they're showing up at more and more receptions and events. Take the crabmeat-stuffed cucumber cups on the right. In fact, take a few. At just about 25 calories a pop, they are a cool, rich-tasting calorie bargain to enjoy at any cocktail party.

3 mini-quiches 360 calories

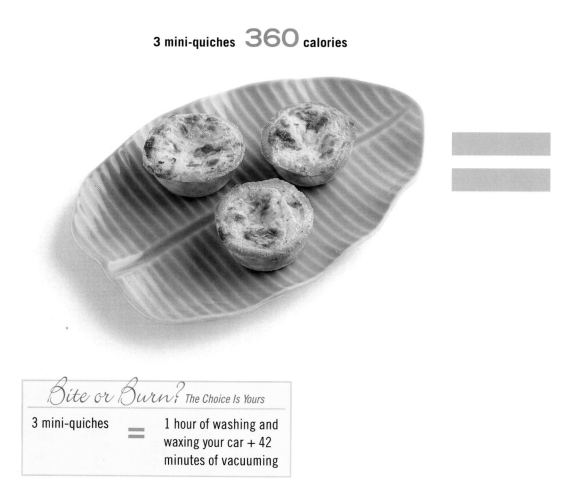

Bite or Burn? The Choice Is Yours

| 3 mini-quiches | = | 1 hour of washing and waxing your car + 42 minutes of vacuuming |

14 cucumber cups filled with crabmeat
360 calories

Vegetable Appetizer

Even a vegetable party appetizer can add calories if it's fried. Frying adds fat as well. An alternative vegetable appetizer offers crudités with a range of dips. While the guacamole and hummus both have fat, it's the good kind of fat—essential for all-around good health. The range of dips has another advantage: It tempts the palate to try different tastes and take in more vegetables at the same time, for bargain prices on calories!

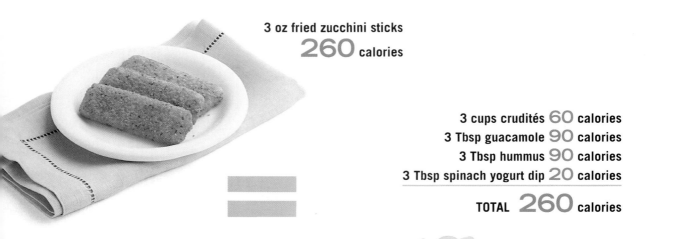

3 oz fried zucchini sticks
260 calories

3 cups crudités **60** calories
3 Tbsp guacamole **90** calories
3 Tbsp hummus **90** calories
3 Tbsp spinach yogurt dip **20** calories

TOTAL 260 calories

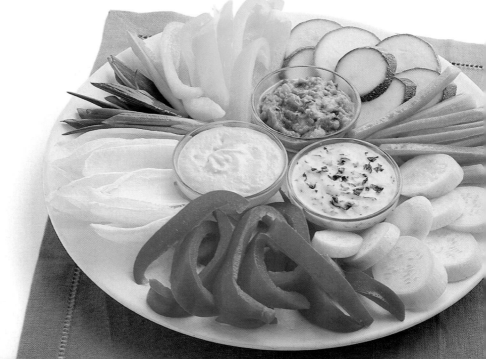

Sophisticated Lady

This tiny bite of foie gras on toast will cost you 370 calories. Want to serve your guests an equally sophisticated hors d'oeuvre for far fewer calories? Have Jeeves pass around this platter of potatoes and blinis with caviar, then down a few—with your pinkie lifted, of course.

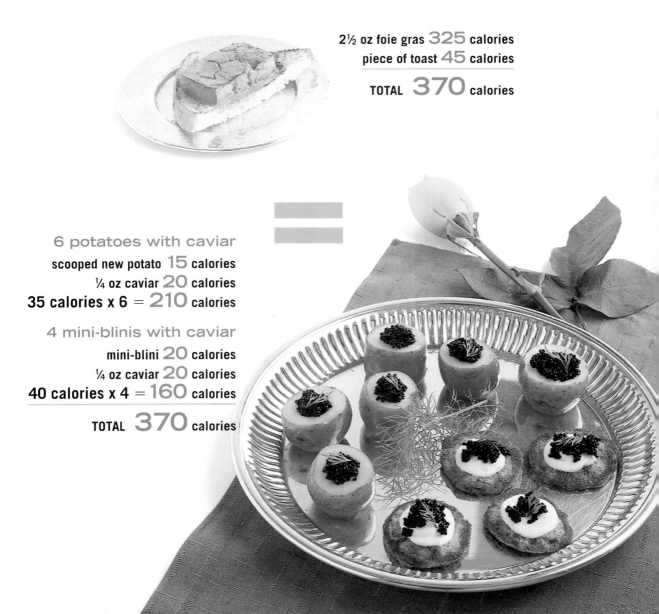

2½ oz foie gras 325 **calories**
piece of toast 45 **calories**

TOTAL 370 **calories**

=

6 potatoes with caviar
scooped new potato 15 **calories**
¼ oz caviar 20 **calories**
35 calories x 6 = 210 **calories**

4 mini-blinis with caviar
mini-blini 20 **calories**
¼ oz caviar 20 **calories**
40 calories x 4 = 160 **calories**

TOTAL 370 **calories**

Getting Liverish from Foie Gras

Foie gras—literally, "fat liver"—is a costly, up-market delicacy served in only the finest restaurants. Its rich taste is pleasing to some, but for the weight-conscious and those concerned about health, even the tiny slice pictured below is a minefield of fat and cholesterol. It contains the cholesterol equivalent of 16 slices of fatty bacon and the fat equivalent of 7 ounces of fried pork rinds. Adding insult to injury, the foie gras production process has been banned in eight countries on grounds of animal cruelty.

3½ oz foie gras
240 milligrams of cholesterol
71 grams of fat

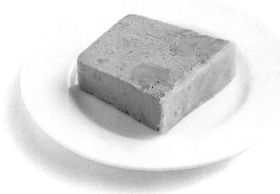
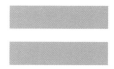

16 slices fatty bacon, 240 milligrams of cholesterol

7 oz fried pork rinds, 71 grams of fat

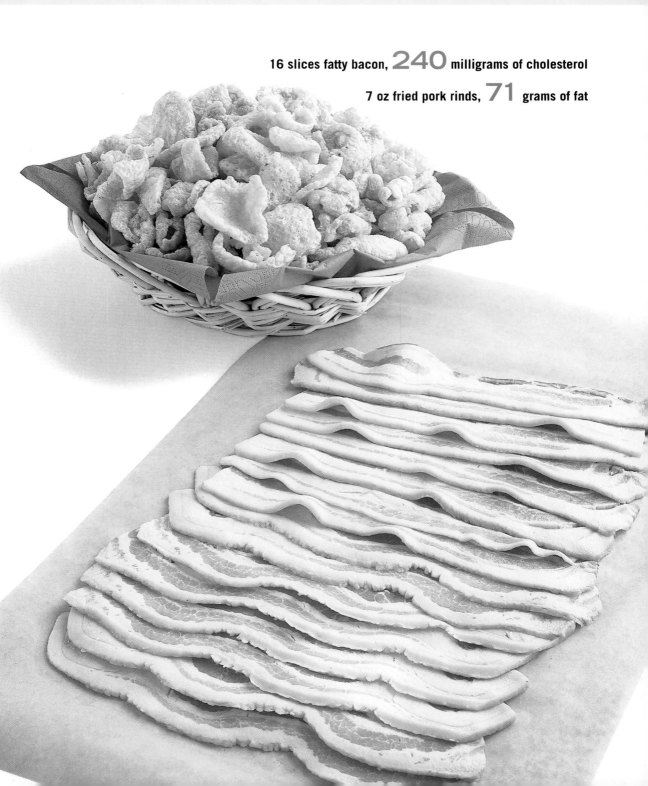

Four to One

More than four to one: Those are the odds by which veggie pâté beats liver pâté when it comes to saving calories.

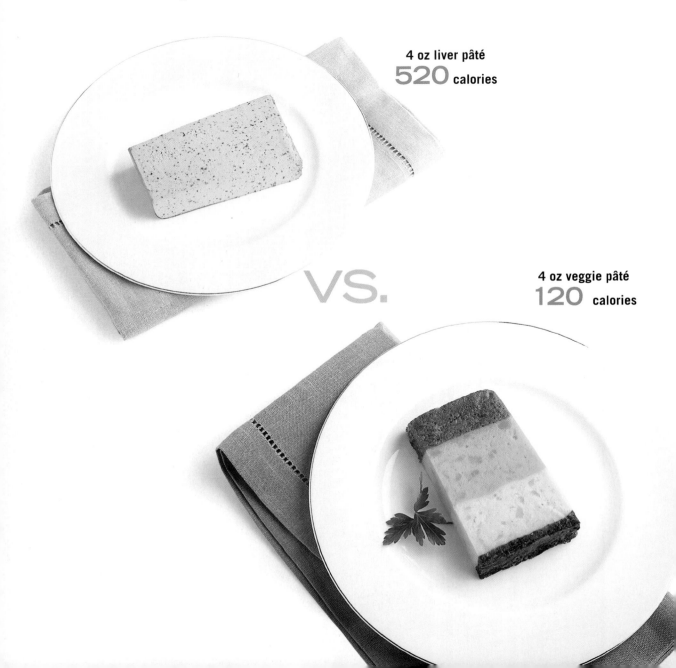

4 oz liver pâté
520 calories

VS.

4 oz veggie pâté
120 calories

Giving Thanks with Relish

Give thanks! It is possible for stuffing to be low-calorie, healthy, and absolutely delicious, as shown here. The bottom line? Relish as much of it as you like, secure in the knowledge that you've made a Picture-Perfect choice that will satisfy your appetite.

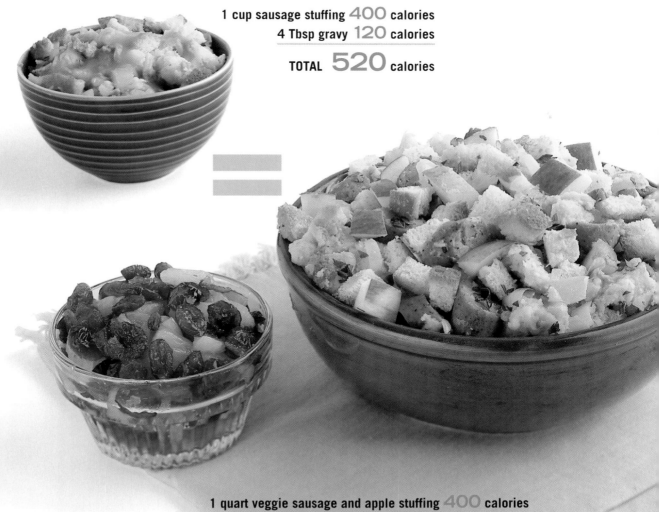

1 cup sausage stuffing 400 calories
4 Tbsp gravy 120 calories

TOTAL 520 calories

1 quart veggie sausage and apple stuffing 400 calories
½ cup pineapple cranberry relish 120 calories

TOTAL 520 calories

Festive Finger Food

Finger food: It's so easy to just keep on eating it. Take the pastry snack on the left. It's a small amount of food at a big cost in calories. Down even a few of these appetizers, and you've consumed a substantial number of calories—before sitting down for dinner. Take in the same number of calories with the choices on the right—all of them—and you do yourself a nutritional favor while getting a jump start on satisfying your appetite.

3 pastry hors d'oeuvres (2 oz) 270 **calories**

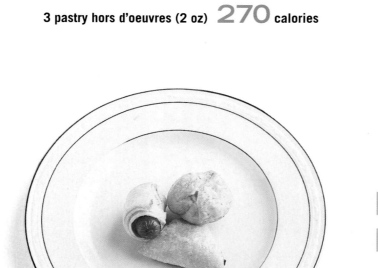

4 oz shrimp with cocktail sauce 140 calories
marinated asparagus wrapped in veggie ham
(9 stalks asparagus and 3 slices veggie ham) 80 calories
6 grilled mushrooms with 2 Tbsp black bean sauce 50 calories

TOTAL 270 calories

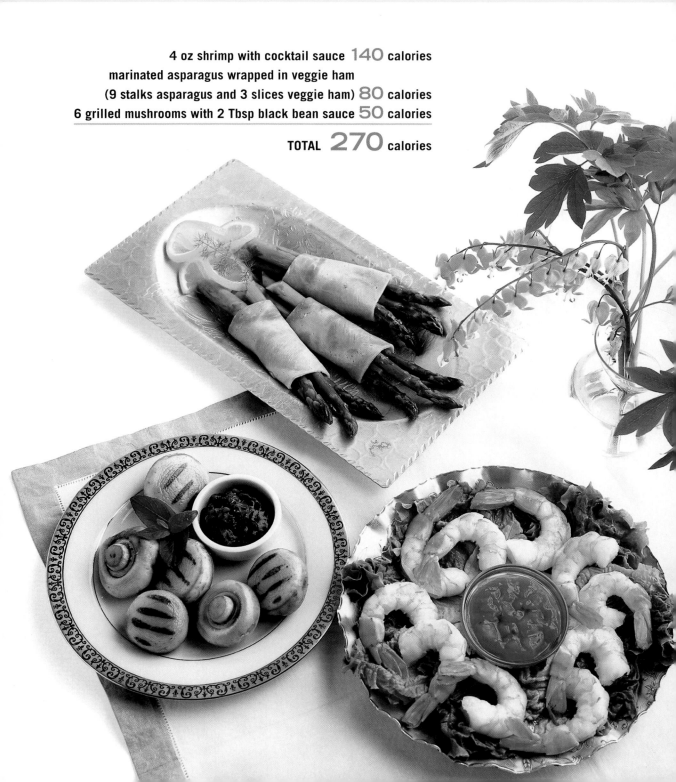

Special Occasion

A special occasion doesn't have to be synonymous with a high-calorie meal. Take a look at this comparison. The meal on the right is every bit as festive as the one on the left. In fact, you could argue that, with lobster and wild mushrooms, the meal on the right is even a bit more upscale. It's also a more intriguing menu—one that is creative and that required real thought and imagination. All in all, it's a very apt offering for a special occasion—at less than half the calories of the "special" meal on the left.

1 cup creamed seafood in pastry shell 400 calories
7 oz roast duck 680 calories
1½ cups long-grain and wild rice
(prepared with herbs and 1 Tbsp butter) 420 calories
½ cup green beans 20 calories
½ cup crème brûlée 280 calories

TOTAL 1,800 calories

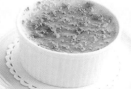

VS.

1½ cups sautéed wild mushrooms 100 calories
8 oz lobster tail 240 calories
1 cup long-grain and wild rice (prepared with herbs, sherry, and broth) 200 calories
1 cup green beans 40 calories
stewed tomato 20 calories
¼ cup citrus dip for lobster 60 calories
1 scoop blood-orange sorbet with orange slices 70 calories

TOTAL 730 calories

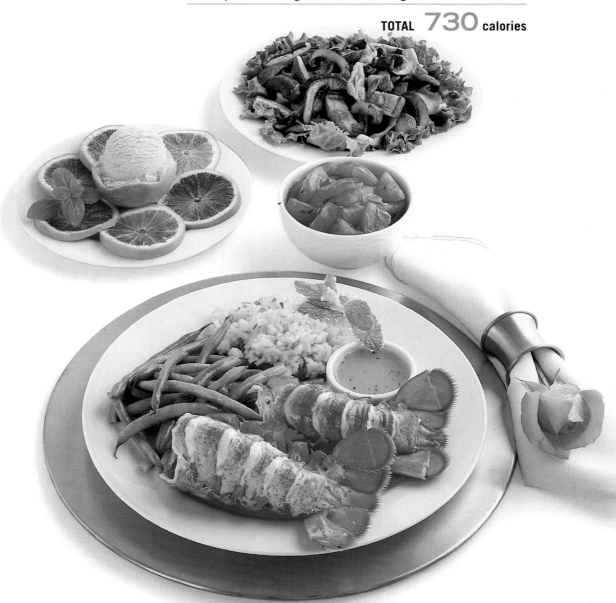

Eager for Eggnog?

To many people, eggnog is as much a part of the holiday season as gifts and decorations. But it's important to be aware of its cost as well as its role in the festivities. And the cost is high, with a heavy concentration of fat, sugar, and alcohol giving eggnog its excessive calorie count. Of course, you shouldn't give up your holiday cheer, but think about saving the eggnog for a very special occasion.

1 cup eggnog 600 calories
fat content equivalent to 5 pats of butter
sugar content equivalent to 6 tsp of sugar
alcohol content equivalent to 3 Tbsp of alcohol

Winter Holiday

Chilly weather outside makes you want something comforting and lush inside. Pecan pie certainly fills the bill, but at an exceptionally high calorie cost. Similarly dark and sweet are such treats as those pictured on the right: fruit cake, dried plums, and figs. A bite of each of these items satisfies both the tastebuds and the craving for comfort—without the high cost in calories.

wedge pecan pie
640 calories

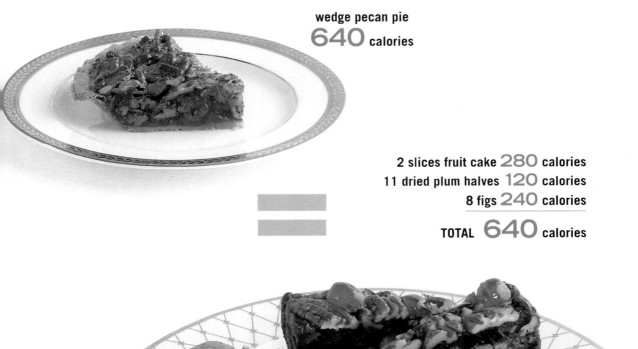

2 slices fruit cake **280** calories
11 dried plum halves **120** calories
8 figs **240** calories

TOTAL 640 calories

Holiday Cheer

Of course, I'm not recommending that you drink everything pictured on the right. But just take a look at how much holiday cheer you *could* imbibe for the same calorie count as one measly eggnog. What's more, the eggnog gets most of its calories from saturated fat—the bad kind of fat. Besides, what says "holiday" better than rich red wine or sparkling champagne?

Bite or Burn? The Choice Is Yours

| 1 cup eggnog | = | 2.4 hours of dancing or 5.4 trips up and down the steps of the Statue of Liberty |

1 cup eggnog 600 calories

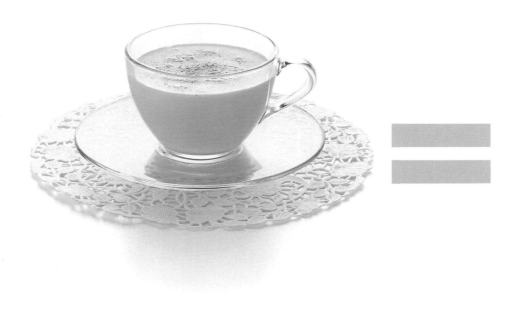

3 4-oz glasses champagne 270 calories
3 4-oz glasses red wine 270 calories
3 4-oz glasses sparkling fruit punch made
with champagne, diet ginger ale, and fruit 60 calories

TOTAL 600 calories

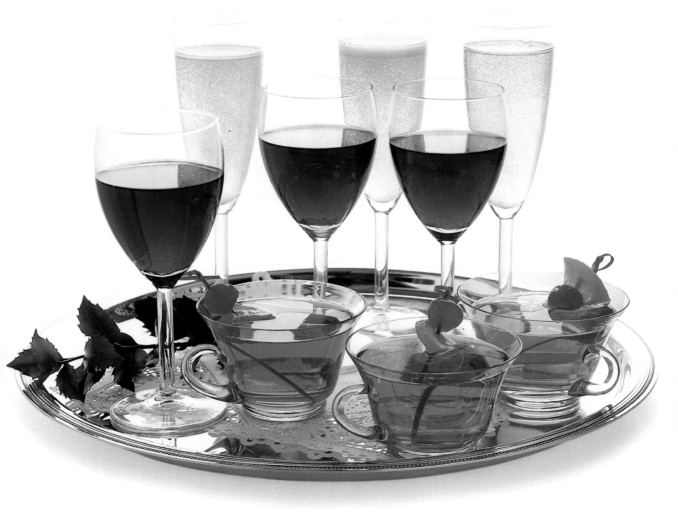

For Special Holidays, Special Treats

Easter means candy—and there are lots of choices. Instead of the traditional Easter egg and jelly beans, there are lower-calorie options like special Easter lollipops. Mix and match for the best combination of special-occasion taste at the lowest calorie cost.

1 Easter egg (1 oz) 120 **calories**
2.8 oz jelly beans 280 **calories**

TOTAL 400 **calories**

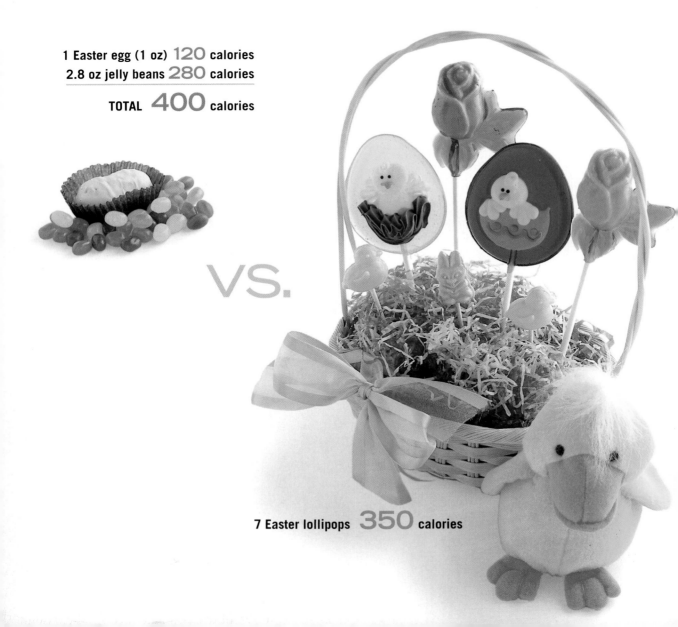

VS.

7 Easter lollipops 350 **calories**

Choosy Chocolates

When you choose chocolate as a special treat for a special occasion, think about something that is both festive and lower-calorie. The chocolate-dipped fruit on the right makes a colorful and impressive display that is more than good enough to eat. There's more of it—and at far fewer calories than you think.

3 chocolate truffles (3 oz total)
420 calories

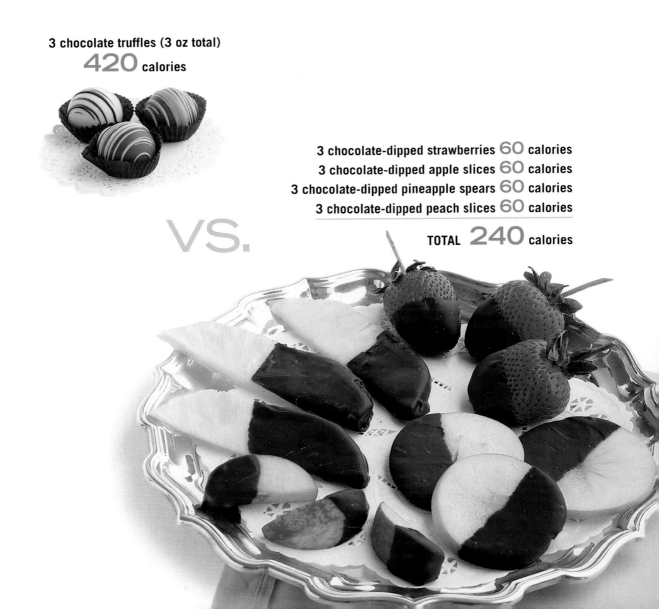

VS.

3 chocolate-dipped strawberries **60** calories
3 chocolate-dipped apple slices **60** calories
3 chocolate-dipped pineapple spears **60** calories
3 chocolate-dipped peach slices **60** calories

TOTAL 240 calories

The Picture-Perfect Weight-Loss Journey

We've come to the end of the 30-Day Plan—but not, as you can see, to the end of this book. What's left? Well, I've said all along that the 30-Day Plan is a way to get you started on a journey. Over the last 4 weeks, you've acquired the equipment you'll need for the journey: You know how to read food labels . . . how to shop for Picture-Perfect Weight Loss . . . how to make different choices for breakfast, lunch, dinner, and snacks . . . how to explore and express your needs. You have empowered yourself—and in the case of children, you have helped to empower your kids—to set out on an entirely new path when it comes to eating.

Like all paths, this new way of eating will have some bumps and potholes. That's what I'll be addressing in the next chapter. For now, however, celebrate! You've successfully turned onto the right road for Picture-Perfect Weight Loss and a lifetime of healthy eating.

Day 30 goals:
- [ ] Weigh in.
- [ ] Celebrate! You're starting down a new road. . . .

PART III

THE DIET-FREE LIFETIME PLAN

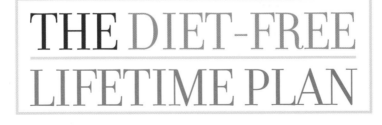

Firefighter Michael Carter lost
80 pounds on Dr. Shapiro's plan.

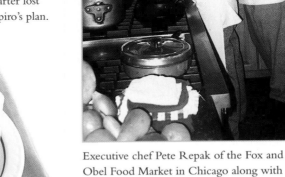

Executive chef Pete Repak of the Fox and
Obel Food Market in Chicago along with
associate Kathleen Perez prepare meals for the
seven people in the locked house featured on
Good Morning America.

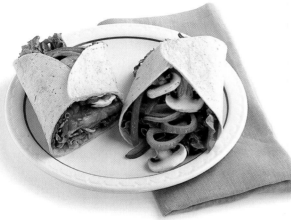

Chapter 11

TROUBLESHOOTING

I've seen it hundreds of times: A patient comes in for an appointment after a vacation of 1, 2, 3 weeks—or even longer. She "knows" she has slipped back into old habits of eating, and she is "certain" she put on weight during her vacation. Yet the scale shows that she has dropped 2 pounds, or 3, or even, as in the case of one patient who was away for a month, 7 pounds! A month's vacation—and a loss of 7 pounds.

Why was this patient so surprised? Why are all these patients who "know" they've slipped so surprised? Because vacation is outside the routine of their normal daily lives. It's time away, a holiday—even from Picture-Perfect Weight Loss! Or so you think. You're off to see new places, do fun things, experience a range of adventures. One of those adventures is eating. Whether you're headed for an exotic destination where you want to test and taste the local fare, or going back to your favorite resort where you know the food is superb, eating well is an integral part of what constitutes a vacation. So why didn't these patients put weight back on?

The answer is because once you have be-

come a Picture-Perfect Weight-Loss eater—once you have learned the principles of Food Awareness Training and have become mindful about your food choices—you never really do slip all the way back to your old habits. You simply can't.

Here's another example: A lot of the firefighters tell me they are certain they will never eat another bagel again as long as they live. I am certain they will. What they won't do—ever again—is start the day with two bagels slathered with butter or cream cheese. In fact, eating a bagel will never again be an issue to the firefighters. It will be a choice—something they reach out for among a range of options, something they enjoy much more than they ever did when they were wolfing down two at a time without thinking. My firefighters, like my vacationing patients, have learned to think differently about food. And that has changed everything.

Picture-Perfect Weight Loss is a journey. There are pitfalls along the way—some hidden hazards, some all-too-obvious difficulties. Whether you realize it or not, you're now fully equipped and totally prepared to deal with all dangers; you're ready to shoot down any trou-

Seafood Vegetable Pasta "El Barrio"

Firefighters typically consume a quarter to a third of a pound of pasta "in a single sitting—with the big guys going back for seconds," says Jimmy Lanza of Ladder Company 43/Engine Company 53 in New York's "El Barrio," the neighborhood also known as Spanish Harlem. That's why his recipe for Healthy and Delicious Seafood Vegetable Pasta is making such a difference for the hearts, health, and waistlines of his fellow officers. "By adding good-tasting, low-calorie ingredients like shrimp, scallops, clams, and vegetables in large quantities, everyone gets to eat enough to feel full," Lanza notes. "At the same time, the ingredients reduce the risk of cancer and the chances of having a heart attack." He's right, and in the process, he has come up with a Picture-Perfect pasta dish. Here's his recipe. Since it will feed 12 to 14 New York firefighters, divide the amounts by 3, 4, 6, or any other appropriate number to come up with portions that make sense for you and your family.

Healthy and Delicious Seafood Vegetable Pasta

1   large red onion, sliced into half-rings

1   garlic clove, minced

4   cans (16 ounces each) white clam sauce

1   can (46 ounces) vegetable or onion broth (or broth made from bouillon cubes)

8   ounces sun-dried tomatoes

1   can (5½ ounces) water chestnuts

2   cans (16 ounces each) chickpeas

5   pounds assorted fresh or frozen vegetables

3   pounds penne rigate pasta

3   pounds sea scallops

1   large red pepper, sliced in strips

Juice of 2 fresh lemons

1   tablespoon lemon pepper

1   tablespoon capers

3   tablespoons grated Parmesan

3   cans (6½ ounces each) minced or chopped clams

3   pounds peeled, deveined shrimp

Italian parsley, to taste

16   ounces large pitted black olives

Grated cheese, Italian parsley, crushed red pepper, to taste

Spray a skillet with Pam. Place over medium heat and sauté the onion and garlic until soft. In a large saucepan, heat the clam sauce, broth, sun-dried tomatoes, water chestnuts, and one can of chickpeas. Add the onion and garlic. If using fresh vegetables, blanch or steam them separately to soften. Start boiling the water for the pasta, according to the package directions. At the same time you add the pasta to the boiling water, add the scallops, red pepper, lemon juice, lemon pepper, capers, Parmesan, and vegetables to the sauce. Pour the second can of chickpeas into a blender and puree; add the puree to the sauce to thicken it. Add the clams, shrimp, parsley, and olives to the sauce. Cook the pasta until it is firm to the bite. Pour the sauce over the pasta to serve; garnish with extra grated cheese, parsley, and/or crushed red pepper to taste.

bles ahead. Let me show you what I mean. We'll start with some obvious obstacles.

The Snack Attack

It's 11:00 at night. You got up from the dinner table 4 hours ago—satisfied with what you had eaten. You are tired and about to go to bed. But unaccountably, inexplicably, you are ravenous. What do you do?

Or, it's 3:00 A.M., and you find yourself sitting bolt upright in bed. So far from feeling sleepy, you feel an irresistible craving for something salty or crunchy. Before you know it, your bare feet have taken you to the kitchen.

Or, it's 4:00 in the afternoon. You ate breakfast, had a quick but hearty lunch, and have been working flat out all day. You could use a pick-me-up—a break for something sweet to keep you going.

How do you get past the snack attack?

You don't. There is no "wrong" time to eat. The idea that the calories in a late-night snack won't be burned off is simply not true. The notion that eating in the middle of the night means you won't sleep well the rest of the night is dubious. The theory that an afternoon pick-me-up is the first step down the slippery slope to weight gain is nonsense.

Actually, you've already started dealing with the late-night or middle-of-the-night snack. It was back in chapter 5, when you went shopping on day 1 of your Picture-Perfect Weight Loss 30-Day Plan. What you bought then represents the food choices available to you when you're assailed by a snack attack at bedtime or in the middle of the night. For that salty or crunchy craving, try a few pretzel rods or a sour pickle. If sweet is what you want, grab a low-

calorie Fudgsicle or Creamsicle, or maybe a sorbet or a fat-free frozen yogurt. And you can always fall back on hard candies or Tootsie Pops.

When the snack attack occurs during the day when you're at the office, you have even more choices—and you know what to do with them. Go for a high-fiber snack like fruit to take the edge off the craving—and to "pick up" your quotient of healthful nutrients.

The Dessert Dilemma

To dessert or not to dessert—it seems always to be the question. And by now you know the answer: The choice is yours. Make it mindfully, and if possible, go for the lower-calorie option. Remember that there are lots of ways to enjoy the special pleasure of dessert, including frozen yogurt, sorbets, fresh fruit, or a cooked fruit concoction like poached pears *flambé* in Grand Marnier—all delicious, all low-calorie.

Some situations, however, make the dilemma even more problematic. Suppose you are a guest at a dinner party. Dinner was delicious, if a bit on the high-calorie side, but you filled up on the vegetables, went easy on the meat dish, avoided the cream sauce, and enjoyed your meal thoroughly. Now the hostess serves a lavish chocolate cake—homemade—for dessert. What do you do?

One reaction is simply to choose to have the cake because you want it. Period. Another is to decide it would be rude to refuse the hostess's offering—an ungracious rejection of her hard work. On the other hand, do you really want the 500 calories the cake represents? And if you have just one bite and leave the rest, isn't that just as much a rejection as saying no to the offer—maybe even more of a rejection?

Tom's Tactics

Firefighter Tom Kontizas applies strategy to mealtime—especially when he is eating a firehouse meal. His tactics make sense for anyone—whether you're preparing your own meal or eating a meal prepared by others—and I'm grateful to Tom for sharing these tactics with my readers.

1. Drink one or two glasses of water before a meal—any meal. It takes the edge off the appetite.
2. Start with a salad, include a wide range of vegetables—whatever is in the fridge, Tom says—and eat a lot of it. Tom's favorite ingredients are Boston and romaine lettuce, red onion, marinated artichoke hearts, and tomatoes. His favorite dressing is either bottled light creamy ranch or his own homemade vinaigrette. It consists of equal parts of extra-virgin olive oil and balsamic vinegar, Dijon mustard, fresh garlic, and salt and pepper to taste. Tom also likes to sprinkle some grated Parmesan over the salad.
3. When eating rice or pasta, combine it with an equal amount of vegetables. Tom's favorite is Goya yellow rice mixed with peas and pearl onions. He uses frozen vegetables, but any fresh or canned vegetable will do as well.
4. For dessert, stick to sorbet and/or any fruit in season.

Tom has also become a highly skilled Picture-Perfect Weight-Loss chef. Here's one of his tasty recipes.

Baked Fish Fillets

4 flounder fillets, about 6 ounces each (or other variety of fish)

1 tablespoon extra-virgin olive oil

2 tablespoons white wine

Chopped fresh garlic, to taste

Chopped parsley, to taste

Fresh lemon juice, to taste

Salt and pepper, to taste

Lemon wedges

Preheat the oven to 350°F. Spray a baking dish with garlic-flavored Pam. Arrange the fillets in the dish and add the oil, wine, garlic, parsley, lemon juice, and salt and pepper. Bake for 10 to 15 minutes, or until the fish flakes easily. Serve with the lemon wedges.

The fact is that it's perfectly easy and not a violation of etiquette simply to say, "None for me, thank you," when the cake comes your way. If further explanation seems desirable, you have a range of possibilities. You can explain that "the dinner was so good I have no room for anything more," or you might suggest that you're "allergic to chocolate" (yes, you react by gaining weight), or you could just say that you're "watching calories." People understand.

Similarly, this is something worth thinking about when you're the one doing the entertaining. Do dinner guests really demand those drop-dead desserts that impress the eye and overload the system with caloric richness? Instead of setting out to strut your stuff with some fabulous dessert confection, your guests might be just as pleased—and possibly extremely grateful—to be served a *macédoine* of fruit with a splash of kirsch, or maybe baked apples stuffed with raspberries, or perhaps cool, clean melon halves with an assortment of sorbets from which to choose. After all, you're probably not the only one who is concerned about nutrition and conscious of calories.

Fruit desserts offer lots of choices and lots of chances for creativity, but I've known patients who try to eat *only* fruit desserts as a way of trying to wean themselves away from their craving for sweets. It doesn't work. In fact, there is no cure for the desire for sweets, and any effort to kill the desire will only come back to haunt you—just like any kind of deprivation. Fruits are delicious and make wonderful desserts, but they don't have to substitute for sweets all the time. On the contrary, it makes sense to include lower-calorie sweets in your diet on a regular basis; that actually reduces the intensity of the craving.

With dessert as with every food, rigidity won't work, and abstinence will only make the heart grow fonder. Don't be afraid of dessert. Approach your dessert options mindfully— then choose the one that's right for you.

The Vacation

You're off to Paris, and there's no way you're not going to sample the culinary highlights of the world's most famous cuisine.

Or, you and your spouse, a real wine lover, are heading to the Napa Valley for a combination wine-tasting tour/second honeymoon. It's absurd to think you're going to "watch what you eat" as you compare Chardonnays on a romantic terrace overlooking a vineyard.

Vacations are the time to indulge yourself, the time to splurge. But indulging yourself and splurging don't necessarily mean reverting to old habits of eating. A vacation is a change of routine, but it doesn't mean a change in the Picture-Perfect Weight-Loss philosophy. It's always possible to experience the special tastes of vacation time within the framework of Picture-Perfect Weight Loss.

My advice is to leave for vacation with a plan in mind. Just as you think about how you'll spend your time, consider also how you'll spend your calories. Just as you lay out different clothes to pack for different weather and varied occasions and events, try to lay out where you might splurge on high-calorie food choices and where you can indulge in lower-calorie choices. Thinking about it ahead of time can at least take the sting out of the high-calorie choices when you confront them. Whatever you do, don't leave for vacation telling yourself you "can't have" certain foods. There's no point in going to Paris to avoid croissants, no sense in steeling yourself to resist cheese with your wine in Sonoma County. You're not avoiding anything; you're just planning where those certain foods will fit in.

One other tip: The vacation eating starts when you get on the airplane, so order a special meal ahead of time, or even bring your own (especially now, when shorter flights often offer no meal at all). The same advice applies if you're driving or taking the train: Don't let yourself get over-hungry, and when there are choices before you, go for the lower-calorie options where possible.

Down in the Dumps

Sometimes, life throws you a curve. It happens to everyone, and whatever it is—job troubles, relationship troubles, illness, a death in the family—it can bring you down. The negative emotions increase your need to eat. This isn't abstract metaphor. The mind and body are connected, and that's how the connection works: Agitation in the mind stirs cravings in the appetite.

There's not much you can do about this, and certainly it's tough enough trying to deal with the issue that's troubling you without worrying about what you're eating as well. But just by being aware of the potential for mind-less eating, you bring the principles of Picture-Perfect Weight Loss to the front of your brain—and that's where they'll do the most good in guiding your eating choices. It's im-portant to try to keep in mind that high-calorie food won't put an end to your troubles or lift you out of your depression. In fact, the mind-body connection can work both ways, so that healthful, low-calorie eating may have as real an effect on your mind as your mind has on your body.

Of course, so can exercise, and this might be the time to try physical exertion as a new ap-proach to the blues. Research has shown, for example, that a "runner's high" doesn't happen only to long-distance runners. Sustained, fo-cused exercise affects certain neurotransmitters in the brain for a kind of "natural Prozac" ef-fect. Besides, it can take your mind off your troubles.

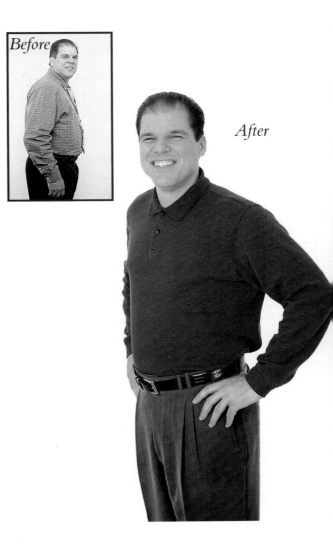

Before

After

Firefighter Dean Pappas lost 28 pounds on the Picture-Perfect Weight-Loss plan. "At first, I thought there was nothing out there I could bear to eat. Then I began to try things I'd never had be-fore: veggie burgers, veggie sausages, popcorn instead of potato chips. I liked them."

At the other extreme, try meditation as a cure for the blahs. Picturing a lovely beach with gently waving palm trees may help lift you out of your funk—talk about the Picture-Perfect way to do things!

Hidden Hazards: Food Saboteurs

In addition to the obvious difficulties along the Picture-Perfect Weight-Loss path, there are also hidden hazards. Among the most potentially damaging of these hazards are food saboteurs. Like saboteurs everywhere, these foods appear to be something they are not. That is, they appear to help you lose weight, when in fact they can actually prompt you to gain weight—mostly because you're enticed by the weight-loss claim to allow yourself to eat more of these foods than you otherwise would.

One category of food saboteurs claims to be "free" of ingredients that add calories or fat or cholesterol or are in some other way associated with weight gain—or they have reduced amounts of these ingredients. These are the fat-free baked goods, the sugar-free cookies, the dietetic candies, the low-sodium pretzels, the no-cholesterol potato chips. Well, no potato chips have cholesterol; potatoes are plant foods, and all plant foods are cholesterol-free. But check out the calorie count on even a minuscule bag of potato chips—it's bound to be high. Also, be aware that the chips may be loaded with trans fat, another kind of "bad" fat that can increase your risk for heart disease. As for eating fat-free baked goods, when you do so, you're exchanging fat calories for just as many refined-carbohydrate calories. What's more, where fat-free muffins are concerned,

you might give yourself permission to eat more muffins than the regular kind. And that, in turn, may actually make you gain weight—the very opposite of what you intend! So beware foods that are "free" of various ingredients; they may imprison you in calories instead.

I call a second category of food saboteurs the "healthy naturals." The packaging of these foods often shows a pastoral scene, and the lettering may be rustic-looking. The aim is to win you over with promises of healthy, farm-fresh eating. A carob bar instead of a chocolate bar, pretzels covered in yogurt instead of white chocolate, potato chips from sweet potatoes, honey-sweetened cookies, muffins made with "natural" fruit juice—you get the picture. What you don't get with the healthy naturals is any break at all on calories, nor any particular redeeming nutritional benefit. A potato chip is a potato chip, whether it's the traditional snack food or a sweet potato chip in a tasteful bag with a higher price tag.

How can you tell if you're being beguiled by a saboteur? You know how: Read the nutrition label. And here's a tip provided by a staff nutritionist in my office: If you would not allow yourself the "regular" version of the fat-free or "natural" food you're considering, don't allow yourself the fat-free version, either. It's quite likely a saboteur, and you're about to rationalize your way into a food choice that you would normally not make. You'll allow yourself to indulge in this rationalized food choice more often, and you'll permit yourself more liberal portions than you would if it were a "regular" food. This is why food saboteurs are the only foods the Picture-Perfect Weight-Loss program suggests you avoid altogether. Find another option.

Hit the Trail—With the Right Snack

Trail mix. It sounds like the out-of-doors, like a good, healthy hike in a pristine wilderness. What could be better for you? And that's just the way trail mix is marketed—as a "health food" with lots of nutritional value. But look closer at the nutritional values. There's plenty of added sugar in that sweetened pineapple and papaya; the banana chips are fried; the yogurt raisins contain both sugar and fat; the coconut is high in fat to begin with, then adds sugar from the sweetening process. The result? Ten ounces are practically a day's supply of calories. Stick to dried fruit snacks. The same quantity of food offers a similar taste and texture at almost half the calories and with even more nutritional power.

10 oz trail mix (coconut, yogurt raisins, banana chips, and sweetened dried fruit)
1,200 calories

10 oz dried fruit tidbits (unsweetened dried fruit: dried plums, apricots, pears, and mango)
700 calories

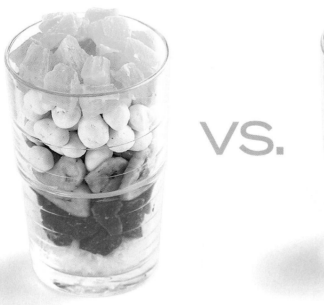

VS.

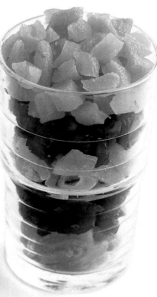

Don't Be Seduced by Reduced-Fat Claims

Don't eliminate sweets, but don't waste calories on "nutritionally correct" quasi-treats like "reduced-fat" cookies. They're no bargain!

11 reduced-fat cookies 660 **calories**

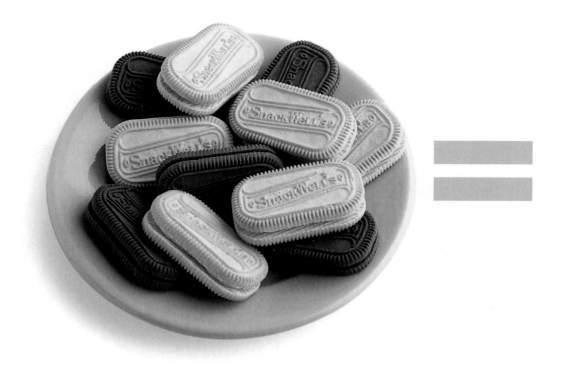

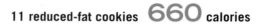

11 scoops fat-free frozen dessert 660 calories

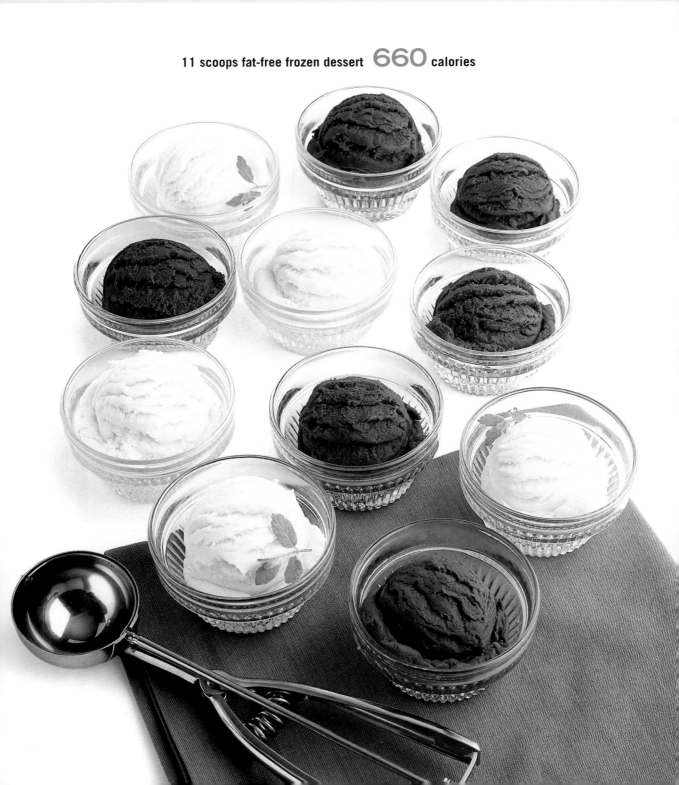

Yogurt Yarn

It's a pretzel, so it's low-calorie; it's yogurt, so it's healthy eating; and it's a tiny portion, so it's "dietetic." Right? Wrong! This demo shows you exactly why. Yogurt pretzels are saboteurs: They sound healthy and look like something a weight-conscious person should have—a weight-reducing way to satisfy a craving for both sweet and salty. Uh uh. Next time you want pretzels, have pretzels—and save enough calories to eat more snacks in the bargain.

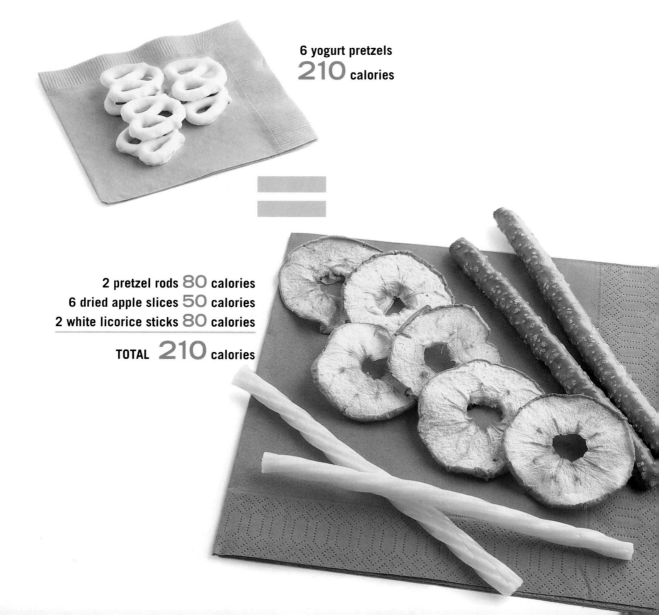

6 yogurt pretzels
210 calories

2 pretzel rods 80 calories
6 dried apple slices 50 calories
2 white licorice sticks 80 calories
TOTAL 210 calories

Fear of Thinness

Even harder to discern among the potholes that can trip you up on the path to Picture-Perfect Weight Loss is the sheer fear of thinness. What makes fear of thinness so hard to see is that it is rooted in an individual's psychology—and it can take many forms. Yet all of the guises in which fear of thinness appears have one underlying similarity: The thing that is frightening is the change from overweight to thin.

There are no two ways about it: Change can be scary—both to the person effecting the change and to those around him or her. It can seem threatening; it threatens to disrupt a way of life that, for good or ill, has become comfortable, manageable, understandable. People resist that sort of disruption—often unconsciously. Amazingly, even the person who wants to be thin can find herself resisting becoming thin.

Rocking a Relationship

Picture-Perfect Weight Loss may change the dynamics of your relationship with your spouse or lover, children, friends, colleagues. In many cases, as my staff psychotherapist Susan Amato puts it, "a person who is overweight serves a purpose in a unit—that is, in a couple or family. When one person in the unit loses weight, the whole unit changes."

Children who were used to a cozy, comfortable, chubby mom may find a svelte, glamorous mother unsettling. As one patient put it to me about her kids: "First they freaked out, then they acted out." Readjustment took time.

A husband or wife may suddenly—and unconsciously—feel insecure over the other's weight loss. Maybe he or she fears it makes the spouse attractive to the opposite sex in a new way—and that makes him or her vulnerable in a new way. The worried spouse may even try to sabotage the other's weight loss—maybe by bringing home "gifts" of candy or sweets, or by urging that the weight loss be "celebrated" at a lavish restaurant, where high-calorie foods are urged on the newly thin marriage partner.

Even friends may be threatened by your weight loss. For one thing, the overweight person is often the unthreatening "universal pal" who is invited to everything. He or she is typically thought of as an easy, restful presence—one who's not going to snag a member of the opposite sex, for one thing, but also someone who can always be relied on to fill the numbers, show up, listen to everybody else's tales of woe.

Lose weight, and your friends start to assume the weight loss has affected your character. "Can I still rely on her?" they may wonder. "Is she now going to be a competitor in the dating arena? Didn't she used to be more fun—back when she was overweight and jolly?"

As the dynamics of these relationships begin to shift, even the person trying to lose weight may hesitate. Consciously or unconsciously, you may feel a reluctance to "disappoint" your children, worry your spouse, unsettle your friends. If so, stop! Picture-Perfect Weight Loss is your decision; you're doing this for you, not for others. Their needs are their responsibility. Your responsibility right now is to you—to your need to lose weight, even if it means change. Good friends and most partners will appreciate your getting control of your life—

and delight in the hitherto undiscovered part of your personality. After all, while it may be a cliché to say so, variety *is* the spice of life. Finding new aspects to a relationship can be exciting—even if it might seem a bit unsettling.

Fear of Intimacy

It's not only your effect on others that you may worry about as you lose weight; you may also have to confront some deep-seated worries of your own, worries that being overweight had kept undercover. Psychologists often talk about the "secondary gain" that some people get from problems that seem, on the surface, to be really disturbing to them. The secondary gain that many overweight people experience is a protection against intimacy. After all, being overweight can take you out of the dating game, can serve as a barrier against the "messiness" of a romantic relationship, can take you out of the running for marriage or a lover or sexual activity. Whew! Now you don't have to compete, take a risk, put yourself out there, maybe get rejected. What a relief! Sex ceases to be an issue; even your own sexual appetite can simply be repressed, stashed away underneath your weight.

Not surprisingly, for some people, weight loss can regenerate all those fears of intimacy that have been allayed for so long by overweight. It's one of the key reasons these people resist weight loss, even though they know somewhere inside themselves that they want to be thin.

Unfortunately, there's no avoiding the risks of intimacy—and no substitute for intimacy's rewards. Relationships with others are messy, but they're worth the effort. Burying the possibility of intimate relationships in overweight

works only up to a point; if it were really making you happy, you wouldn't now be undertaking Picture-Perfect Weight Loss. Stick with it. It will open up a whole new, exciting world that you will now have the courage to enter.

Fear of Exposure

Fear of thinness really comes down to fear of exposure. It's the fear of getting attention, the fear of how others perceive you, the fear of being seen through, the fear of having to compete with everyone else—a kind of performance anxiety. It makes people uncomfortable. Staying overweight is so much safer.

In fact, staying overweight can be an eternal excuse:

You didn't get that last job promotion? It wasn't your job performance; it was your weight, you reason.

Someone else got the part in the play? You console yourself with the thought that it wasn't that you have no talent; it was that you didn't "look the part"—that is, you weren't thin enough.

A delightful patient of a few years ago was an opera singer, a job in which overweight is not traditionally considered a shortcoming. Yet Sharon never got the good jobs, never did well in auditions. "It's because of my weight," she kept insisting. But the truth was that Sharon's voice, although pleasant, didn't have the power or range or distinctiveness that her chosen field demanded. And as long as she remained overweight, she avoided facing that truth.

Sure enough, as Sharon lost weight, she had to come to grips with the fact that she wasn't going to make it as an opera singer, not because of her weight, which was now no longer an issue, but because she really didn't have what it takes. It was a tough lesson, but having learned it, a new, thin Sharon was eventually able to get on with her life. She has changed careers, and for the first time in her life, she really feels successful.

Sabotage! By Others—And by Yourself

When confronting their fears of thinness, many people sabotage themselves. Usually unconsciously, sometimes with subtle deliberateness, they put themselves in positions where there are no choices except high-calorie ones. While such situations do exist, they're the exception, not the rule. So when patients tell me of being in such situations over and over again, I suspect self-sabotage—born of a fear of thinness—at work.

Some of my patients have tried so many diets and failed so many times to keep off the weight that their self-doubt has turned into a self-fulfilling prophecy. "I'll never be able to keep this up," they say. "I've failed at so many diets before. I've done this hundreds of times, and it has never worked."

But of course, Picture-Perfect Weight Loss is not a diet. It's not like anything you've ever done before. And you *can* keep it up—for a lifetime. After all, the whole idea of Picture-Perfect Weight Loss is to make changes. At this point, 30 days into the program, you've made considerable changes already. That means you're already successful.

You've come this far. You're not going to let a few potholes slow you down, are you? There are too many rewards up ahead to stop now. Keep going. You have all you need to stay on course for Picture-Perfect Weight Loss.

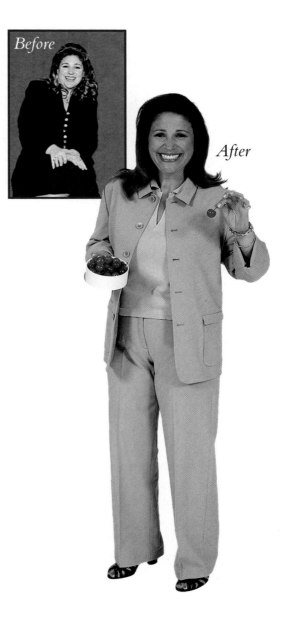

Before

After

"My generation didn't grow up with mothers who work out and have good eating habits. But I want my daughter to," notes the Chicago 7's Joanne Rusch.

Chapter 12

PICTURE-PERFECT WEIGHT LOSS FOR LIFE

Mike Carter, an official of New York's Uniformed Firefighters Union, lost 80 pounds as a result of changing his eating habits to follow the principles of Picture-Perfect Weight Loss. As of this writing, he has kept the weight off for 2 years.

Police detective Dorothy Mellone, who first came to me in 1995 after her second pregnancy brought her weight to 170 pounds, went down to 118 pounds—and has stayed at that weight ever since.

The Chicago 7 have lost a total of 282 pounds as this book goes to press; all continue to lose weight as they continue to make Picture-Perfect Weight Loss their eating norm.

None of these people have changed their lives. Mike Carter still goes to lunches and cocktail parties with politicians and lobbyists. Dorothy Mellone still goes on stakeouts. The Chicago 7 still have the jobs and families and responsibilities they had before they began Picture-Perfect Weight Loss. What they have changed is their relationship with food and their eating habits.

At cocktail parties in the state capital, where legislators and citizens meet and mingle, Mike Carter waits for the shrimp hors d'oeuvres to be passed around. Dorothy Mellone takes fruit to a stakeout, not the potato chips and fried foods her colleagues bring. David Taylor of the Chicago 7, who used to "load up on meat and have almost nothing else," has "flipped the ratio"—turned it on its head. Now, he loads up on soup, salad, and vegetables, and makes meat the small side dish in his meal. Firefighter Dean Pappas never used to eat fruit. "Now, I eat it every day," he says. What's more, Dean carries a bottle of light salad dressing with him when he goes to a restaurant, and he carries what he calls his "pacifier" Tootsie Pops all the time.

Changes—in mindset, knowledge, understanding. Additions to the mental menu—the kinds of foods they think about eating. Flipping the ratio. Carrying light salad dressing. Waiting for the shrimp. Little changes such as these have made a big difference to all these Picture-Perfect Weight-Loss veterans.

They haven't changed their lives. They've changed their relationships with food, and they've made the change an integral part of their lives. How did they do it? One meal at a time.

A Week
of Ready-Made Menus

In a way, the Chicago 7 had it easy. Because they could spare only a single week to learn Picture-Perfect Weight Loss, we had to give them a total-immersion course. That's why we locked them in a house, and it's why we devised, prepared, and served three Picture-Perfect Weight-Loss meals a day. The seven didn't have to shop for themselves or cook for themselves. They didn't even have to set the table. All they had to do was sit down at it and sample the menus before them.

In that single week, they all tried foods they had never even thought of trying before—veggie meats, Egg Beaters, light bread, tofu—all beautifully cooked for them by executive chef Pete Repak of Chicago's Fox and Obel Food Market, all combined in ingenious ways to create healthful, appetizing, low-calorie menus.

They also had a personal trainer who took them through exercise routines they could do at home easily. In addition, they had a personal nutritionist—the chief nutritionist from my office in New York—and their own personal counselor, psychotherapist Susan Amato, also from my New York team, who helped them deal with some of the issues that had kept them stalled at weights that had been making them unhappy.

Those issues—in fact, seven separate lifetimes of perceptions and habits—got locked into the house with the Chicago 7. Tia and Jim Chisholm admit that they were literally afraid of trying new foods. "We just automatically didn't bother to try anything new," says Tia. Debbie Davis struggled with a divorce and "a sense of self-pity about failure at marriage." Dick Johnson spoke of well-meaning

but hurtful comments about his weight by people who had seen him only on TV and only from the neck up. At the center of a whirling storm of family activities and demands, Heidi McInerney felt she could find time for herself only after everyone else's needs had been met, late at night, when the comforting thing to do was to eat and snack and nibble until the wee hours of the morning.

Getting help for the not-so-simple process of beginning to address these fears, problems, and issues was an important step taken by the seven, as important as the exercise, the supermarket shopping tour, the discussions and food demonstrations. That's because, as the seven learned, these issues played a role in shaping their old eating habits. If they were going to change their eating habits, these issues would have to be addressed.

Certainly, though, the meals we prepared for them were an education in themselves. The carefully designed menus got the seven thinking, not just about new foods to eat, but about the appetizing meals they could create, the nutritious and tasty meal plans they could invent on their own.

For example, the Saturday morning breakfast served to the seven consisted of cantaloupe; a vegetable omelette made with Egg Beaters and flavored with onion, peppers, mushrooms, and tomatoes; a bialy with jam or light cream cheese; and of course coffee, tea, or diet hot cocoa. That's a very hearty breakfast. It's a very tasty breakfast. It's also a breakfast that let the seven start the day with fruit and vegetables for a nutrition turbo-charge. Total calorie count? About 300 calories per person, depending on how much each ate.

"Dear Diary": What They *Used* to Eat . . .

Here are three food diaries from the "before" side of the equation—that is, before these three members of the Chicago 7 changed their relationships with food.

Tia Chisholm

Time	Food (Preparation, Serving Size)
9:15 A.M.	2 eggs scrambled with Monterey Jack cheese, 2 slices white toast with grape jam, 1 12-oz can of Classic Coke
2:45 P.M.	6 oz Cherry Coke
4:45 P.M.	12 Triscuits with Monterey Jack cheese, 12 oz Cherry Coke
8:15 P.M.	12 oz Classic Coke
8:45 P.M.	12 oz Classic Coke, 1 piece chocolate mint pie

Tia rarely sat down to a meal. Instead, she nibbled away all day at very high-calorie foods. She also drank a lot of calories, consuming a number of sodas throughout the day. Her typical "before" way of eating was fairly mindless, definitely high-calorie, and almost entirely devoid of healthful nutrients—a surefire path to overweight and health problems later on.

Jim Chisholm

Time	Food (Preparation, Serving Size)
6:00 A.M.	1 cup of coffee with 1 tsp sugar, 1 plain doughnut
12:10 P.M.	24 oz Diet Coke, 3 eggs with Cheddar cheese and ketchup, 4 oz potatoes and onions with Cheddar cheese and ketchup, 8 oz steak and ketchup
7:20 P.M.	6 oz fried ocean perch and ketchup, 12 oz Diet Coke, 2 servings macaroni and cheese
10:35 P.M.	1 bowl of Cap'n Crunch and skim milk

Jim is a big man with a big appetite, but his "before" regimen was low on fiber and heavy on high-fat foods and on frying, the most fattening of food preparation styles. For Jim, the issue was to learn to satisfy his hearty appetite with vegetables, fruit, and protein from fish, soy, and legumes—the foods at the base of the Picture-Perfect Weight Loss Food Pyramid.

Dick Johnson

Time	Food (Preparation, Serving Size)
7:00 A.M.	1 glass orange juice, 1 banana, 1 cup coffee with sugar
8:00 A.M.	1 cinnamon raisin bagel with butter, 1 cup coffee with sugar
1:30 P.M.	McDonald's cheeseburger with ketchup, Gatorade
2:30 P.M.	1 roast beef sandwich on natural wheat bread with 1 tsp of mayonnaise and 1 slice provolone cheese, 1 Pepsi
7:00 P.M.	½ serving of lasagna, Caesar salad, garlic bread, 2 glasses of Merlot
9:00 P.M.	1 bowl of Häagen-Dazs ice cream

As a TV anchorman, **Dick** works long days, and he used to simply eat all day long. Except for his salad at dinner, vegetables played a minuscule role in his daily intake, which featured high-calorie foods every few hours or so.

Another breakfast featured fresh raspberries, light waffles with light syrup, and a side order of veggie sausage links—plus coffee, tea, or diet hot cocoa. Total calories? 380.

Sunday lunch for the seven started off with minestrone soup, centered on pizza with tomato sauce and assorted vegetables, and finished off with a cooling slice of watermelon. The average calorie intake? 400 calories. Wednesday's lunch was seafood salad on Boston lettuce, marinated cucumbers and tomatoes, a seeded roll, and tangerines for dessert. 380 calories.

Dinners? Their first night in the house, the Chicago 7 dined on jumbo shrimp cocktail, penne pasta with eggplant and zucchini, and Italian ices for dessert. Even big eaters took in only about 500 calories. Tuesday's dinner was stuffed tomatoes, couscous with either curried chicken or tofu, and a dessert of berries with whipped topping. Another dinner consisted of marinated asparagus, grilled salmon with dill, herbed cauliflower, and poached pears in red wine. Total calorie count: about 420 calories per meal.

To see the complete menu, turn the page. Does this look like "diet" food? Like the kind of eating that makes you feel deprived? Not at all. In 7 days of such eating—not to mention snacks from the Anytime List at any hour—no one left the table feeling hungry or unsatisfied. And in 7 days of such eating, everybody expanded their range of food choices—and everybody lost weight.

Executive chef Pete Repak proved to the Chicago 7 how delicious-looking and -tasting low-calorie foods could be. You can prove it, too. Try Pete's recipes starting on page 310.

A Week of Meals with the Chicago 7

	Day 1	Day 2	Day 3
Breakfast	Sliced orange Choice of Cheerios, Raisin Bran, Special K, or oatmeal Light yogurt English muffin or light toast with jam or light cream cheese Choice of coffee, tea, or diet hot cocoa	Cantaloupe Vegetable omelette made with egg whites or Egg Beaters, with onion, peppers, mushrooms, and tomatoes Bialy or light toast with jam or light cream cheese Choice of coffee, tea, or diet hot cocoa	Raspberries Light waffles and light syrup (Log Cabin or Aunt Jemima) Veggie sausage links (such as Yves or Morningstar Farms) Choice of coffee, tea, or diet hot cocoa
Lunch	Black bean soup with chopped onions and salsa Mixed field greens with light balsamic vinaigrette Sesame bread sticks Sliced mango	Veggie salami sandwich on light bread with lettuce and mustard Assorted pickles Sliced tomatoes Low-calorie Creamsicle	Minestrone Pizza with tomato sauce and assorted vegetables Watermelon
Dinner	Jumbo shrimp cocktail Penne pasta with eggplant and zucchini Italian ice	Marinated asparagus Grilled salmon with dill Herbed cauliflower Red wine poached pear	Hot-and-sour soup Chinese vegetables with shrimp and scallops with hoisin or black bean sauce Steamed brown rice Pineapple and fortune cookie

Day 4	Day 5	Day 6	Day 7
Sliced banana Choice of Wheatena, oatmeal, or quinoa or choice of cold cereal Raisin squares Light yogurt Choice of coffee, tea, or diet hot chocolate	Fresh fruit and cottage cheese Light pancakes with light syrup and figs Choice of coffee, tea, or diet hot chocolate	Honeydew melon Veggie Canadian bacon and egg on English muffin Choice of coffee, tea, or diet hot chocolate	Sliced fresh fruit Light French toast with light syrup and blueberries Choice of coffee, tea, or diet hot chocolate
Vegetable plate with baked Idaho or sweet potato Sorbet with fresh cherries	Vegetable-lentil soup Light tuna salad on light bread with lettuce and tomato Fresh peaches	Seafood salad on Boston lettuce Marinated cucumbers and tomatoes Seeded roll Tangerines	Tomato-vegetable Florentine soup Sloppy joe made with soy crumbles on bun Low-calorie Fudgsicle
Texas-style chili made with soy crumbles Mesclun salad with light ranch dressing Baked apple	Stuffed tomato Couscous with curried chicken or tofu Berries with whipped topping	Fresh fruit cup Veggie Salisbury steak with mushrooms Whipped potatoes Whole green beans Lemon ice	Dinner out at a restaurant

Tomato-Vegetable Florentine Soup

2 tablespoons olive oil

1 cup yellow onions, diced into ¼-inch pieces

2 tablespoons fresh minced garlic

½ teaspoon cracked fennel seed, toasted

¼ teaspoon cracked coriander seed, toasted

½ teaspoon black pepper, freshly ground

½ teaspoon dried oregano

¼ teaspoon crushed chile flakes

1 dried bay leaf

2 tablespoons kosher salt

½ cup celery, peeled and diced into ¼-inch pieces

½ cup carrots, peeled and diced into ¼-inch pieces

1 cup button mushrooms, diced into ¼-inch pieces

½ cup fresh fennel, diced into ¼-inch pieces

¼ cup Italian parsley, coarsely chopped

2 cups canned tomatoes, chopped

1 cup canned tomato puree

½ cup dry white wine

3 cups vegetable stock, tomato juice, or water

8 ounces frozen chopped spinach, thawed (squeeze out excess liquid)

¼ cup Parmesan cheese, grated

2 tablespoons good-quality balsamic vinegar

Heat the oil in a 2-gallon pot over medium–high heat until just barely smoking. Add the onions and garlic and stir well to prevent sticking. Add the fennel seed, coriander seed, pepper, oregano, chile flakes, bay leaf, and salt. Stir well and sauté for 1 minute.

Add the celery, carrots, mushrooms, and fennel to the pot and stir well. Add the parsley, chopped tomatoes, tomato puree, and wine to pot. Bring to a boil over high heat.

Add the stock, tomato juice, or water to the pot. Simmer uncovered over medium-low heat for 30 minutes.

Add the spinach, Parmesan, and vinegar. Taste soup and adjust seasonings as desired. Serve immediately.

Makes 5 servings

Texas-Style Chili

¼ cup canola oil

2 cups white onions, diced into ¼-inch pieces

1 tablespoon fresh garlic, minced

1 pound chili-style soy crumbles

2 teaspoons ground cumin seed, toasted

1 teaspoon ground coriander seed, toasted

1 teaspoon dried oregano

½ teaspoon black pepper, cracked

2 tablespoons chili powder

1 tablespoon kosher salt

¾ cup dark beer

2 tablespoons Worcestershire sauce

½ cup orange juice

2 cups fresh tomatoes, chopped

2 cups canned San Marzano tomatoes

1¼ cups salsa, any style

1 can kidney beans, drained

4 cups vegetable stock, tomato juice, or water

½ cup fresh cilantro, coarsely chopped

¼ cup fresh lime juice

1 cup green onions, sliced, for garnish

Heat the oil in a large cast-iron Dutch oven or pot over medium-high heat until almost smoking. Add the onions and garlic and sauté until soft.

Crumble the soy and add by handfuls to the pot, continuously stirring and breaking up the crumbles as you go. (This product will stick and burn if you don't pay close attention and keep stirring until fully cooked.) You may need to add additional oil.

Add the cumin seed, coriander seed, oregano, pepper, chili powder, and salt to the pot. Stir well.

Add the beer, Worcestershire, orange juice, and fresh tomatoes to the pot. Stir well and bring to a boil.

Reduce the heat and add the canned tomatoes, salsa, beans, and stock or tomato juice or water to pot.

Simmer over low heat for 1½ hours.

Stir in the cilantro and lime juice. Serve in bowls garnished with green onions.

Makes 5 servings

Red Wine Poached Pears

2	bottles red burgundy or Rhône-style wine	4	cinnamon sticks
1	cup port	2	teaspoons whole allspice
1	cup sugar	¼	teaspoon kosher salt
1	tablespoon whole black peppercorns	1	orange, sliced
10	cloves	5	pears, seasonal best, almost ripe
1½	tablespoons star anise pieces	1	orange, sliced into thin rings
1	teaspoon whole fenugreek seeds	5	scoops fat-free frozen vanilla yogurt

Find a pot that is wide enough to just barely hold five pears lying down and deep enough to completely cover them with 6 cups of poaching liquid. In the pot, combine the wine, port, sugar, peppercorns, cloves, star anise, fenugreek seeds, cinnamon, allspice, salt, and sliced orange. Bring to a boil. Reduce the heat and simmer until the mixture equals 6 cups.

Carefully peel the pears. Using the small end of a melon baller, carefully scoop out the bottom of the pear and work your way inside the pear to remove the seed and core. Immediately place the pears in the simmering poaching liquid.

Lay the pears down on their sides in the poaching liquid. Shingle the thinly sliced orange on top of the pears to help keep them submerged.

Simmer the pears in the poaching liquid until they are tender and deep ruby in color, but not mushy. This could take anywhere from 15 to 40 minutes, depending on the pears.

When the pears are tender, remove the pot from the heat. Remove 15 ounces of the poaching liquid and pour into a saucepot. Let the pears cool in the remaining poaching liquid.

Over medium-high heat, simmer the poaching liquid until it is reduced to about 8 ounces. Be careful not to burn. Transfer the reduced liquid to a smaller pot and reduce until 3 ounces remain.

To assemble, slice the pears—warm or at room temperature—in half from top to bottom. Make sure that no seed or core remains. In the bottom of five shallow bowls, place two pear halves, top with a scoop of frozen yogurt, and drizzle with a little warm reduced pear poaching liquid.

Makes 5 servings

Breaking the Cycle, Forging New Habits

Despite their intense training, once back home, each of the Chicago 7 had to find his or her own way of putting Picture-Perfect Weight Loss in place. It took time. After all, the seven were challenging the assumptions of a lifetime, blazing uncharted territory in the supermarket and at the stove, shattering some old habits and replacing them with new ones. It doesn't happen overnight.

Still, Debbie Davis, who grew up steeped in her family's Southern background, eating just about everything fried without ever thinking about it, now sautés vegetables in Pam and thinks "constantly" about "the healthier foods I love to eat, about extending my options."

Joanne Rusch, who "used to knock off a whole bag of reduced-fat Oreos" and assume she was "watching her weight," now shops for snacks—and everything else—off the Anytime List. When she wants a sweet snack, she reaches for a Tootsie Pop. When a salty craving sets in, she grabs a handful of peanuts.

The seven also learned to make exercise a habit. Heidi McInerney walks outside at least three times a week. Being "outside" is important. With three young kids, it's helpful to get away from the hustle and bustle in the house and dedicate this time to herself. What's invigorating for the body turns out to be refreshing for the mind as well.

But more than this, in choosing exercise at the end of her evening "workday," Heidi has broken the cycle of putting everyone else's needs first. For Heidi, it's a major breakthrough, a giant step. The homemaker in her family, she has also typically been the giving center of a close-knit extended family—her own parents, siblings, and other relatives, who all spend huge amounts of time together. With all this family interaction whirling around her, Heidi tended always to put herself last. No more. Of course, she still loves and cares for her kids, her husband, and the other relatives who gather around just about every day. But by taking an hour in the evening for a brisk walk with friends, Heidi has also taken a chance on stepping out of the center. By thus breaking the cycle, she has empowered herself. Cobwebs cleared and cardiovascular system revved, Heidi is more ready than ever to deal with family, job, friends—and new menu options for new eating habits.

For Dick Johnson, a self-styled "Dairy Queen freak," the cycle that needed breaking was an addiction to DQ's famous milk shakes. It was as if his car were on automatic pilot, he told psychotherapist Susan Amato, as if a recording in his head were telling him to pull into the parking lot every time he drove past the Dairy Queen outlet. "I can't imagine passing it by," he admitted during an early counseling session in the house.

As time went by, though, Dick came to understand that he could change all sorts of habits. He learned to reach for a butterscotch candy when he felt the urge for something sweet, not for a pint of ice cream that gave him, he realized, "maybe a 10-minute boost" and a lot of calories. He also found he could "grab an apple or an orange to take the edge right off the craving" for something sweet. In fact, says Dick, his pockets are constantly filled with hard candies, and "my car trunk looks like a produce market."

"I never understood the concept of 'toxic people.' But I would often find myself with such people, and I see now how I used to give in to them, go eat, and feel powerless. Now I just choose not to be in their company," says Heidi McInerney, a member of the Chicago 7.

Before

After

In addition, he discovered that he could simply change his environment when a craving for high-calorie foods seized him. Just getting up and going into another room, or taking the dog for a walk, or turning to a different kind of music on the radio—anything that changed the circumstances of his surroundings, no matter how temporary—could "break the cycle," in Dick's words. Once broken, it no longer held Dick prisoner.

That's why he can now drive right past Dairy Queen. He has reprogrammed the recording in his head. These days, the recording sends him to McDonald's, where he pretends he's ordering for a child and asks for a Happy Meal shake. "It's five sips," Dick says, and for those of us who know him, it's a funny image: this tall, powerful guy with his kiddie portion of shake. But it works. It does the trick for him. He hasn't denied himself the taste he yearns for, but he has taken away the power of that appetite to rule his actions. He's in charge now. He is figuratively as well as literally in the driver's seat. With this minimal change, Dick has made a huge difference—and shed 51 pounds in the process. "I got it," Dick says of his new consciousness in choosing. "It's all something of a mind game, and I finally got it. I finally understood that I could eat well and eat foods I like and still lose weight."

David Taylor is a deeply religious man who lacked faith in his ability to discipline himself. He worried that he would simply not be able to replace the habits of a lifetime with a new way of eating and a new commitment to exercise. He'd been on diets before—with only temporary results. He had joined a health club but couldn't seem to find time in his busy schedule to stick to an exercise routine. A handsome man with a football player's build, David was nevertheless self-conscious about his appearance—unwilling to wear short-sleeved shirts that, in his eyes at least, revealed ample, slack-muscled arms.

Despite the obstacles he faced, David is the "high performer" among the Chicago 7, the leading scorer in weight loss with 52 pounds shed in 8 months. Ask him if he knows why, and he's reluctant to attribute his success to self-mastery; he'll say only that he's "a work in progress." Yet closer questioning makes it clear that discipline is exactly what is at the root of David's weight loss. He has completely changed his eating habits, and while he still finds it hard to get to the health club, he now works out three times a week on the Nordic-Track in his condo.

Success, David has found, is its own motivation, reinforcing the tentative new practices of eating and exercise until they become firm habits. Especially when the success is noticed—when it's public and social, when members of his church mention it, when women seem to be paying more attention. Most important of all, David is paying more attention. David has made changes, and he likes the changes he has made. The Chicago 7 began Picture-Perfect Weight Loss with "Lock the Door, Lose the Weight" on *Good Morning America* in the fall of 2000; by the spring of 2001, David Taylor was confidently donning his short-sleeved shirts.

New options, new habits, revolutionary re-sults. No one says it won't take some time. But for your health, your appearance, and your sense of yourself, you need to take the time. And now is the time to do it.

You've spent years becoming overweight—and being unhappy about it. Like the Chicago 7, give yourself the time you need to undo those old, bad habits and to forge new, healthy habits of eating and exercise for life.

Firing Up a New Relationship with Food

Check out the "before" and "after" food demonstrations of the firefighters' meals starting on page 318. The difference between then and now is staggering. As one of my patients put it, "If these guys can do it, anybody can."

"These guys" are people who bear perhaps a bit more than their share of life's stresses. In addition to the normal pressures of mortgages, kids, working spouses, and sharing housework, their 15- or 24-hour shifts include a fair amount of downtime, as they wait . . . and wait . . . and wait. They're not in control of what will happen or when it might happen, but when it does, they can be pretty certain they will face danger—sometimes extreme danger. Then, carrying upwards of 75 pounds of equipment on their backs, they trudge up several flights of stairs through smoke and flame just to find the problem and start the job of fire fighting.

They're a close-knit fraternity. They share traditions, values, a culture forged in helping one's brother in times of danger. It is not, as one of them said to me, "a tofu crowd." In fact, the firefighters who have undertaken Picture-

Perfect Weight Loss deserve a special badge of courage, for they have battled not only their own lifetime eating habits but also the derision and downright baiting of the other guys in the firehouse. At least at first.

"I'm going to eat a doughnut every day in your face," one of my firefighters was told by a snickering colleague the week he began his Picture-Perfect Weight-Loss program. Another said he was the target of catcalls every time he stepped into the gym to work out. One admitted to me that the "kidding could be cruel, but then, firefighter humor tends to be perverse because we see so many difficult situations." In his case, the perverse humor consisted of "guys bringing in elegant desserts to tempt me or having pancake parties with eggs and bacon." Did the kidding work? In a way. "It encouraged me," this firefighter said, "because now it was a matter of winning, and firemen don't like to lose."

After a few weeks of Picture-Perfect Weight Loss, when the pounds started sliding off, the firefighters found that a lot of their derisive brothers were now interested in their progress. Instead of jeering, they wanted to know how it works; in place of mockery, they asked for suggestions. They could see what anyone could see: Making a habit of Picture-Perfect Weight Loss is a way of eating well, getting healthy, becoming and staying thin.

And as Mike Carter says: "It's easy."

It's Easy

This is the key—the real secret to Picture-Perfect Weight Loss: It's easy, although it may be easy for different people in different ways.

Mike Carter says it's easy to "find an alternative to the high-calorie choice." Instead of "a deluxe cheeseburger with onion rings, it's a portobello mushroom sandwich." Instead of a bag of potato chips "eaten mindlessly," it's a piece of fruit. Does he miss the "before" meals? Has he sacrificed taste? "I haven't sacrificed a thing in terms of taste," he says. "I certainly don't miss the grease. I don't miss the cheeseburgers at all; they just made me feel fatigued."

Mike is a fairly typical case study. When he left the firehouse to become "a desk jockey" in the union office, with lunches and cocktail parties and dinners all part of the job, he gained a substantial amount of weight. He tried diet after diet, and sure enough, he lost weight through deprivation, but he couldn't sustain it. "It made me miserable," he recalls. As a union official, he was also aware that "heart attacks are the number one killer of firefighters in this country," and he was pretty sure that the typical firehouse menu was a contributor to that. The philosophy of Picture-Perfect Weight Loss made sense, however, so Mike "made the commitment, then started eating."

For the first 3 months, he couldn't believe his own food diary. "Sometimes I ate six times a day. I was certain I was gaining weight that week. But at every weigh-in, I was losing weight."

He grew to love veggie burgers, waffles with light syrup, and the steamed sea bass with ginger and scallion and the vegetable-filled dumplings at his favorite Chinese restaurant. When he has a beer or two at the end of the day, it's light beer, with microwave-popped light popcorn. "I now weigh what I weighed 20 years ago," says Mike, "and I'm in better shape."

The bottom line after losing 80 pounds and keeping them off? "It's been so simple that it's frightening," he says.

It was easy for firefighter Tom Kontizas, too—easy to "become more interesting in my tastes" and enjoy red beans and coleslaw for lunch and stacks of fruit with his morning cereal. No problem for Lieutenant Larry Quinn Jr. to have "changed my tastebuds" and "literally changed the foods I eat." "If you can eat a certain way and it's beneficial, why would you do anything else?" questions Larry. Why, indeed? Where's the sacrifice in it? In the words of Father John Delendick, who was "always heavy" and who lost a total of 83 pounds on Picture-Perfect Weight Loss: "I've lost a lot—of weight, that is; I've given up nothing."

I'll give the last word on this subject to Dorothy Mellone, the New York City cop who spends her days on the streets fighting organized crime and narcotics. She doesn't have a lot of time to sit around and plan menus. Fortunately, she no longer needs much time. "I constantly think about what I eat," Dorothy says, "but I don't notice any more that I'm thinking. It is a normal routine. It has simply become part of me to watch what I eat."

For Dorothy, as for the firefighters featured in this book, the Chicago 7, and the thousands of patients I've treated successfully, Picture-Perfect Weight Loss has become a habit. Not a program, not a project, not a special event. It's a way of shopping for food, cooking, and eating that has become a way of life.

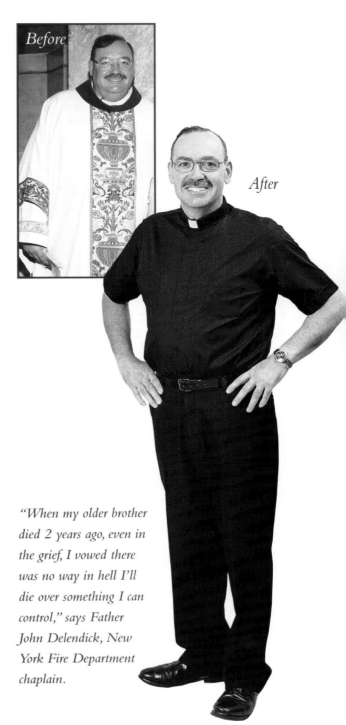

Before

After

"When my older brother died 2 years ago, even in the grief, I vowed there was no way in hell I'll die over something I can control," says Father John Delendick, New York Fire Department chaplain.

The New York Firefighters' Breakfast: Before and After

Before they began Picture-Perfect Weight Loss, the New York City firefighters used to stoke up hard at the firehouse, taking in enough calories and fat to add unhealthy weight and a real burden on the heart. Today's breakfast for "graduates" of the program is a model of nutritious, low-calorie choices—and a very hearty meal to kick off a hard day of work.

BEFORE

2 bagels with butter 1,400 calories
2 doughnuts 500 calories
1 slice pound cake 420 calories

TOTAL 2,320 calories

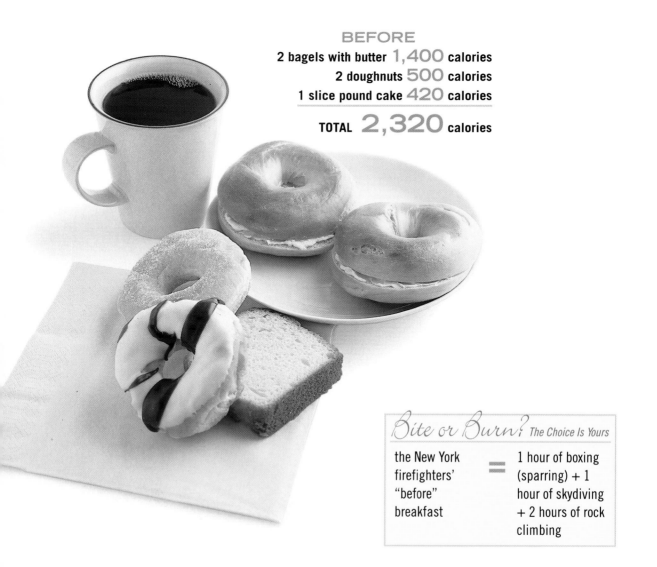

Bite or Burn? The Choice Is Yours

| the New York firefighters' "before" breakfast | = | 1 hour of boxing (sparring) + 1 hour of skydiving + 2 hours of rock climbing |

AFTER

2 English muffins with jam	300	calories
2 bialys	320	calories
1 apple	80	calories
1 banana	90	calories
1 pint mixed fruit	100	calories

TOTAL   890 calories

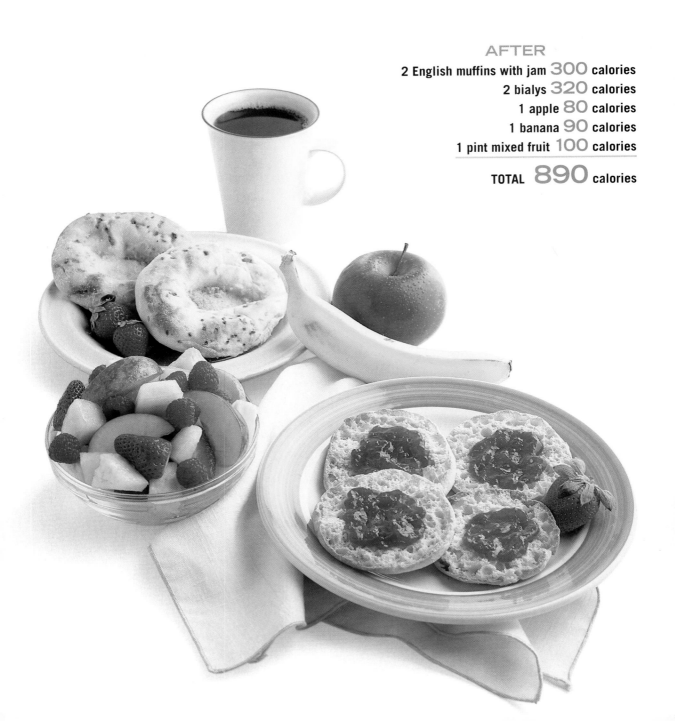

The New York Firefighters' Lunch:
Before and After

It was always so easy to run around the corner from the firehouse and pick up a couple of slices of good New York pizza, explained the New York City firefighters who took on Picture-Perfect Weight Loss. Now they've discovered that it's just as easy to pick up a bowl of soup and a sandwich. It's just as easy, much healthier, and far, far better for the weight-conscious.

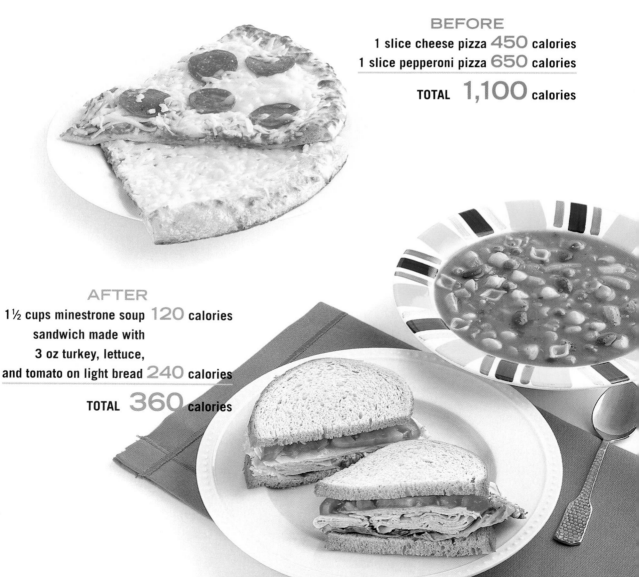

BEFORE
1 slice cheese pizza 450 calories
1 slice pepperoni pizza 650 calories

TOTAL 1,100 calories

AFTER
1½ cups minestrone soup 120 calories
sandwich made with
3 oz turkey, lettuce,
and tomato on light bread 240 calories

TOTAL 360 calories

The New York Firefighters' Take-a-Break Snack: Before and After

Instead of wolfing down a bag of high-calorie potato chips—laden with fat—the trim veterans of Picture-Perfect Weight Loss snack on pretzel rods and keep hard candies handy for when they feel a craving for something sweet.

BEFORE
3 oz potato chips
450 calories

AFTER
3 pretzel rods 120 **calories**
3 hard candies 60 **calories**
TOTAL 180 **calories**

The New York Firefighters' Dinner:
Before and After

Think of it this way: Guys who thought there was no alternative at all to the meal on the left have learned that there are lots of alternatives. Further, these alternatives are delicious, satisfying, and filling. A perfect example of this is the meal on the right, with its range of textures, its life-enhancing nutrition, its palette of tastes ranging from spicy to starchy to rich to cool, and its appeal to the weight-conscious.

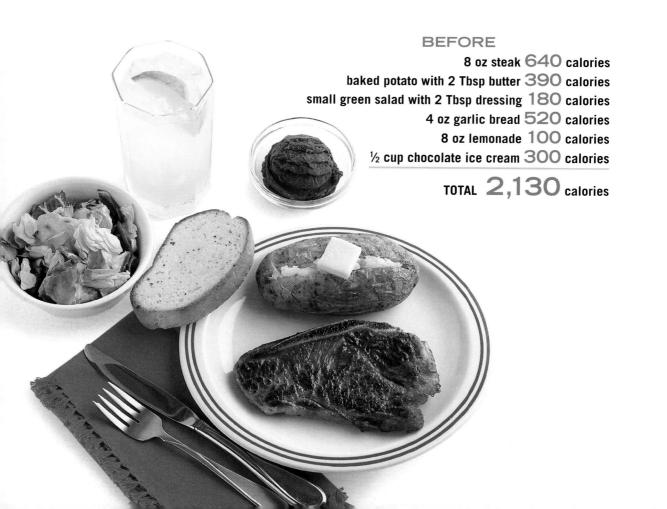

BEFORE

8 oz steak	640	calories
baked potato with 2 Tbsp butter	390	calories
small green salad with 2 Tbsp dressing	180	calories
4 oz garlic bread	520	calories
8 oz lemonade	100	calories
½ cup chocolate ice cream	300	calories
TOTAL	**2,130**	calories

AFTER

4 oz shrimp with cocktail sauce 140 calories
seafood pasta marinara
(2 oz pasta, 4 oz seafood,
and ½ cup marinara sauce) 350 calories
portobello mushroom 20 calories
2 cups marinated vegetables 80 calories
roll (1 oz) 80 calories
3 scoops sorbet 180 calories
fruit and whipped topping 40 calories
8 oz diet lemonade 0 calories

TOTAL 890 calories

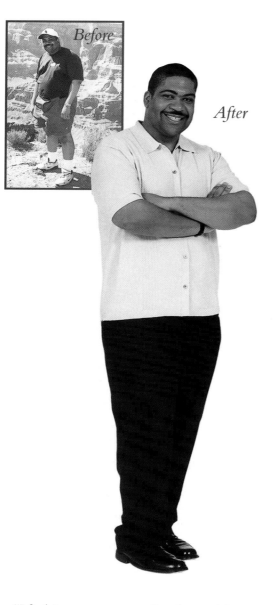

Before

After

"I find it easy now to run for a bus, and I can dash up the four flights of stairs to my condo," says David Taylor, *who was featured on* Good Morning America *as a member of the Chicago 7.*

Commitment to Change

For New York's firefighters, the bottom line on the "before" meals pictured on the previous pages totaled an oppressive 6,000 calories per day. The "after" eating comes to a manageable 2,300. Easy—once the men had made the commitment to change. Let's say it one more time: "If you do what you did, you get what you got."

You had enough of what you got, and you were determined to stop doing what you did. You chose to buy this book and to undertake Picture-Perfect Weight Loss. You chose change. And deep down, you understood that it was a choice for life.

Are you committed? You've spent 30 days making changes. Some of the changes have been small, some big. You've introduced new foods into your daily menu and new physical activity into your weekly calendar. You've also introduced new thinking into your brain: You have new attitudes toward old standbys like dairy products and recent innovations like soy-based products; you have a new awareness about calories and nutrition. You've even let yourself deal with some emotional issues concerning your view of yourself and your needs—and maybe you've begun to exorcise some old demons.

It sure sounds like you've made a commitment. In fact, when you think about it, you've done a lot, and you've come a long way. Up ahead is the big prize: the new, trim you—looking good, feeling energetic, choosing a gorgeous bounty of low-calorie, healthful, nutritious foods day after day for life.

My prescription? Don't stop now.

It's a Wrap

Wraps have become an extremely popular choice for lunches and snacks, but some can be quite high in calories despite their modest size. The vegetable wrap beats the Brie wrap by a mile in calorie count and healthfulness, making it a great way to take in your vegetables.

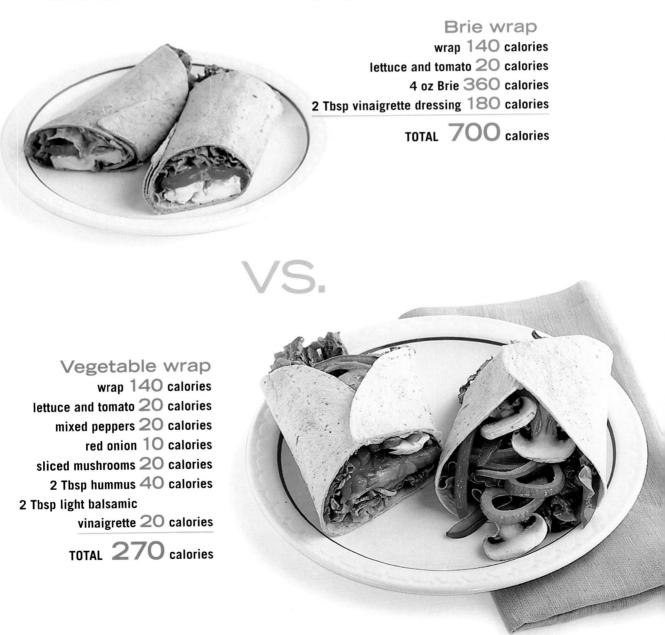

Brie wrap

wrap 140 calories
lettuce and tomato 20 calories
4 oz Brie 360 calories
2 Tbsp vinaigrette dressing 180 calories

TOTAL 700 calories

VS.

Vegetable wrap

wrap 140 calories
lettuce and tomato 20 calories
mixed peppers 20 calories
red onion 10 calories
sliced mushrooms 20 calories
2 Tbsp hummus 40 calories
2 Tbsp light balsamic
vinaigrette 20 calories

TOTAL 270 calories

Index

Underscored page references indicate boxed text and tables. **Boldface** references indicate photographs and illustrations.

326

D

T

W

Conversion Chart

These equivalents have been slightly rounded to make measuring easier.

VOLUME MEASUREMENTS

U.S.	Imperial	Metric
¼ tsp	–	1 ml
½ tsp	–	2 ml
1 tsp	–	5 ml
1 Tbsp	–	15 ml
2 Tbsp (1 oz)	1 fl oz	30 ml
¼ cup (2 oz)	2 fl oz	60 ml
⅓ cup (3 oz)	3 fl oz	80 ml
½ cup (4 oz)	4 fl oz	120 ml
⅔ cup (5 oz)	5 fl oz	160 ml
¾ cup (6 oz)	6 fl oz	180 ml
1 cup (8 oz)	8 fl oz	240 ml

WEIGHT MEASUREMENTS

U.S.	Metric
1 oz	30 g
2 oz	60 g
4 oz (¼ lb)	115 g
5 oz (⅓ lb)	145 g
6 oz	170 g
7 oz	200 g
8 oz (½ lb)	230 g
10 oz	285 g
12 oz (¾ lb)	340 g
14 oz	400 g
16 oz (1 lb)	455 g
2.2 lb	1 kg

LENGTH MEASUREMENTS

U.S.	Metric
¼"	0.6 cm
½"	1.25 cm
1"	2.5 cm
2"	5 cm
4"	11 cm
6"	15 cm
8"	20 cm
10"	25 cm
12" (1')	30 cm

PAN SIZES

U.S.	Metric
8" cake pan	20 × 4 cm sandwich or cake tin
9" cake pan	23 × 3.5 cm sandwich or cake tin
11" × 7" baking pan	28 × 18 cm baking tin
13" × 9" baking pan	32.5 × 23 cm baking tin
15" × 10" baking pan	38 × 25.5 cm baking tin (Swiss roll tin)
1½ qt baking dish	1.5 liter baking dish
2 qt baking dish	2 liter baking dish
2 qt rectangular baking dish	30 × 19 cm baking dish
9" pie plate	22 × 4 or 23 × 4 cm pie plate
7" or 8" springform pan	18 or 20 cm springform or loose-bottom cake tin
9" × 5" loaf pan	23 × 13 cm or 2 lb narrow loaf tin or pâté tin

TEMPERATURES

Fahrenheit	Centigrade	Gas
140°	60°	–
160°	70°	–
180°	80°	–
225°	105°	¼
250°	120°	½
275°	135°	1
300°	150°	2
325°	160°	3
350°	180°	4
375°	190°	5
400°	200°	6
425°	220°	7
450°	230°	8
475°	245°	9
500°	260°	–